# The EFT Coach

**Emotional Freedom Technique™** for the **Professional Coach**

Mary L.R. Jones BSc Psychology, MSc, AMT Practitioner & Trainer, Personal Coach, NLP Practitioner

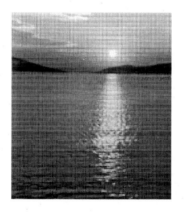

**1st Edition, March 2004**

**The EFT Coach:**

**Emotional Freedom Technique™ for the Professional Coach**

First Edition March 2004

Copyright © The Future Starts Now 2004

Cover design © The Future Starts Now 2004

Cover photo © M.L.R. Jones. Sunrise over Skyros Island, Greece.

Published by:

The Future Starts Now, Ipswich, Suffolk, UK.

www.thefuturestartsnow.com

ISBN: 0-9547361-1-7 (softcover)

Printed and bound by Antony Rowe Ltd, Eastbourne

**Disclaimer:**

Neither Emotional Freedom Technique™ or coaching should be used as a substitute for medical treatment or psychotherapy. Where treatment is required for a specific psychological or clinical disorder, you should use EFT, if at all, only under the supervision of a qualified health professional.

The use of EFT within coaching is recommended only on the assumption that a coaching client has not been diagnosed with any clinical psychological condition, including but not limited to schizophrenia, clinical OCD, bipolar disorder, dissociative disorder or any other psychological disturbance likely to produce extreme or dangerous emotional reaction.

While EFT has produced excellent results for many people, success is not guaranteed either by the author of this book or the originator of EFT. By applying the techniques in this book you agree to take full responsibility for your emotional and physical well being.

Mary L.R. Jones has no medical qualifications and offers the material in this book only in her capacity as a personal coach, psychology graduate, licensed practitioner and trainer of EFT and a licensed NLP practitioner.

*"Even though I wrote this book, I deeply and completely accept myself."*

# Acknowledgements

The contents of this book would not have been possible without the inspiration of many people.

Head of the list, of course, must be Gary Craig, the originator of EFT, whose persistence in publicising EFT and provision of training materials at low cost has made this remarkable technique available to so many people. In particular I want to acknowledge not only his technical contribution to energy healing, but in setting the tone amongst the many practitioners he has influenced. Gary believes in self-empowerment - a value also highly prized amongst coaches – and perhaps no accident since he is himself a Performance Coach. His generosity in making his technique accessible and affordable has been taken on by the energy healing profession and is reflected in the generosity and openness which characterises the field of Energy Psychology.

Next comes Silvia Hartmann, co-founder of the Association of Meridian Therapies UK, designer of the Meridian Therapies Certification programme, creator of the EmoTrance protocol, and author of many books on EFT and other energy protocols. Most significantly I acknowledge her creation of Adventures in EFT[3] and Advanced Patterns of EFT[4], both of which were a significant inspiration in the writing of this book and which demonstrated the value of mapping out and organising particular uses and patterns of EFT. For a new continent (or perhaps galaxy in Silvia's case) to be "conquered", it is not enough to say *"Well, it's very, very big - you can go anywhere and do almost anything you like"*. To open up the infinite potential of new lands, someone has to go out there, do a lot of noticing, take meticulous records, conduct a proper survey and draw a map so that others may follow with confidence. Silvia is just such an adventurer in the domain of energy healing. If this book manages to do a similar job for the field of coaching - if only to allow a safe beach landing for now - it owes Silvia a debt for showing the value of solid cartography.

Of course, this book is as inspired by coaching as it is inspired by EFT. I wish to acknowledge the depth and quality of training provided by the Coaches Training Institute and in particular the Co-active Coaching Model on which their trainings are based. From the very start, I knew that here was a set of people who not only knew their craft, but also came from a solid ethic based on personal integrity and - most importantly to me - on the absolute assumption that each person has value and deserves total respect and esteem. This integrity permeated not only the trainings themselves, but was manifest in every tutor. This ethic, as well as the set of tools they teach, are presented in the book Co-Active Coaching[2] from which this book draws extensively.

I also wish to acknowledge the significant contribution of NLP to this endeavour. Although it is mentioned but rarely in these pages, it has been a silent but steady influence in my thinking and in many of the ideas contained here. In particular I acknowledge Ian McDermott and Wendy Jago's book, The NLP Coach[5] and the NLP Coach training programme in general. While everyone and everything else seemed to be saying *"Don't combine coaching with therapy"*, the field of NLP Coaching stood out as a beacon, telling me strongly that it **is** possible to combine disciplines, provided an underlying ethic is defined and adhered to. NLP can of course be used therapeutically - but its use as a valid coaching tool (or set of tools) goes unquestioned. It was perhaps fortunate that NLP was not originally called "Neuro-Linguistic Therapy" or we may never have seen NLP and coaching put together.

I also wish to acknowledge and thank Dr Pat Carrington for her Choices technique[7]. With one simple pattern, Dr Carrington transformed the possibilities of EFT to not only take away the negative but to embrace the positive. From this single pattern sprang my belief that EFT could be successfully applied to coaching.

I also acknowledge the few (but ever growing number of) pioneering coaches, who have managed to gracefully include EFT into their repertoire of coaching tools. In particular, I thank them for not only proving that EFT need not confuse the coaching relationship, but giving me permission to explore the murky region of "therapy vs coaching", a taboo amongst many coaches.

On a personal level, I acknowledge the following people:

Ananga Sivyer - my practitioner trainer who provided much encouragement.

Silvia Hartmann (again) for creating the Project Energy protocol which was instrumental in turning this book from a "backburner project" to a concrete reality within a few weeks.

Marysia Appleton for being my first energy coach, long before I ever heard of EFT or thought of becoming a coach myself. Only from this vantage point do I fully understand her role in my journey.

Hazel Lacohée, friend and supporter whose influence was what I needed to start me off on this journey 6 years ago.

Andrew Simensen, for his unwavering belief in me and all my scatterbrained plans and schemes over the past two years, as well as his practical assistance in bringing this book to publication. If most of the value of coaching is in having someone who believes in you 100%, then Andrew has been by far the best coach I ever had.

I make use of several variations of EFT, and discuss several innovative concepts, developed by other practitioners and researchers. As well as referencing them in the text, I expressly acknowledge the origin of the following:

| The Standard EFT pattern | Gary Craig in [1] |
| The Conflict pattern | Silvia Hartmann, Phd in [3] |
| SLOW EFT | Silvia Hartmann, Phd in [4] |
| Guiding Stars | Silvia Hartmann, Phd in [4] |
| The Choices Technique | Dr Pat Carrington in [7] |

Finally, I thank the following practitioners and coaches for their help in reviewing this book and their moral support:

| Dr Christina Elvin | Psychotherapist, Consultant, AMT Trainer and Coach. OEAssociates, UK www.oesassociates.co.uk +44 (0)1604 768343 |
| Milena Galbraith | MA, LMHC. Counselor, Psychotherapist and Coach. Aurora Holistic Counseling, New Hampshire. aurora-holistic@aol.com +1 603-654-6287 |
| Marion R.R. Jones | BA, PGCE, Dip.ION. Nutritional Therapist and Allergy specialist Rayleigh Allergy Clinic, UK. +44 (0)1268 741288 |

# Contents

# 1   Introduction

Coaching and EFT have always coincided for me - both in time and in spirit.

I began my formal coaching training just a month after first downloading Gary Craig's EFT Manual[1]. I applied it straightaway to a couple of personal issues - and was astonished to find that it worked. Determined to find out as much as I could - purely for my own reasons - I ordered the complete set of Gary's training videos. By the time I finally sat down to watch them thoroughly, several months later, I had completed my coaching training. From the very beginning, then, I viewed EFT - its potential and its power - through a coaching lens.

When I completed my AMT practitioner training it seemed at first that I had destined myself to double frustration. When I was coaching, I would often find myself frustrated at finding a clear EFT issue - but not feeling able to use it because I feared it was "therapy" (I question this in depth below). But when I was doing an EFT session with someone for a specific emotional issue, I would also become frustrated, knowing that there was so much more in their life that could benefit from coaching. I seemed to be at an impasse. Both disciplines seemed to be crying out to be combined in some way - and yet the training and books I had read thus far seemed to either explicitly prohibit it, or simply not mention how that might be possible.

Whenever I come across an apparently black and white issue that's causing me friction, I turn to Synthesis. I started asking myself over and over: "If EFT and coaching **could** be combined in an ethical way, what would that be?"

I am grateful for the journey that answering this question began. It has deepened my own understanding of the core of what coaching is really about and its central ethic and purpose, instead of the more superficial aspects of "what tool to use" and judgements based on (perhaps) professional indemnity insurance definitions. And it has led me to discover and develop whole new uses for EFT that arise specifically in a coaching context. Perhaps most importantly of all, it has led me to see the deep threads of coinciding viewpoint and assumptions about clients that tie the two disciplines together.

This book tracks my journey and makes available the insights and discoveries I made along the way. Increasingly I am noticing coaches and EFT practitioners combine their skills. Clearly many other people around the globe are feeling the same way as me. I hope this book provides additional grounding and support for these pioneers.

At the end of Adventures in EFT[3], Silvia Hartmann asks the reader to pledge the following:

**Keep on using EFT.**
**Try it on everything.**
**And tell everyone about EFT!**

This book is my way of fulfilling that request.

# 2  Aims and Audience

EFT Coaching seems to straddle a notional division between therapeutic goals and coaching goals. Although this division is examined and questioned later on, this division creates dilemmas for coaches, EFT practitioners, their clients and self-help users alike.

For a coach/practitioner who has not worked through the "coaching versus therapy" issue, using EFT within coaching can set up a feeling of internal incongruency about using EFT, fearing that EFT is therapy – although I say why this is not so later on.

And for a self-help user wanting to make positive life changes but coming across fears and blocks, it can be confusing whether to seek "therapy" to address the blocks (and the past events that formed them), or whether to find a coach to help achieve their goals.

My aim in this book is to demonstrate an approach and provide techniques to show how it is possible to remain firmly in the domain of coaching while benefiting from EFT along the way. In so doing I hope I am giving birth to a new breed of coaching, which makes full use of the power of EFT to produce required energy shifts, while still remaining true to the purpose and spirit of coaching, that of focusing on "what next" and moving the client towards achieving their goals.

When I began writing this book I originally intended it to be aimed primarily at the practitioner who is already trained as a coach and is already familiar with EFT. But as the book progressed it became clear that it could serve a useful function to anyone with any level of interest or training in either coaching or EFT. The sections below outline how each type of reader can benefit from this book.

However, although of interest and use to people at any level, it does not aim to teach you how to be a coach, or how to be an EFT practitioner. There are numerous coaching training institutions worldwide, and prospective coaches are encouraged to seek formal training through one of these. If you wish to add EFT to your coaching practice you are strongly encouraged to seek training in EFT, and in particular to do practitioner training through the Association of Meridian Therapies (AMT) if you are in the UK. A list of reading and training resources for EFT is provided towards the end of the book.

## 2.1  Coaches with EFT Training

Assuming you already have coaching and EFT training separately, this book will show you how to combine the two disciplines in an effective way and it will give you some concrete ideas for additional uses of EFT that you might not have thought of.

A particular challenge for many coaches is to personally resolve issues of personal integrity and ethics around bringing in techniques previously thought of as "therapy tools" into a coaching context. Therefore, a particular emphasis of the book is how to use EFT in the service of the coaching - just as some coaches already use NLP or other standalone techniques to enhance their repertoire of coaching tools or to make their conventional coaching tools more powerful. The ethics of coaching are examined and principles for using EFT within coaching are proposed as a basis for ethical EFT Coaching. The practical issues of incorporating EFT into your coaching are also covered.

## 2.2  Coaches without EFT Training

If you are a trained coach you may have come across the increasing numbers of other coaches started to advertise EFT as one of their primary tools. In a relatively young and fast-developing industry, it's natural for coaches to be curious and interested in new areas of specialism and new tools to improve the effectiveness of coaching.

But virtually all the information and resources available about EFT, concentrate almost entirely on its therapeutic applications - because that is where EFT originated and because the applications there are so clear.

So the coach who is intrigued by EFT and interested in integrating it into their practice may start working through the available resources and find themselves in pretty scary therapeutic territory, seeing hypnotherapists, acupuncturists, psychotherapists, abuse counsellors and medical doctors talk about applications for EFT which clearly would not be relevant to a coaching context. It can take (as it took me) a great deal of time to extrapolate from the therapeutic examples of EFT and realise the potential for benefit within a coaching context.

The **great thing** about EFT is that it seems to have almost limitless application to any type or variety of emotional disturbance.

And the **problem** with EFT is that it seems to have almost limitless application to any type or variety of emotional disturbance. Which means really knowing how and when it can be applied can take some time to grasp, unless you are given lots of real examples.

It's a bit like being shown an aeroplane and being told you can go anywhere you like in the world. If you don't know certain destinations even exist, then no amount of examining the fuselage or the wings will get you there. And no amount of understanding the intricacies of how EFT works and seeing it applied to a hundred trauma cases will help you know that EFT can help you decide if your life goals are correct, or help you maintain professional detachment with a client.

If you are a coach wondering whether to include EFT in your practice, what you probably really want to know is when and how EFT can assist coaching - what types of issues it can address, whether it can be combined with your existing conventional coaching techniques, and whether there is anything about EFT that might be particularly applicable to your own coaching specialism. And you would probably like to know about this **before** you invest a lot of time and money on training.  If you are in this category, this book is for you.

## 2.3   EFT Practitioners without Coaching Training

Many people from therapy training and backgrounds (counsellors, psychotherapists, hypnotherapists etc) are increasingly being drawn into coaching as a profession - and EFT practitioners (many of whom will also have additional therapeutic training) are no exception.

If you already have formal EFT practitioner training you will probably already have some awareness of the potential for the use of EFT in coaching applications. Gary Craig's Palace of Possibilities training set focuses very much on such applications. Gary himself is a Performance Coach and often speaks about the potential of EFT to improve performance in all sorts of areas from business to sport.

But, the challenge for EFT practitioners coming into coaching is somewhat different to that for coaches learning about EFT. Apart from the challenge of acquiring more general coaching skills (to which the answer is coaching training with a good coach training academy or institution), there are two particular challenges.

Firstly, they may wonder whether and how a coaching session with EFT differs from a "therapy" session with EFT. If it's the same, then why call it coaching? If it's different, how is it different?

Secondly, they may want help in shifting focus from the usual list of therapeutic EFT goals (eliminating fear, anxiety, trauma and physical ailments) to a new set of coaching goals.

This book addresses both these challenges, by examining core coaching fundamentals from an EFT point of view, by addressing the issue of focus and primary goals between the two contexts, and by explicitly listing and explaining uses of EFT for coaching purposes. It also mentions types of therapeutic EFT usage to be avoided in a coaching context.

# 2.4  Self-helpers

Although I originally aimed this book at existing practitioners and coaches, I am well aware of the growth of both self-coaching and self-healing amongst people who are non-practitioners. The numerous books offering do-it-yourself coaching techniques, not to mention the growth of EFT self-help workbooks and web forums, are testament to the existence and needs of this audience. This book should therefore also be of interest to those who perhaps have used EFT for self-help and want to expand their application of EFT to self-coaching goals.

The book is also a primer for prospective clients of the EFT Coach. For such readers this book serves to expand their knowledge of what is possible using coaching and EFT - which should help a prospective client of either coaching or EFT decide which methods they find appealing and therefore what sort of coach or practitioner they want to seek out.

# 3  How to use this book

Many elements of this book interconnect in ways which do not prefer one order of presentation over another. For instance, having described generally how EFT can assist with visualisations as a coaching technique, it then becomes necessary to refer to this again when talking about how visualisations can be used to deal with a particular situation within coaching.

I have therefore begun with the lowest level elements first (principles, skills and techniques), before moving on to wider applications and situations within coaching. This means that when the larger coaching applications are discussed the reader will already have some familiarity with many of the concepts already.

In order to help convey this interlinking of material, many sections include a "Related sections" list which refers you to sections covering terms and topics mentioned in that section. This allows you to immediately see whether there are other sections you might want to read to complete your knowledge - or whether you have already read them.

For the reader with only coaching or only EFT experience (or neither), it is recommended that you read from the beginning in sequence, as this will familiarise you with the elements of both EFT and coaching in reasonably bite-size pieces which are built on later in the book.

If you are already well versed in both coaching and EFT, you will be able to use this as a reference book, dipping in at whatever level of detail is appropriate to you at a given moment. For instance you may be about to conduct a Peak Experience exercise with a client and you may wonder how EFT could be used to assist that exercise specifically. Or you may be working with a client on some specific blocks, and you may want some ideas about how EFT could help with that.

In the "how to" chapters (7, 8 and 9) I have deliberately included as many fictional examples of setup phrases as possible. Although I have attempted to explain the thinking and possibilities around each application in words, ultimately one example can be the key to understanding how to use EFT in a particular context, or be the trigger for the practitioner to come up with an adaptation that fits the current circumstance. As with EFT itself, the theory is interesting, but it's the practice that matters and which makes the difference.

# 3.1  Linguistic conventions

- I use both "he" and "she" throughout the book to refer to both client and coach at different times. I believe this reflects the random appearance of different genders in life and I prefer it to any more arbitrary or formalised way of referring to an example person. It goes without saying that either client or coach may be of either gender.

- I capitalise terms which have specific meanings within EFT such as "Aspect" or "Reversal", and specific coaching concepts and techniques such as "Peak Experience" or "Future Self". I do not capitalise terms which also have a much more everyday meaning such as "fear", "block", "belief", "value" or "goal" and for which the everyday meaning is adequate to allow full understanding.

- In "related sections" listings, each section listed is followed by either an up arrow ( ⇧ ) or a down arrow ( ⇩ ) to indicate whether the section is earlier or later than the current reading point. This is to aid navigation and perhaps help the reader know if they have already visited that section.

- In places I have re-used examples or ideas which have appeared in many of the works mentioned above. Rather than simply steal these examples or leave them out when they are so relevant, I therefore reference them, when they occur, with a superscript numeral e.g. [1] The reference section lists all these sources.

# 4  Glossary

| AMT | Association for Meridian Therapies |
| CTI | Coaches Training Institute |
| EFT | Emotional Freedom Technique |
| ICF | International Coaching Federation |
| PR | Psychological Reversal |
| TFT | Thought Field Therapy (forerunner of EFT) |

# 5  Ethics and Principles

*"Everyone should carefully observe which way his heart draws him,*
*and then choose that way with all his strength."*

*Hasidic saying*

In this chapter we address most of the likely doubts or objections that you may have or may come across when thinking about how to use EFT within coaching. If you have no doubts or objections at this stage, you may be able to skip this section. But it is likely that you may be asked about some of these issues by fellow coaches or even clients - so it is useful for you to have some answers to hand.

In all that follows, I have presented what works for me and my personal integrity. I do not want or require that all coaches using EFT adopt any of the following simply because it says so here. Principles followed blindly without being rooted in personal integrity are better than nothing but they are not the best that you can achieve or model for your clients. Each coach and practitioner needs to work out what works for them. My aim in what follows is to show you the thought process that I went through so that you might accelerate your own process of working through the issues. If you come to a different conclusion because of your own background or circumstances, then follow it with all your strength.

## 5.1  EFT isn't (Psycho)therapy

In the discussion that follows, I will be contrasting "coaching" with "therapy". It's important that I define what I mean by "therapy", since I believe it means many things to many people. But as is so often the case when a word triggers controversy, the problem can lie as much in the differences of assumed meaning as with the actual thing to which it refers. This is especially likely when a technical term has been present in everyday language for a long time.

Everyone thinks they know what "therapy" means, even if they have never had any. Just as many people will use "Freudian" as an adjective without ever having read anything by Freud. "Therapy" has become an everyday term. So it's not unusual for trainee coaches, without a background in psychotherapy, to be told to "avoid doing therapy" but to really have no idea what it is they are trying to avoid.

When coaches say "coaching isn't therapy", they mean it (in my experience) in the sense of "lie-on-the-coach-and-tell-me-about-your-childhood-type-psychotherapy" or "seeing my analyst" aimed at "coming to terms" and "understanding why". And this is the idea of "therapy" that I am referring to below.

Taking this definition of what "therapy" is, EFT isn't "therapy". It is a technique which is applied to any client intensity or belief, **without analysis** by either client or practitioner, and which results in the release of energetic disruption.

Indeed it is possible to conduct a successful EFT session without the client even telling the practitioner what the issue is. (In fact you will see Gary Craig do this on a number of occasions on his training CD's when someone in a workshop prefers not to discuss particular aspects of their issue). Usually the client does tell the practitioner - but this is only to enable the practitioner to formulate effective setup statements using the client's own language, and to help the client apply the technique to the various aspects of the problem in an orderly and thorough way. And although sometimes memories are recalled along the way, this is not necessary. Sometimes the issue is resolved without the client ever knowing "why".

The fact that EFT can be successfully self-applied, once the mechanics have been learned, further demonstrates the status of EFT as a technique, and not (psycho)therapy. One cannot perform counselling or any type of psychotherapy on oneself, because of the inherent dynamics of these as therapies.

I ask the reader to bear all this in mind in what follows. Where I discuss possible objections to the use of EFT on the grounds that it might be therapy, I am not saying that I think it is therapy - I am reflecting a fear that others **may** have that it **might** be so.

Related sections:

6.1.10    The Client Has the Answers ⇩

6.2.1    The Cause of Negative Emotions ⇩

# 5.2  Internal and External Ethics

If you have signed up to a code of ethics or conduct for your profession, then clearly this needs to be your baseline for making more specific ethical decisions.

In some parts of the world, especially the US, these ethics may even have legal force restricting how you operate your practice - and none of what follows is intended to suggest or imply that you should ignore any legal requirements that apply to you.

In the UK, many of these areas are largely unregulated, and so adherence to ethics rests primarily upon the codes of conduct and requirements of professional associations and on the ethics of individual practitioners.

But when it comes to ensuring truly ethical behaviour in a profession like coaching or any type of therapy, adherence to a set of external professional standards is not enough. A truly ethical standpoint is achieved only by combining external professional obligations with internal personal integrity.

In this section I examine both the external ethics of the coaching profession, and the role of personal ethics.

## 5.2.1  The ICF code of conduct

There are coaches who strongly believe that "therapy should never be combined with coaching". I believe this approach is genuinely motivated and comes from an ethical desire to avoid overstepping the bounds of the coaching relationship.

Indeed, as a member of the International Coaching Federation, I take such considerations very seriously and for a long time also avoided the use of EFT within coaching sessions because I assumed (incorrectly - see above) that EFT should be classed as a sort of therapy.

However I increasingly felt this restriction to be unnecessarily limiting in terms of the needs of the client. I had assumed that what other people had written about not allowing coaching and therapy to ever be combined, must be based on the ICF code of conduct.

I decided to look for myself, to check in what ways the inclusion of EFT as a coaching tool could be in contravention of any items of the code - but on examination I could not find anything which indicated that.

(The ICF code of conduct can be viewed in full at: http://www.coachfederation.org/abouticf/standards.htm)

The following items from the ICF code seemed relevant:

1. **I will ensure that my coaching client understands the nature of coaching and the terms of the coaching agreement between us.**

2. **I will not intentionally mislead or make false claims about what my client will receive from the coaching process or from me as their coach.**

3. **I will not give my clients or any prospective clients information or advice I know to be misleading or beyond my competence.**

Having considered these items carefully I believe is it completely acceptable to use EFT as a coaching tool (in the same way that some coaches use NLP and other techniques within coaching) provided the following practices are followed:

1. It is made clear to the client, from the outset of the coaching relationship, how and when EFT will be used. EFT needs to be explicitly mentioned in the coaching agreement and explicitly discussed as part of "designing the alliance" in the intake session. (Providing them with a copy of this book may be useful to help ensure clients understand how you intend to use EFT within the coaching relationship).

2. The status of EFT as a technique in terms of what it can and cannot do, its success rates and so on, need to be made explicit to the client at the outset of the coaching relationship. This in fact is the same information that any responsible EFT practitioner should make available to a client in any case, but this emphasises the point.

3. The practitioner makes his/her experience and qualifications in EFT explicit so that the client can have full awareness of the coach's competence at using EFT. In addition the coach must be ready and willing to refer the client to another more experienced practitioner if necessary. An EFT Coach should be as willing to suggest a client consult with another EFT practitioner as they should be to suggest consulting a financial advisor, legal advisor, psychotherapist - or even another coach - if it is clear that the client's interests are best served in that way.

In listing these practices I believe I have honoured both the spirit and the letter of the ICF code of conduct to the best of my ability. In particular, by making them explicit to myself (or yourself) it then becomes possible to make them explicit to the client too, so the client can make an informed choice when choosing a coach.

Related sections:

5.1        EFT isn't (Psycho)therapy ⇧

## 5.2.2   Personal Code of Conduct

In coaching, as in many professions where the success of the outcome depends on the authenticity of the professional, you do not achieve a state of "ethical grace" by simply avoiding doing what has not been done before in case it oversteps an ethical boundary. I believe that once you have assured yourself that you are not doing anything overtly in contravention of your professional obligations, the rest is a matter of personal judgement based on your own personal integrity and your understanding of what will best serve the client's needs.

Having satisfied the spirit and letter of any external code of conduct, all your other decisions need to be based on a far more detailed personal code of conduct. Most coaches run their practices in a way that has been modelled for them by their coach training school, mentor coaches or in what they read in coaching manuals. Few coaches, in my experience, actually examine and set out explicitly for themselves what their own personal code of conduct will be.

The effectiveness of coaching, as with much therapy, depends critically on the personal qualities of the coach or therapist and the degree to which they "click" with their client. "Clicking" can be helped along with learned rapport-building techniques, but ultimately finding the right coach or therapist is as mysterious a process as falling in love or making new friends. The fact is, the power of a coach lies in their authenticity - the degree to which they can be fully themselves in the presence of the client. It is inescapable therefore that coaches base their practice on their individuality and on their fearless expression of that individuality.

Even conventional, "no therapy here" coaching schools allow for coach individuality.

> "There are no cookie-cutter coaches. The principles, contexts and skills of coaching are valuable for understanding what to do, but there is no magic coat of coaching that you can put on and be assured of success…. Coaches too come in a variety of forms with… different ways of getting from here to there. The fact is, there is no infallible recipe to make you a perfect coach. So instead, **bless all the differences**. They make life interesting and create more ways for more people to enjoy the power of a coaching relationship" [2]

Unless you aim to be a "cookie-cutter coach", you will almost certainly be unique in your practice in some way or another - specialising in a particular type of client or domain, having strong preference for some coaching tools rather than others, or simply by having your own sense of mission and vision which inevitably creates an agenda for your practice. Indeed, as the number of professionally trained coaches grows, the trend is towards coaches making themselves more specialised and more "special" as a general marketing strategy.

I therefore believe it is important that all coaches - as soon as they start to feel themselves defining their own niche and style to differentiate themselves from other coaches - think explicitly about their own personal code of conduct.

Coaching - and being a coach - can be distilled down to one thing: integrity. That is, assisting your clients to live in integrity and demonstrating and living in integrity yourself as a person and as a coach. Ultimately, where a particular coach chooses to draw the line must, once any explicit professional code of ethics has been satisfied, be a judgement call by the coach, with the ultimate benchmark being what is in the client's interest.

What follows in this section presents you with many of the key issues involved in a personal code of conduct, as well as suggesting a set of principles covering the use of EFT specifically.

The rest of this book shows you how to use EFT as a coaching tool whenever you decide it is appropriate and in keeping with your own integrity and personal code of conduct.


# 5.3  Objections and Counter-objections

The following sections deal with possible objections to using EFT as a coaching tool. They cover objections I have actually seen or heard either in coaching manuals or expressed by individuals. If you don't have these objections yourself, you may want to arm yourself with the accompanying counter-objections in case you find yourself questioned by colleagues or even clients.

By the way - I do not mean the following to imply or assume that you as a reader subscribe to all or any of these objections - or even that I think all or most coaches do. But since I have come across every single one of them first hand, clearly some do.

## 5.3.1 "Coaching and Therapy Shouldn't be Combined"

The central objection to using EFT within coaching is that coaching is not therapy and therefore the two should not be combined. This, of course, is based on a more general assumption that EFT is a type of therapy which, as I have asserted already, is not the case and I have given some general reasons why this is so.

However, many people assume it is and therefore have objections based on that assumption. I have also said that the term "therapy" is misunderstood by many people. And in what follows below, I examine several specific misunderstandings or mis-definitions of therapy which are or could be used as the basis for objections to using EFT, and show how even accepting those assumptions does not preclude the use of EFT.

Related sections:

5.1         EFT isn't (Psycho)therapy ⇧

### 5.3.1.1 "Therapy is About the Past, Coaching is About the Future"

The distinction that is often used regarding coaching and therapy is:

Therapy is about "what happened?" – reviewing the past and coming to terms

Coaching is about "what's next?" - making plans, taking action

At first sight this looks like a neat and clear divide: therapy is about the past, coaching is about the future.

But coaching clients are never blank slates who turn up at the session with no past. The way they make choices and their problems achieving goals are **totally** about what they believe is possible for them based on their past experiences. Even if coaching doesn't involve spending time talking about the past (because you've told them to "Bottomline" their issue without telling you the story), the past is still there in the background, lurking, influencing the client's thinking and feelings about their goals and about what's happening in the coaching session itself.

In fact, the past is frequently visited even within conventional coaching. Some basic coaching techniques such as Peak Experiences depend on the coach and the client revisiting the past in order to learn and gather resources.

Another clear way that the "past" is dealt with in coaching occurs simply as a result of the ongoing coaching process. Most coaching relationships last at least a few weeks, and can go on for 6, 12 or 18 months. This means that the coach and client will be, quite correctly, wanting to look at events from the client's recent past – even if it is only to find out how the client did with their homework last week. Although this may seem like an absurd argument, my point is this: What is the difference in examining what happened to the client last week, and what happened to them 10 years ago? Why is last week's experience acceptable to include under "coaching", while the other must be seen as "therapy"?

I believe the past/future distinction between what defines therapy and what defines coaching is simplistic and misleading. I believe that it is not **where in time** you visit that defines therapy versus coaching, but what you **do** while you're there.

To take a geographical metaphor, one person may visit a seaside hotel in order to recharge their batteries, enjoy the peace and quiet and fresh air and to feel inspired while they plan the next stage of their lives. Another person may be in the next room in the very same hotel in order to escape a violent relationship, and write a history of their abusive past. The choice of location in time and space is the same. The focus of attention and intention of the two people are entirely different – and it is this which makes the distinction between "What happened" and "What's next", not whether the current place of learning is the past or the future.

I strongly believe that if the coaching relationship is set up correctly from the outset, with coaching goals clearly defined, then it **is** possible and acceptable to spend time looking at the past when it is plain that these issues are holding the client back from achieving their coaching goals.

Related sections:

6.1.2        Coaching the Client's Whole Life ⇩

6.1.12       Coaching the Past ⇩

6.1.21       Bottomlining ⇩

8.1.12       Peak Experiences ⇩

## 5.3.1.2   Client Confusion about Therapy versus Coaching

One of the biggest reasons given for avoiding therapy within coaching is the fear that clients can get confused about which is which. (As I have already stated above, "therapy" is a technical term which has entered everyday language and which is therefore widely misunderstood by clients and coaches alike).

For "talk-based therapies" such as counselling, psychotherapy, cognitive behavioural therapy or other techniques based primarily on dialogue between client and therapist, I would agree that the client is going to find it hard to distinguish when they are being coached and when they are receiving "therapy".

But, even if you think that EFT is a therapy (which I don't, for reasons already stated), one of the beauties of EFT is that it is **very** clear to the client when it is taking place!

If you are doing a setup statement, tapping on the points and checking intensity levels you are doing EFT. When you stop and continue the conversation, you are coaching. It's true that there sometimes needs to be discussion between rounds of EFT to check intensity levels or deal with insights and root issues that might come up - but it is obvious that this discussion is following on from a round or leading to another round of EFT.

Because of the explicit nature of EFT, it is also very easy to obtain informed and meaningful consent from the client. The client can't "drift" into doing EFT on an issue without realising it, in the way that might occur with counselling or psychotherapy.

In short, using EFT within coaching, even for issues that might be regarded as "therapeutic" purposes (i.e. dealing with the past), is a very "clean" approach. It is clear to the client when it is happening and this provides awareness to both client and coach about what is happening and when.

Related sections:

5.1        EFT isn't (Psycho)therapy ⇧

## 5.3.1.3 Primary Focus of Attention

Even though EFT isn't itself a therapy, it is used by many therapists (psychotherapists, hypnotherapists, acupuncturists, counsellors, even doctors and nurses) for issues that are normally considered as "requiring therapy". I will refer to this use of EFT as "EFT in a therapy context".

Carrying out EFT with a client in a therapy context has some distinct differences to using EFT as a coaching tool, even though the technical application of EFT, when it is used in either case, is identical.

It is this rather subtle change of "flavour" and "contextual atmosphere" that can be hard to grasp initially - and was something that I grappled with in my practice for some time. One key difference is on the "primary focus of attention" in the two contexts.

When using EFT in a therapy context, the primary focus is on the client's problem and the use of EFT to clear the emotional charge the client feels in relation to it. The goal is to fix the presenting problem, defined as achieving zero intensity for the specific problem(s). There is no need for reference to wider life goals within the session, even if there turns out to be a long term impact on the client. Where an EFT practitioner does consider wider ecological impact on the client's life (e.g. when dealing with addictions or behaviours which have dominated a client's life for many years), this is only as a precaution to check for possible negative impacts which either need to be dealt with as part of the EFT, or which affect the pace at which the work proceeds.

In contrast, when using EFT as a coaching tool, the primary focus is on the client's stated coaching goals. The client wants to achieve one or more goals, such as making a big life change, completing a project or increasing their level of fulfilment. This primary focus makes EFT just one of many tools and techniques within the coach's repertoire, along with visualisations, life purpose exercises, balance wheels and so forth. In a coaching context, the coach decides to use EFT, or some other technique, only if at that point EFT seems to be the best way to move the client towards their goal. This affects what EFT gets applied to. The client may have a significant emotional issue – but if it is not related to or getting in the way of achieving the coaching goal, then it won't be addressed during the coaching using EFT or anything else.

Holding the client's coaching goals as the "primary focus of attention" is a way to ensure that EFT is used only as a coaching tool, and not a therapeutic one. In coaching terms, it requires the coach to "hold the client's agenda" and not allow the coaching to be side-tracked.

Related sections:

| | |
|---|---|
| 5.1 | EFT isn't (Psycho)therapy ⇧ |
| 6.1.13 | Holding the Client's Agenda ⇩ |
| 8.2.8 | Ecology Testing ⇩ |

## 5.3.1.4 Therapy Goals and Coaching Goals

Another key difference between EFT in a therapy context and EFT as a coaching tool, is the definition of the "goal".

When EFT is used in a therapy context, the "problem" is whatever the client is experiencing as distressing or negative in their life. This would typically be a relatively severe issue causing the client ongoing and noticeable distress. It is the distress which has prompted the client to seek help. Examples would be a recognisable list of EFT-able issues: trauma, grief, phobias, PTSD and so on. The "goal" of EFT in a therapy context is therefore to relieve the distress and restore emotional balance.

Within a coaching context, the "problem" is whatever is blocking the client's progress towards their stated coaching goals. The ultimate "goal" of EFT as a coaching tool is therefore identical to the overall coaching goal – with subgoals of removing whatever emotional blocks to progress may be found. This change of context can result in using EFT for much milder issues which the client may never have even have thought about as being a particular problem before and which probably would never have prompted seeking professional help to solve.

For instance, suppose a client's goal is to start their own business and they have hired a coach to help them achieve this goal. In the course of working through what needs to be done to achieve this goal, the client and coach may discover that the client has a dread of filling in forms, is nervous about making phone calls to people she doesn't know, and has a block when it comes to understanding basic finance. These issues don't stop someone from living a happy life - but become major issues in relation to the larger life goal. "Problems" in a coaching context are therefore defined according to what emotional issues are preventing the client from moving towards their goals.

The fact is that emotional state and goal achievement are tightly coupled. Sports psychology demonstrates this explicitly. To be asked to coach without having recourse to one of the fastest and safest ways of managing emotional state yet discovered, is really to put arbitrary professional boundaries above the needs of clients.

Like many of our belief systems, the distinction between coaching and therapy may have been valuable once. But our knowledge of human performance and the interaction of the human energy system and human behaviour has moved on and expanded. Coaching needs to expand its view of itself to keep up. As a "content free" and client-led technique, I believe that EFT offers the perfect tool for bridging this gap between the need to address emotional state and the ultimate focus on goal achievement.

**Note:**

It may well be that the problems that turn up within coaching are of the more severe type - in which a qualified practitioner of EFT may legitimately offer to deal with it. It's also possible that what starts off looking like a fairly mild block (e.g. disliking calling unknown people on the phone) may lead to uncovering childhood traumas and fears. In these cases it is important that the coach maintains clarity about EFT as coaching tool and EFT in a therapy context. If the issue that comes up is sufficiently big, in the coach's opinion, it is advisable to put the coaching relationship on hold and book specific sessions to deal with and fully clear the issue before resuming coaching. It remains an option at all times to refer the client to a different therapist or practitioner for that issue, especially if it may involve specialist experience. Ultimately, coach and client need to agree explicitly what is happening and how the coaching will be affected.

### 5.3.2  Fixing versus Changing

Although coaching does not aim to "fix" a client (because they are assumed to be Creative, Resourceful and Whole), nevertheless, whatever definition of therapy or coaching you prefer, coaching does (and should) result in client **change**. In my opinion, it is the linguistic confusion between the idea of someone being changed and someone being "fixed" which is really at the heart of many coaches' discomfort or worry about the therapy/coaching divide.

To be comfortable knowing that one is not "doing therapy", requires coaches to be clear about what sort of change can occur **within** coaching, even when there has been no sniff of "therapy" at any stage.

Client change has occurred whenever:

- Self-concept is expanded
- Values are honoured more
- Fears and doubts are honoured less
- The idea of what's possible is expanded
- Self-belief is expanded

- Behavioural flexibility is increased

- Action towards goals is easier

All of these changes are changes in the clients "way of being" (although they may also show up in what the client "does"). But nothing needed to be "fixed" in order to achieve that. What happens in client change is a realisation of potential, through changes in perspective and self-understanding, and an alteration of the choices that the client is making.

All of these changes produce positive results in client's lives. And yet, undergoing coaching, with or without EFT, to bring about these changes, is not seen as "fixing" the client - it's just seen as the outcome of good coaching. And these remain exactly the sort of changes or outcome that are being aimed for but which might be achieved more quickly with EFT-assisted coaching

I may seem to be labouring this issue. But since the coaching versus therapy issue is so problematic for many coaches - and especially for coaches with therapeutic backgrounds - that I have considered it useful to come at the issue from as many angles as possible. Only by considering the issue in many different ways is it possible for each individual to deal with the complexity of an issue which is so often presented in black and white.

Related sections:

6.1.1      The Client is Creative, Resourceful and Whole ⇩


## 5.3.3   "Using EFT in coaching is an easy way out"

This objection is rooted in the "No pain, no gain" philosophy that characterises so much of our "very gainful and very painful" culture. Whether you want to blame it on centuries of religious conditioning about the "holiness of sacrifice", or whether you think we feel unworthy of success unless we've "paid" for it by being unhappy first, the fact is, Pain isn't necessary for Gain - at least not in the field of energy psychology.

That doesn't mean you don't have to work, be persistent, show up consistently and so forth in order to achieve results. It's just that the process of working, being persistent and showing up needn't be unpleasant - and without the presence of inner conflict and "reversals", it should actually be experienced as satisfying and fulfilling.

Coaches should be as interested in the client's Process (their ongoing state of being) as in their results. A client who goes through hell to achieve a particular goal is probably going to think twice before doing it again. A client who starts out feeling unequal to their chosen goal but who achieves it with relative ease and pleasure is a client who is more likely to feel confident about tackling more changes or projects in the future.

The job of any coach is surely to make the achievement of the client's goal easier (quicker, bigger, more sustainable) than it would be if she did it by herself.

Coaches take the trouble to attend coaching school, to learn coaching techniques and to get plenty of practice, so that they can find the **easiest** way of getting the client from stuck to unstuck, from failure to success, from dream to achievement. Any additional tool that makes any of these aspects easier is a complement to existing coaching tools, not a negation of them or of coaching in general.

This objection also implies concern about whether the client benefits fully from the learning that is involved in coaching at "normal speed". I deal with this as a separate objection below.

Related sections:

5.3.3    "Anything that works that fast must be superficial" ⇩

6.1.7    Process Coaching ⇩

6.2.3    Psychological Reversal ⇩

## 5.3.4   "Coaching should be about results, not about making clients feel better"

*"If you're going to fight a war you have to feel very well".*

*General Montgomery*

This is another objection rooted in "no pain, no gain", "if it's not hurting it's not working" thinking. These seem to be core beliefs of Western society - and they are severely self-limiting beliefs at that.

The fact is, if your clients start achieving the results they want in their lives, there is a pretty substantial risk that they **will** feel good about it.

It's also a fair bet that when your clients come to you they feel bad about something - such as  not achieving something yet, or not feeling fulfilled - and they want your help to not feel bad any more. They are trying to feel better via achieving a certain goal. And that's not confined to coaching - that applies to any reason anyone ever has for doing anything.

There are numerous coaching behaviours and skills which are expressly aimed at making the client feel better in order that they continue to make progress (e.g. celebrating with the client), increasing the client's feeling of resourcefulness (e.g. tapping into Peak Experiences in order to connect with resourceful states) and so on.

"Feeling better" is at the heart of coaching - it is central to the process and it is an inevitable outcome of its success. You can't get a client from stuck to unstuck without involving them feeling better about the thing they feel stuck with. Basically, feeling stuck feels bad. Getting unstuck - realising there are options and a way forward, even if the solution hasn't yet been found or the goal been reached - feels better. Suddenly there is hope, optimism, a sense of progress and possibility that wasn't present before. Feeling good is therefore not a luxury - it's at the heart of all significant and sustained achievement. EFT and other energy-based techniques simply encourage the client's awareness of their emotional state as a tool to move them forward.

Related section

8.1.1    Resourceful States ⇩

8.1.12   Peak Experiences ⇩

## 5.3.5   "Anything that works that fast must be superficial"

Some coaches believe that working through a client's obstacles to achievement is a process which must take significant time or else "the lessons won't be fully learned". Somehow, "fast" is equated with "superficial". And the idea of removing lifelong fears or blocks to progress in a single session, or even in two or three sessions, invites suspicion that something has been "missed" or that the client's new "way of being" cannot possibly be sustained in the long term because the results can't be very deep, real or permanent.

This attitude exactly mirrors the reaction of the psychotherapy profession when Roger Callahan first began using TFT (a forerunner of EFT) with his psychotherapy clients and began publishing his results.

Callahan (and his student Gary Craig who developed EFT as a self-help version of TFT), observed that even though the results were often fast, they also seemed to be permanent. Clients who were previously water phobic (or spider phobic or flying phobic) and who were released from their phobia, did not "relapse" back into their phobias later on. Clients who suffered severe anxiety and distress while thinking about past traumas and who became able to retell their stories without a flicker of anxiety, did not reacquire their distress for that story later on. They observed that the only times a client would notice distress for an issue that had been worked on with EFT was when they were presented with some aspect of the feared object, or some element of the story which had not come up during the EFT session and therefore had not specifically had EFT applied to it.

The reason that results seem to be permanent lies in the assumption that EFT makes regarding the cause of negative emotions.

What's important here is to bring into consciousness, and then question, the assumption (belief) that things **must** take a long time only because they **did** take a long time in the past. If you are a coach then you will be comfortable with the idea of questioning beliefs, thinking about where they really come from and being prepared to try out a new perspective.

I will observe that the "rate of change" that occurs with EFT, tends to happen at a speed appropriate to the client and their own particular requirements. There appears to be something self-regulating about how quickly or how slowly different clients release different problems and make progress towards goals. If you are a coach you will be familiar with this natural variation between clients already. Although EFT can accelerate many processes within coaching, I do not believe it is possible for a client to move faster than is useful or constructive for him. I cover the issues of Beliefs about the Rate of Change and Changing Beliefs Safely in more detail below.

If this objection is one that is a problem for you, I urge you to deal with it not at the level of belief or as an intellectual exercise, but at the level of practice and results. Try it for yourself. Try it with your friends. Get hold of Gary Craig's training materials and see the results of EFT in action. In fact I recommend this in any case as part of the practice integration process.

Related sections:

6.2.1       The Cause of Negative Emotions ⇩
6.1.16     Action and Learning ⇩
8.1.11     Locking in the Learning ⇩
9.5.3       Changing Beliefs Safely ⇩
9.5.5       Beliefs about the Rate of Change ⇩
11.1         Practice Integration Process ⇩

## 5.3.6    "EFT doesn't respect the uniqueness of each individual client"

This objection is rooted in the observation that EFT appears to be a simple "one size fits all" protocol. This is then compared against coaching's regard for each individual as a unique human being.

It's true that EFT involves tapping the same set of meridian points for every issue and every person. It's also true that the general form of the setup statement has the same structure for each application of EFT. But that's where the truth of the objection ends.

Each application of EFT is totally customised to the individual based on:

- Their actual intensity rating at the start
- The problem being worked on
- The words the client uses to describe the problem
- The related memories or insights the client has mentioned

In fact, a great deal of the practitioner training is spent exactly on the issue of forming the right setup statement for each client and each issue, learning how to find and use exactly the right terms that "do it" for the client.

An EFT session is rather like going to be fitted for a suit. The tailor may start out with a very general pattern and taking some standard overall measurements. But to really get a well fitting suit requires minute adjustments, creative solutions to be found for "non-standard" body shapes and extremely close attention to the **client**, rather than the suit.

In a room full of suited people it may appear that "everybody is dressed the same", but for each suit to really fit has required totally individual attention. Successful and effective use of EFT requires the same level of personalisation and is very far from being a "one size fits all" solution.

I may finally note not only the existence of "standard" coaching tools (such as wheel of life, Peak Experiences or Future Self) but also the proliferation of "coach-yourself" books which cannot possibly hope or claim to be providing an individualised service. And yet these tools and these books have value - because the client comes along and provides the content of his own life and experience which suddenly make the exercises uniquely relevant to each reader. These "standard" coaching tools and exercises provide a structure within which the individual can work in a unique way - and EFT is just the same.

# 5.4  Suggested Principles of EFT Coaching

Having satisfied ourselves that EFT need not contravene any existing coaching ethics and that many common objections to EFT are not well founded, it is still useful to define a set of principles to guide how it **is** used within a coaching context. This is because even though EFT can be applied in a way that avoids a "therapy" context, there are still many therapeutic uses for EFT which would not be appropriate in a coaching context (just as for some NLP interventions).

I am not advocating carte blanche use of EFT on anything and everything that might occur within a coaching session – I am advocating selective and conscious use of EFT in specific ways and within a defined framework. The following principles are offered as a suggested framework for ethically using EFT within coaching. They are offered because they have worked for me - you are free to adopt your own set of principles of course. Most of the following principles have already been hinted at in the previous sections.

## 5.4.1  Principle of Informed Permission

It's a central principle of coaching - especially co-active coaching - that everything that occurs within the coaching - choice of tools, choice of area to explore - is done only with the permission of the client. Nothing is imposed or prescribed and the client is never obliged to take part in any exercise, process or discussion if they do not want to.

I believe strongly that the same should apply to the use of EFT within coaching, and not just because of the general principle of respecting the client's wishes and building trust.

Forcing a client to do EFT is likely to set up a Psychological Reversal to the process, which will prevent it from working. If you are a confident coach and you have built up good rapport with your client, then the chances are that a client will "comply" with a request or suggestion to use EFT. But it is especially important to understand your power in this matter and to make it very explicit to clients that (a) they don't have to use EFT except when they want to, and (b) if they get to a point in the process of using EFT where they want to stop, that they can do so.

Permission in the form of compliance is not good enough. The client needs to give **informed** permission. This means that they need to be educated enough about what EFT can do, and about the alternatives available, that agreement to use EFT on a specific issue can be a conscious choice. This issue of choice and education of the client should be covered explicitly when designing the alliance with the client. But it is also the coach's job to remind the client whenever he perceives a risk of overstepping the boundaries of the client's true wishes.

Related sections:

6.2.3      Psychological Reversal ⇩

6.1.4      The Designed Alliance ⇩

## 5.4.2   Principle of Personal Ethic

This principle can be expressed as:

*"If I would go here with conventional coaching, I can also go here with EFT"*

So, if in conventional coaching you absolutely avoid ever exploring the past with a client, then you will not be in personal integrity to start going there with EFT. But if there are specific times when you do already consider it useful and in the client's interests to visit the past (e.g. for learning and reference), then using EFT in that context does not contravene your existing ethic.

In other words, this principle says that instead of wondering whether to use a particular tool (*"Is it OK to EFT here?"*), the question becomes one of territory and objectives of the coaching (*"Does exploring this issue further the client's coaching goals?"*).

I discussed above the need for coaches to develop their own personal code of conduct in addition to any professional code of conduct they have signed up to. This principle shows the practical usefulness of doing so, since it allows ethical decisions to be made much more easily concerning the use of new tools.

## 5.4.3   Principle of Goal Furtherance

This principle can be expressed by the question:

*"In what way will using EFT now, get the client closer to his goal?"*

I am suggesting that the appropriate way to use EFT within a coaching context is in direct furtherance of the client's agreed coaching goals. This principle is a powerful and easy way to avoid getting side-tracked into a client's other emotional issues, even if it is obvious that the client's current emotional issue could be addressed using EFT.

This is in keeping with coaching's viewpoint on client emotions generally. It is not the purpose of coaching to be led by the client's current emotional state or emotional response to the coaching. **Managing** the client's emotional state is not the purpose of coaching. But **noticing** the client's emotional state is required in order to know where the client is, and to understand what obstacles may be in the way of achieving the client's goals. The focus of attention is always and ultimately on getting the client nearer his goal.

Related sections:

5.3.1.3    Primary Focus of Attention ⇧

## 5.4.4  Principle of Congruent Motivation

The principle of congruent motivation addresses the question

*"What is a proper motivation for using EFT in my coaching?"*

With so many coaching academies and so many brands, breeds and specialisations of coaching, it can be hard to select which type of coaching you want to do - or what additional tools (NLP, EFT etc) you want to bring into your offering as a coach.

With coaching burgeoning as a profession, coaches are increasingly being urged to find ways to differentiate themselves from other coaches or to "find their niche". Unfortunately, the goal of "finding your niche" can turn into a fairly superficial marketing exercise, instead of being what it should be – a way of asking yourself hard questions about who you really want to be as a coach and how your coaching fulfils your purpose as a person. At this particular moment in time, EFT looks like a great way to stand out from the coaching crowd - just as NLP did for some time - but that is not why I included it in my practice, and it probably shouldn't be your motivation either.

I use EFT simply because I fell in love with it. It worked for me personally. I became fascinated by its possibilities. And I found myself becoming frustrated when I was working with clients, knowing that at particular points EFT would be a highly efficient tool and would undoubtedly fast-track my client towards their goals, but I felt unable to use it because of various "cannots" and "should nots" that I picked up as a new coach.

Do not add EFT to your coaching because you think it is "fashionable" or because you fear you might be "left behind" by other coaches. Neither should you add EFT to your coaching because you fear that coaching by itself is lacking (or worse, that **your** coaching is lacking). The truth is, you don't **need** EFT to be an excellent coach.

Only add EFT to your coaching if you feel strongly drawn to it, and feel inspired by the possibilities that might be possible for **your clients** if you do. As with all coaching, a big part of your power as a coach lies in the degree to which you can model congruence for your client - they get to experience you in a state of personal integrity and acting congruently with your true self, unafraid to express that and given in service to the client's goals.

Doing EFT with a client because you think you "ought to" use new methods, or because you fear that your other coaching techniques aren't good enough on their own, will be picked up by the client, at least unconsciously. The correct reason to use EFT at a particular point within your coaching is because at that precise moment in time, you feel with all your intuition, heart and mind that of all the techniques available to you, EFT is the perfect one to use.

(Notice this criteria also means you get to choose a non-EFT technique if you feel that is what is required, even if you "know" that the issue is an EFT-able one.)

## 5.4.5   Principle of Integration with Integrity

It is important that the way that you go about learning EFT and integrating it into your practice should build and enhance your own feeling of integrity about using it with clients.

Making any change to your coaching practice, whether it be changing your charging structure, changing how you advertise and enrol clients or adopting new techniques into your repertoire, requires one specific thing to make it work:  and that is to make whatever changes congruent with your professional standards and ethics and with your personal sense of honour.

I have covered the issue of professional ethics as regards coaching above. But since each person's personal standards and sense of honour are based on different criteria, what recommendation can be made that will address these - and yet still leave the final decision in your hands as a professional?

I believe the answer is to follow a process that ensures your personal and direct experience of EFT as a self-help user and as a client of an experienced practitioner, and to avail yourself of the best quality training available to you in your area. In section 11 I give a step-by-step process for experiencing EFT and building up your knowledge in a congruent way which is intended to help fulfil this principle.

Related sections:

11.1        Practice Integration Process ⇩


## 5.4.6   Principle of Client Responsibility

This principle is a re-emphasis of a coaching principle: that the **client** is responsible for his own progress and the **client** does the work. (It also mirrors an EFT fundamental that clients are responsible for their own wellbeing).

This principle means avoiding any use of EFT in which the coach "does EFT to or for" the client.

There are therefore a few varieties of EFT which I personally have decided **not** to use within a coaching context:

- Surrogate tapping - where the coach taps on themselves in place of the client - either during or between sessions.
- Proxy tapping - where the coach remotely taps on the client - either physically or by mentally imagining tapping on the client - either during or between sessions.

I believe that proxy or surrogate tapping for a coaching client is as inappropriate as praying for them, sending them angels or worrying about them in between sessions.

If you strongly feel the need to be tapping on your client's behalf then you may have a self-management issue that you need to deal with. For instance: *"Even though I feel responsible for the client…"*.

Even if you feel a strong desire to proxy tap your client and even if your client **asks** you to do so, it is ill-advised. To do so without their knowledge violates the principle of permission. To do so **with** their knowledge is to set up a emotional dependence on you, which is totally counter to the object of coaching - which is to help clients develop their own resourcefulness and power over their own lives.

If you still feel strongly drawn to providing a proxy tapping service, then you need to rethink the label you choose for your service. There are many people providing "remote healing" of various kinds, and EFT could well be one of them - but this is **not** coaching.

Although proxy tapping and surrogate tapping when the client is not present is not recommended, this does not mean that the coach must never tap themselves while coaching. There are occasions when a coach may tap for their own issues, or to maintain rapport with a client or to work on shared issues - these occasions are covered elsewhere in the book (Avoiding Burnout and Co-active Tapping).

Much has been written about the apparent improvement in results when two people work on an issue together perhaps with one tapping the other, compared to one person working alone - and I do not dispute this effect. When I am doing EFT with a client, I always tap along as a matter of course - but not to deliberately increase the effect, but to maintain my rapport (an accepted and desirable coaching goal) and to help me tune in to what is happening with the client.

Please understand that surrogate or proxy tapping will not cause harm to your client in terms of their emotional or physical wellbeing. The harm is to the fundamental principle of coaching - that the object is to help the client become a resourceful and empowered person.

I have included direct physical tapping of the client under the definition of proxy tapping, even though direct tapping is a common practice amongst practitioners. Although it does not violate the Principle of Permission (you can easily obtain permission from the client), it does violate the principle of Client Responsibility. Barring physical disability there is not normally any reason why a client cannot tap themselves. To do a client's tapping for them creates a dependence which I believe is inappropriate for a coaching context.

Related sections:

5.4.1      Principle of Informed Permission ⇧

6.2.13    Clients are Responsible for their own Wellbeing ⇩

7.1.7      Avoiding Burn-out ⇩

8.2.2      Co-active Tapping ⇩

# 5.5  Key Points

- Ensure you examine and maintain concordance with the ethics of any professional body you are currently a member of. For ICF members I believe this means: (1) Making your use of EFT clear to clients when they sign up; (2) Making the status and expected results of EFT clear to clients; and (3) Making your qualifications in EFT explicit to clients.

- It is advisable to develop a personal code of conduct on top of any external ethical obligations. This personal code of conduct will enable you to avoid being a "cookie-cutter coach" - to develop your own distinct style, specialism or use of innovative coaching tools without feeling hampered by poorly defined ethics.

- The divide between "therapy" and coaching is not as simple as the distinction between the past and the future. The past is a valid place to visit within coaching, and clients never begin coaching with a "blank slate". It's not visiting the past which defines the process as "therapy" - but your reason for going and what you do when you are there.

- The nature of EFT is that it is very clear when it is happening - enabling the client to easily avoid confusion between coaching and EFT. This contrasts with traditional talk therapies where client confusion can more easily arise.

- When EFT is used in a therapy context the primary focus of attention is on the client's emotional intensity and what factors (Reversals or Aspects) are contributing to it. There is no attention on wider life goals or life purpose. In coaching, the primary focus of attention is on the client achieving their coaching goal(s) - only emotional issues which are preventing progress towards the agreed goal are relevant to address with EFT.

- The "goal" of EFT in a therapy context is to remove emotional distress - which would typically be significant enough to prompt the client to seek help. The "goal" in EFT Coaching is the client's overall coaching goal and its purpose is to remove any emotional blocks to progress - which may be very mild in emotional intensity.

- EFT is not "an easy way out" in a coaching context. EFT teaches us that it is not necessary for a client to experience pain or struggle in order to achieve meaningful goals. The purpose of coaching is to unstick clients and help them move towards action and success - EFT simply offers one more tool to help that process of unsticking clients.

- Coaching isn't just about getting results - it's also about the client's state of Being - and that critically includes them feeling better. Feeling better is a valid goal within coaching, both at the start of the process - when the client experiences new hope and confidence about achieving his goals - and at the end, when they can enjoy their achievement.

- EFT enables fast change - but it is far from superficial. Changes resulting from EFT tend to be permanent. The speed of change also seems to be naturally self-regulating according to client belief and need.

- EFT is a highly individualised technique, requiring the practitioner to take account of each client's vocabulary, contributing Aspects and Reversals in order to achieve results. This makes EFT entirely compatible with a personalised process such as coaching.

- Coaches are urged to develop their own principles for using EFT or any other modality in conjunction with coaching, but the following principles are offered:

- Principle of Informed Permission: Clients should be sufficiently educated about EFT and its uses that informed permission can be obtained by the coach whenever it is used. Passive compliance is not sufficient.

- Principle of Personal Ethic: Whatever principles you apply to your coaching in general should also apply to your use of EFT. Using EFT should never result in you exploring areas you would not explore using conventional coaching techniques.

- Principle of Goal Furtherance: The proper use of EFT within coaching is to further the client's progress towards their agreed coaching goals. This principle avoids coach and client getting side-tracked into other emotional issues not connected with the goals.

- Principle of Congruent Motivation: Your personal motivation for using EFT within coaching should be congruent with your personal experience of EFT. It should not be motivated by external pressure such as fashionability or finding a niche. Incongruent use of EFT at specific times or in general will be felt by your client.

- Principle of Integration with Integrity: You need to integrate EFT into your personal life before you can integrate it into your practice with integrity. This means following a staged process of exploring and using EFT for yourself and satisfying yourself of its efficacy, before using it with clients.

- Principle of Client Responsibility: Avoid any use or pattern of EFT which involves "doing to or for" the client. This includes avoiding surrogate or proxy tapping, or physically tapping the client yourself.

# 6 Fundamentals

This chapter looks at some key fundamentals of both EFT and coaching. As stated at the start, this book is not intended to teach you how to coach or how to be an EFT practitioner. Nevertheless it is useful to introduce some fundamental concepts of both which underpin what follows, especially since they are referred to later on in this book. If you are a coach who is already very familiar with EFT, then you may skip this section - although you may enjoy seeing just how compatible coaching and EFT are in terms of their philosophy of the client.

The purpose of presenting these fundamentals is twofold:

Firstly, it is a way to introduce some basic concepts to readers who perhaps are familiar with EFT but not coaching (or vice versa) and who therefore would benefit from a primer in one or the other.

Secondly, it serves, for those readers who are familiar with one or both fields, to talk about the degree to which coaching and EFT fundamentals are compatible. It's important when you are grounded in a discipline with strong ethics to be sure that if you are to add a modality to your work that the new modality does not contravene your existing ethical framework, or to be assured that the new discipline reinforces those principles.

The more I closely examined the underlying principles of coaching and the practical features of EFT, the more I became convinced that the two methods are extremely close in philosophy and practice. The following explores this relationship in some depth. If by some chance you find it hard to integrate coaching with EFT on grounds of ethics or principles after reading this, then at least you will know on what point(s) you object, which I hope will be helpful to you in coming to a decision based on your own integrity.

## 6.1 Coaching Fundamentals

In this section we examine many fundamental ideas and principles that exist within the coaching profession to see how the nature or use of EFT relates to them. Sometimes EFT directly and obviously supports these fundamentals. Sometimes there seems to be a contradiction - which needs examination and resolution. And sometimes it's not clear what the relationship is - and finding a relationship helps to build an overall picture of the relationship between EFT and coaching.

### 6.1.1 The Client is Creative, Resourceful and Whole

*"From a co-active coach's point of view, nothing is wrong or broken, there is no need to fix the client. ...When they look inside with the help of a coach, they'll find they know themselves, their strengths and their limitations."* [2]

One of the four cornerstones of the co-active coaching model is that the client has nothing wrong with them and does not need to be fixed. However, the client does have things in their life they would like to achieve or improve.

One of the common distinctions often drawn between therapy and coaching centres on this point: that therapy is about "fixing" a client who needs it, while coaching is about working with a client who is already "whole". The more I have worked with both coaching and EFT the more I have come to reject this distinction and indeed this view of the "therapy" client.

At first sight, the idea of using EFT within coaching to "clear negative emotions" seems like a violation of this assumption. Having wrestled with this apparent "contradiction" for some time in my own practice, I want to offer a perspective I have come to which has synthesised the two viewpoints in myself and which now allows me to use EFT as a coaching tool with complete personal integrity and fully honouring the Creativeness, Resourcefulness and above all Wholeness of all my clients.

The solution to this paradox lies in the standard EFT setup statement:

> "Even though I have this problem, I deeply and completely accept myself".

In this statement are held two important implicit ideas:

- That "the problem" is a separate thing to "I" - expressable as "I am not my problem, I am me".
- That the "I" remains completely acceptable (perfect and whole), regardless of the currently experienced "problem".

Indeed, many practitioners and self-help users of EFT have varied the final part of the setup statement to more accurately reflect their own particular form of self acceptance such as:

> "Even though I have this problem, I'm OK"

> "Even though I have this problem, I love myself"

> "Even though I have this problem, God loves me"

> "Even though I have this problem, I'm a worthwhile person"

to give but a few examples. It would therefore be completely valid to create a new setup statement which goes:

> "Even though I have this problem, I am Creative, Resourceful and Whole"

To me, the fact that such a setup statement can be created, means that EFT need not in any way be a threat to the assumption of client creativity, resourcefulness and wholeness. Indeed EFT can be a way to explicitly and powerfully emphasise that fact to both coach and client.

EFT is premised on the assumption that underneath all the various energy disruptions that might be present in the client, is - and always has been - a whole, creative, resourceful being. In fact it is a notable and replicable feature of the effect of EFT that removal of emotional disruptions tends to bring out spontaneous expressions of all these aspects of the person.

In my experience, the effects of EFT in revealing the true client to themselves is very similar to the effects of using conventional coaching exercises which allow the client to connect with resourceful states, discover creative solutions to their problems or experience themselves as worthy and complete human beings. It's just that EFT can often get clients to these states somewhat faster, and that with EFT the effect tends to be sustained over a much longer period, if not permanently.

Holding your client as Creative, Resourceful and Whole is one thing - but getting your client to hold **themselves** that way is the ultimate in client empowerment. And for me, nothing beats EFT for getting clients in touch with that state fast and in a very experiential way - perhaps because the very structure of EFT draws this to the client's attention.

As Silvia Hartmann notes:

> "*EFT does not install anything new that was not there before,... There is no such thing as rubbing in positives during EFT... and this is not how the emergence of positive results comes into being. ...What EFT does is to get blockages out of the way which allow the* **natural abilities, functions and actualities of achievement** *inherent in the person who is using this to shine through and become activated.*"[3]

In other words, underneath the client's current set of negative thoughts, memories, stresses, blocks and all manner of other disturbances, the client **is** Creative, Resourceful and Whole. The job of the EFT practitioner, like the job of the coach, is to help this underlying client to be revealed. Michelangelo once claimed that when he sculpted a statue from a piece of marble, he wasn't creating something, he was only revealing what already lay within. In my view both coaching and EFT resonate perfectly with that principle. Using this metaphor, we can now view EFT as a particularly useful sort of chisel to help reveal the client to themselves.

## 6.1.2   Coaching Addresses the Client's Whole Life

The idea behind this second cornerstone of co-active coaching is that there is no part of the client's life that isn't able to benefit from coaching, or which might not need to be looked at in order to achieve goals in another area.

Conventionally, a person's "whole life" is intended to mean "all domains of a person's current existence" such as work, home, family, friends, health, finance, hobbies, relationships, spirituality etc. This is often represented in two dimensions by the ubiquitous coaching Balance wheel (or "Wheel of Life") with many spokes, each spoke representing an area of the person's life.

However, there is another dimension to the idea of someone's "whole life" which can sometimes be left out in coaching for fear of delving into "therapy" territory - and that is the time dimension.

For me as a person, "my whole life" includes every experience I've had from the moment I was born, including but not limited to all the aspects of my life right now such as work, home, family etc. Not only that, but since I do not expect to drop dead in the next 5 seconds, "my whole life" also includes a yet-uncreated life in the future. In fact, probably 99% of the concerns and issues I have about my current life only have any relevance in relation to an anticipated future life.

At first sight, EFT may seem to be focussed almost exclusively on the past - because it is often applied to past traumas and memories which have given rise to negative emotions and beliefs. But in fact, within an EFT session, the most consistently referenced and examined point in time is **right now**. It's a fundamental part of the EFT procedure that the practitioner needs to keep checking out the client's **current** intensity of feeling in order to track progress and know when the issue is cleared.

As an EFT practitioner, I am not very interested in knowing about what happened in the past. I may ask the client to tell the story of what happened, but only in order for the client to tune into how she feels about it **now**. I don't even want to know how she felt back then - I only want to know how she feels right **now**. The client's **current** intensity and quality of feeling is the **absolute compass** by which the EFT practitioner navigates. In other words, the past is only a place of reference - all the work occurs while focussed on the present. In fact, it is so irrelevant to the EFT practitioner to know what happened, that it is entirely possible for the client to tell themselves the story, without telling the practitioner, and simply report the ratings they get after each round of EFT.

For me, EFT allows a particularly powerful way of tying together the client's past influences with their future goals without having to get into "therapy" about it. I believe it is all too easy for a "therapy phobic" coach to push forward on a client's goals even when it is clear that there are emotional obstacles to progress or success that are rooted in the past. EFT offers a way to release these obstacles without getting caught up in lengthy stories about the client's past, examining how they felt back then or any of those other "therapy" type interactions. Only by allowing in the client's full experience of their past, their present and their future can a coach claim to be "addressing a clients whole life".

Related sections:

5.3.1.1   "Therapy is about the Past, Coaching is about the Future" ⇧

6.1.12    Coaching the Past ⇩

## 6.1.3   The Agenda Comes from the Client

*"In a co-active coaching relationship the agenda comes from the client, not the coach.
...They set the agenda. The coach's job is to ensure the agenda doesn't get lost."* [2]

This is the third cornerstone of the co-active coaching model. In EFT also, both the starting point and end point of the work is determined completely by the client.

I recently took part in a weblist discussion on the role of forgiveness in healing. There were some on the weblist who had experienced abuse in childhood and were expressing extreme resentment at some types of therapy which "required" the client to achieve forgiveness of their perpetrators in order for the healing to be "done". This is a case of the therapist deciding the agenda for the client and imposing it on them.

In EFT, there is no prescribed endpoint. The client is "done" when they decide they are. Indeed, it is quite possible to achieve partial results with EFT and for clients to choose to stop at that point if that's the result they want for the moment - just as in coaching a client may decide on goals which a coach may believe are well below what is possible for the client, but which the client wants to limit themselves to right now, for their own reasons.

In EFT as in coaching, it is the client who decides what the "goal" is - and defines what "success" means to them.

*"...just asking the client up front what their fears and reservations might be, and asking them also how they would like to proceed, and where they would like to start, is the very best, and most ecological and most profoundly appreciated way of responding to any form of conscious or unconscious client resistance".* [4]

It is therefore completely possible to envisage using EFT as a tool in the service of the coaching, only to the degree that the client wants it and to the degree that it assists in the achievement of the coaching agenda.

Related sections:

6.1.8     Big Agendas and "little agendas" ⇩

6.1.14    Holding the Client's Agenda ⇩

## 6.1.4   The Designed Alliance

*"In co-active coaching, ...clients play an important part in declaring how they want to be coached. ... Clients learn that they are in control of the relationship and ultimately of the changes they make in their lives."* [2]

This is the fourth and final cornerstone of the co-active coaching model. It refers to the mutual responsibility and activity of client and coach to move the coaching forward and achieve the client's goals.

Since both hold equal responsibility for the outcome of the coaching, they need to agree at the start of the coaching relationship how they plan to work together, who will do what, how they will communicate with each other and so on.

So even though the client has come to the coach "for help", the relationship is conducted in such a way that empowerment is handed straight back to the client.

This closely mirrors the way that EFT practitioners work. EFT was originally designed specifically as a self-help tool. Gary Craig intended to make it so standard and straightforward that people could learn it quickly and apply it to themselves with relatively little in the way of training. EFT practitioners have spent time learning the depth and range of what EFT can be applied to, additional variations for specific situations, the theory behind the technique, a multitude of failsafes and ways to unstick the process, safety issues and more. But ultimately they never forget that once the client has learned the basic technique, they are fully empowered to apply it whenever they want to whatever they want. Not only that, but **within** a session, the client is fully able to direct the course of action and suggest different words to use for the setup statements, come up with new lines of enquiry and so on.

In Advanced Patterns of EFT, Silvia Hartmann talks about the concept of "client avidity"[4], contrasting this with compliance (where the client goes along with the practitioner because the practitioner is the expert) and defiance (where the client resists the practitioner for whatever reason). She says:

> "EFT…is a co-operative venture between client and therapist in every sense of the word, and so it is important that both are positive, excited and proactive about what is to come next… What we are looking for is a forward pointing state in which the client aligns with us and both of us really put our hearts, minds and souls forward to resolve the problem with volition and desire". [4]

That surely sounds like a co-active relationship to me!


## 6.1.5   Fulfilment Coaching

> "The definition of what fulfilment means to the client is always intensely personal. …It may include, especially at first, outward measures of success: a great job, enough money, a certain lifestyle. In most cases the coaching will quickly progress to a deeper definition of fulfilment. …what fills the client's heart and soul." [2]

This idea of Fulfilment in coaching closely mirrors the unfolding of an EFT session or series of sessions.

Initially, the client is looking for what might be called "hygiene factors" from the EFT - to sort out troubling emotions, to get the basic emotional functions in order and working smoothly again - just like getting the material functions of life in order during the early stages of coaching.

But as one emotional issue after another is laid to rest, clients start to realise the wider range of what's possible for them, not just emotionally, but in terms of their potential for enjoyment and fulfilment. For example, the client who has just released a lifetime's fear of flying now begins to make plans to visit all the places that she's only dreamed of visiting up till now. And then she realises that if she can fly, she might be able to work or live anywhere in the world that she chooses.

Another example might be of someone who has a dread of paperwork and finance. A client may seek out EFT in order to get him to a state that he can avoid getting nasty letters from the Inland Revenue because his bookkeeping is non-existent and his tax returns are late. But once these blocks are disposed of, he realises that he can do more than just keep on the right side of the taxman. Perhaps now he could start his own business. Or go for that management position he dreaded until now. Just like coaching then, EFT has the effect of expanding the client's idea of what fulfilment means while also helping them achieve it.

Related sections:

8.1.6        Fulfilment Clarification ⇩

## 6.1.6  Balance Coaching

*"Balance is a fluid state, always in motion, because life itself is dynamic"* [2]

Balance coaching is about looking at all parts of a client's life to ensure that all the areas that matter to them are receiving at least adequate attention. As the co-active coaching book says *"It is no service to clients…..to excel in one area of their lives without caring for the rest."* [2]

Where EFT comes into the picture is in understanding - and helping the client come to terms with - the true nature of what Balance really is. It is not a fixed state of affairs that can be achieved and then forgotten because it is "done". It is not much more useful to unstick the client from one fixed, habitual way of life, only for them to get stuck in a new fixed, habitual way of life, even if, like a freshly painted room, the new way of life looks marvellous to start with. This is because life - and especially a fulfilled life - is essentially about growth and change.

To allow a client to really "get" the true nature of Balance, involves more than shifting them from one state to another state - although that's usually a good place to start. To really empower a client to achieve ongoing Balance long after the coaching has ended, involves shifting the client's reasons for getting stuck in the first place - and this relates to the client's need for control.

Having life ordered, predictable and comfortable (i.e. stuck) makes people feel safe. Having things in a permanent state of flux makes many people feel unsettled and unsafe. (Even if you are the kind of person who enjoys change and flux more than most, I guarantee you that even you will have some threshold beyond which more change and flux is unpleasant for you.)

Suggesting to a client that to achieve this thing called Balance means they have to essentially keep reviewing and keep changing, can bring up a variety of negative feelings in many people: from general fear of change, fear of being out of control or even just downright discouragement and despair (*"You mean I can never really achieve this?"*). Perfectionists in particular can have a very hard time with this idea - needing to feel that something is "completed" is essential to them and is simply another way of achieving a feeling of being in control.

To understand how EFT can help with this need to "control", you need to also understand where the need for control comes from. Control derives from fear. The only reason you would ever need to control anything is because there is something you fear happening if you fail to control it. Or to put it another way - if the consequence of **not** having control is something that causes you no fear or concern, then why would you even think about controlling it?

Understanding that fear and the need for control are at the root of successful Balance coaching offers many ways for EFT to assist in that process.

Related sections:

8.1.7        Achieving Balance ⇩

9.2.4        Fear of Change ⇩

## 6.1.7 Process Coaching

*"The coach's job is to notice, point out and be with clients wherever they are in their process"* [2]

An important element of the co-active coaching model is the idea of life as Process. It's not just about the end results. Life is an ongoing process consisting of minute by minute Beings and Doings, which **together** make up the fabric of your life and your overall sense of satisfaction with it.

Process is the element of the co-active coaching approach which stops the coaching being **only** about achieving results (or Doing). It's the element that addresses the Being aspects of the client's life. Not only **what** the client achieved, but **how** she achieved it, **who** she had to become in order to do so, and what states of Being did she pass through along the way. By having a coach who is not only there but pointing out along the way, the client gets to more consciously understand their own Process - noticing their own patterns, making connections and getting insights into how they **are** which deepens their learning about themselves as a person and serves as a resource for later.

EFT also strongly emphasises paying close attention to the minute by minute changes in a client's state of Being as they work through the process of applying EFT to their problem. In fact it is only by closely following the in and outs, the surprises and resolutions of the client's process that a successful resolution can be reached.

One of the features of EFT I find particularly appealing is that even though the procedure works predominantly at the level of physical and emotional release, the client's conscious, rational mind gets to engage fully in the process and to have full awareness of what is happening. Someone didn't just come along and wave a magic wand (dangle a crystal, stick in a needle, lay on their hands or whatever) and "cause" the results to occur, leaving the client wondering what happened, how it happened and what the problem really was anyway.

With EFT the client gets to see and examine **for themselves** the insights, the connections and the process of release. And as the client becomes familiar with the process of EFT, this builds confidence and courage to attempt deeper work and bigger results for themselves - just as Process does within coaching.

Related sections:

8.1.8    Supporting Process Coaching ⇩

## 6.1.8 Big Agendas and "little agendas"

Coaches are trained to identify and distinguish between a client's "Big Agenda" and "little agenda". A "Big Agenda" is the client's coaching goal(s), as agreed at the beginning of the coaching. A "little agenda" is what's on the client's mind right now. Even though a client may be very focussed on an issue, it's the coach's job to notice whether or how this issue relates to the overall coaching goal(s).

For instance, the client's "Big Agenda" might be to achieve better Balance. Along the way there may be a "little agenda" involving the client's irritation with his boss. If the boss issue is affecting the degree to which the client is balancing his work with his family, then the "little agenda" is part of the "Big Agenda". If the client isn't having trouble taking time off work then the boss issue may be something that could or should be parked - or at least identified as a separate issue to be worked on later.

The EFT practitioner adopts a similar role in an EFT session. The client usually has one central problem (e.g. a phobia or a traumatic memory) they want to get rid of – but along the way many different Aspects and Reversals may come up which need to be dealt with in order to clear the overall problem. Or unrelated issues may come up. It is the practitioners job not only to keep track of progress with respect to the overall problem (The Big Agenda), but also only allow time to be spent on related Aspects and Reversals (the little agenda) if they are in service of the Big Agenda.

In EFT Coaching, once the overall coaching goal is agreed, and EFT is understood to be in the service of that goal, then the coaching Agenda and EFT Agenda become perfectly aligned – making the job of identifying any "little agendas" along the way no more difficult than in normal coaching, or normal EFT.

Related sections:

6.2.3      Psychological Reversal ⇩

6.2.12    Aspects ⇩

## 6.1.9  Coachability

Clients are described as "coachable" if they are ready and able to focus on "what's next" in their lives (rather than on "what happened"), and are willing to make the changes necessary to achieve their goals.

But I believe looking at the definition of "uncoachable" is also revealing. What are the reasons that a person isn't able to look at "what's next" or is having difficulty making changes in their life? To describe a client as "uncoachable" is actually often code for saying "the client needs therapy".

But looking at the definition of "coachability" in energy terms produces some interesting observations. More importantly (and encouragingly for the field of coaching) I believe EFT offers a way to expand the set of people who can be "coachable clients" by dealing with many of the issues that might otherwise mark a client out as "uncoachable".

Curiously, it's as important for an EFT client to be "EFT-able" as for a coaching client to be "coachable". There are some attitudes which will prevent EFT working - such as profound disbelief on the basis of existing scientific or religious conviction. But above all, if a client does not want to lose a particular problem, then EFT really won't budge it, even if it may take the edge off to some degree. Similarly in coaching, there needs to be a level of commitment to change from the client, or the best coach in the world isn't going to achieve much with this client.

To illustrate, let's take some examples.

### 6.1.9.1  Example 1

Suppose there is a woman who comes from a background of childhood abuse and low self-esteem. Let's also suppose that she starts a family very young, her marriage fails and she brings up her family alone and with very limited means and very little education. Now let's suppose she gets to her mid-thirties or forties, with children almost grown and she starts to yearn for a life of her own. She wants to improve her financial situation. And she is drawn to finally getting an education so that she can fulfil her talents.

This woman turns up at your office looking for coaching to help her make the transition from down-trodden mother to self-sufficient career woman. It's clear at the first session and as you learn about her history, that this is a woman of immense strength who has endured all that life has thrown her way and survived - not to mention bringing up her children. It is also clear that while she yearns for her new life, the traumas of her past and her low self-esteem are painfully near the surface.

Is this woman coachable? Does she have significant emotional issues which will be an impediment to her as she starts to make changes in her life? Yes. Does she have the strength of character to carry through a long-term project and succeed despite emotional challenges? Again, yes.

So, **is** she coachable?

Many coaches would suggest that a person with such emotional issues should first seek "therapy" to resolve or at least make manageable her past traumas, before beginning coaching.

If this client is eager to make life changes, should she be required to put these plans on hold while she deals with her past? If a coach decides that she should, what does it tell this woman about her ability to take charge of her own destiny when even the person she wants to hire to help, responds by making a judgement that she isn't capable yet?

(Of course, any coach who feels unable to deal with a person of this nature should properly refer them elsewhere rather than take on something they can't handle. But there is a world of difference from saying *"I'm not the right coach for you, I can't provide you with the support you need"* which is a judgement about the coach; and saying *"You, as a person, are uncoachable"* which is a judgement about the client.)

But if you are an EFT Coach, it's possible to view this situation in a different light. With EFT as a coaching tool, it suddenly becomes possible to take on this client as a coaching client, to help her achieve her goals, with the knowledge that **if** any of her past emotional issues arise along the way, they can be effectively dealt with. This may or may not mean thoroughly clearing the past trauma that occurred. But it definitely does mean that any issues which are preventing her from achieving her **goals** will be cleared along the way.

### 6.1.9.2    Example 2

Suppose there is a man who is going through a messy divorce and custody battle. At the same time, he wants to achieve a promotion at work - partly because he wants it for himself, and partly because it will ease his new stretched financial situation.

He turns up at your office seeking coaching to help him prepare for his promotion. He is late for the first session after a long and painful meeting with his solicitor regarding the divorce. He is clearly distracted and all enquiries about his home situation produce great agitation and barely suppressed grief and anguish. Nevertheless, he insists that he must get this promotion and really needs your help in preparing for it.

Is this man coachable? Does he have significant and pressing emotional issues which are making it hard to focus on his work or even attend coaching sessions on time? Yes. Does this man deserve to maximise his chances at achieving a promotion that will help not only him but allow him to meet his new financial obligations? Yes.

So - **is** this man coachable?

Some coaches might legitimately say that a man whose life is in such disorder that even attending coaching is a challenge, is not ready for coaching. But if you are an EFT Coach, you are in a position to minimise the emotional turmoil so that he can focus on his career aims. Again, you need not intend to fully clear every issue surrounding his divorce and his relationship with his children - but you can help them be dealt with sufficiently to allow this client to access resourceful states when he needs to in order to achieve his goals.

### 6.1.9.3    Redefining Coachability

It should be clear from these examples that clarity between coach and client is absolutely vital. It becomes necessary when using EFT in this way to be very explicit with the client and seek agreement such as *"We can do some EFT to get these feelings under control so you can concentrate on your promotion – is that something you'd like to do?"*.

Once the client knows the EFT procedure, you can even agree that he will do 5 minutes of EFT prior to each coaching session to bring himself into a calm state and ready to focus on the coaching. To repeat what I have said many times: EFT is to be used in the service of the coaching – and that means allowing it to be used in whatever way the client wants and derives benefit from – there is no fixed formula and each coach-client pair are free to come up with whatever works for them.

So here is my final word on Coachability. If a client sincerely wants to be coached, then I believe he is coachable. I also believe that a client is to be held as coachable until proven otherwise. Only by entering into the initial stages of coaching can either coach or client really know whether the client can benefit from coaching. All coaches reserve the right to terminate coaching relationships whenever they feel that the client isn't benefiting from the coaching. The only difference EFT makes to that is to extend the range of tools and resources available to allow that benefit to occur.

## 6.1.10 The Client Has the Answers

> "The primary building block for all co-active coaching is this: Clients have the answers or they can find the answers." [2]

It is a fundamental tenet of most if not all coaching models (with the exception of domain specific coaching such as sports or education) that it is the client who ultimately is the best determinant of the solutions for his own life. (Because they are, after all, Creative, Resourceful and Whole).

What this means is that the coach takes extreme care not to advise or instruct the client what they should do, or to plant suggestions based on the coach's own opinions or agenda. The coach's role is to be guide, questioner and skilled technician, applying tools and techniques to the coaching dialogue to help clients discover their own solution.

How is this viewpoint affected by the use of EFT as a technique? I believe this tenet is strongly upheld when using EFT, provided that the words used in the setup statement are generated by the client. EFT practitioners are trained to tune into the client's language, notice the words and phrases they use and to use setup statements based **only** on these words.

> "It is essential not to filter what a person says or to put a different spin on it by accident... the prime directive of formulating opening statements is that they must be in the client's own words and that ONLY the client can know the right words to say." [4]

Sometimes, just as in coaching, it is permissible and even useful for the coach to voice her own intuitions about the client's situation. These can always be voiced as questions so as to invite the client to consider and then agree or disagree.

One area in which the coach often needs to provide more guidance is in the creation of Choices statements. This is partly because clients often feel less confident initially about what format they are looking for, and partly because the coach is often more aware than the client about the need to avoid negatives, and ways to make the statement more powerful.

But even here, it is essential that the creation of a Choices statement be a co-active process. The coach is looking for a form of statement which is not only efficacious in structure, but which makes the client say *"Yes - that's it! That's it exactly!"*. In this situation, it's a case of the client not so much knowing the answers, but recognising them when they see them.

Related sections:

6.1.1    The Client is Creative, Resourceful and Whole ⇧

6.2.8    The Choices Technique ⇩

7.2.3    Intuition ⇩

## 6.1.11 Coaching the Real Client

The aim of coaching is to talk to and coach the "Real" or "Authentic" client, as opposed to the fearful, unresourceful client, or worse still, one of his Gremlins! Some coaches will even say to the client who is expressing fears or doubts *"Am I talking to my client or am I talking to the Gremlin right now?"*

But what or who **is** the Real client? Assuming the client doesn't know yet, then often it's down to the coach to notice when they seem to be coaching what isn't the Real client. And what the coach decides to notice as "not Real" can all too often be down to the coach's judgement (or in its least worst case, the coach's intuition) about what behaviours signal "not Real".

Usually "not Real" is signalled by the client expressing a negative thought or emotion in relation to achieving their goal (e.g. fear, self-doubt). But EFT tells us that our perception of what is a negative thought and what is actually true is often inaccurate. For instance, if a client says *"This goal is going to be really hard"*, the coach may agree with him, because he also would find it hard, or he may disagree and decide the client is expressing self-doubt.

To use Gary Craig's language, if the client and coach have similar "writing on their walls" about what is "hard", then it's likely that they will simply agree that it **is** hard and the opportunity for the client's perception of the difficulty of the goal to be tested and re-evaluated will have been lost.

From an EFT point of view, by "straightening out" any disruptions to the energy system that exist within the client in relation to the goal, the client's true attitude and feeling towards the goal will be revealed. But it does this without making any pre-judgement about whether the client's attitude is "factually correct" or simply an emotional disruption.

EFT therefore offers the coach a valuable way of testing which ideas are coming from the client's "Real Self" (i.e. in the absence of an energy disruption) and which are the result of negative thinking, Gremlins or whatever else.

Once again we have an application of EFT within coaching that is in no way "therapy", but simply revealing the client to themselves as they really are right now, for the purpose of making progress in their lives. In the sections that follow we will see this use of EFT several times when testing for the validity of goals, values and beliefs.

Related sections:

6.1.17    Gremlins ⇩

9.1.2     Validating Goals ⇩

9.5.9     Testing Values ⇩

## 6.1.12 Coaching the Past

> *"For example, if you are thrown into a feeling of childlike inadequacy when someone at work uses a particular tone of voice, you might want to identify what old experiences this connects with and sort them out."* [5]

All human beings - and therefore coaching clients - are "works in progress". They are the product of 20, 30, 40 or more years of conditioning. Even if coaching is about "what's next", all coaches should understand that the raw material they are dealing with (the client) is never a "blank slate".

Even as you focus your client on their current feelings and future actions, each thought, each response is the result of the client's past. (The object of coaching, of course, is to get beyond the conditioning, so that new thoughts, new responses, new actions and therefore new results become possible.) In the sense that all clients are products of their own pasts, coaches are literally "coaching the past".

It is quite possible - and valid - to coach the past. In fact, it is almost impossible to conduct coaching without visiting the past at some point - simply because, as noted above, the client's current reactions, desires, fears and concerns will **always** be informed by their past.

This fact is acknowledged in the quote above from The NLP Coach[5], in which exploration of past influences on current behaviour and feelings is explicitly encouraged. (Unfortunately it doesn't tell you how to "sort them out" - but clearly EFT would be one way.)

But when it comes to coaching the **content** of a client's past, for many coaches this is the primary trigger for worrying about "Is this therapy?".

It is not always the case that visiting the past is in order to heal some terrible trauma. Most clients will have areas of their past which are **not** traumatic or requiring healing as such. But their pasts do hold useful information about the client's current way of behaving, their recurring behaviour patterns and styles of thinking. It is also a great place to visit to gain learning and insight. As the motivational speaker Nigel Risner says *"The past is a place of reference, not a place of residence"*. Failing to refer to the past is missing out on a large resource available to client and coach.

In my view, the ability to effectively coach the past - with or without the assistance of EFT - is part of addressing the client's whole life.

There are many conventional coaching tools which can make a visit to the past well worth taking if it changes the client's level of empowerment to deal with the present. Perspectives work can totally transform how a client decides to view and interpret the past. Visualisations of how the client might choose to handle a past situation can significantly empower the client to feel able to handle similar events in the future. And of course, revisiting Peak Experiences can allow a client to reconnect with a resourceful state or "way of being" that she would like to bring into her present. Ways for EFT to assist in these situations are covered below.

Related sections:

5.3.1.1    "Therapy is about the Past, Coaching is about the Future" ⇧

6.1.2      Coaching Addresses the Client's Whole Life ⇧

8.1.3      Perspectives ⇩

8.1.12     Peak Experiences ⇩

8.1.18     Visualisations ⇩

## 6.1.13 Holding the Space

Ideally the coach creates and then "holds" the space for effective coaching to happen. Different coaches think of this in different ways and may mean one or more of the following, or even other ideas unique to them:

- Creating a conducive atmosphere using tone of voice, style of language or other rapport techniques.

- Holding the intention prior to and during the coaching that an effective coaching will occur.

- Mentally visualising a space (e.g. a dome or bubble) which the client and coach "inhabit" for the duration of the coaching, including deliberately expanding the space as necessary to allow the client to expand into it.

- Noticing and handling any intrusions or interruptions to the "space" (such as background noise, phones ringing) and ensuring they are either gracefully included or effectively excluded, such that the coaching is not damaged.

What I find interesting about the concept of "holding the space" is that it is essentially an energy technique. Although "holding the space" can often occur quite naturally without the coach ever knowing what they are doing (humans are natural energy manipulators even if they don't realise it), that does not mean that they are controlling the energy any less effectively.

Any coach who already understands how to "hold the space" and what that feels like when it works, is likely to feel more comfortable with the idea of a technique which can target the client's energy and manage their own energy, in more explicit ways. Indeed, an essential part of "Holding the Space" is for the coach to properly establish his own energy state. All the self-management techniques listed further on are all ways of using EFT to contribute to the ability of the coach to hold the correct intention, and therefore "hold the space" effectively.

Related sections:

7.1        Self-management Skills ⇩

## 6.1.14 Holding the Client's Agenda

Although a coaching relationship may last many weeks or months and cover all kinds of territory, it is the coach's job to ensure that the goal(s) agreed at the beginning of the relationship are not forgotten and remain the ultimate focus of attention and activity.

There is a similar function that occurs when using EFT on a particular client problem. It is normal for clients to have many different Aspects which all need to be dealt with before the main problem is fully resolved. Without training it is quite possible for a self-help user of EFT to start working on an issue and follow the chain of thoughts and emotions which are brought up along the way and never fully resolve the main issue because they got side-tracked into Aspects which, while connected, were not relevant.

Exactly the same risk applies to coaching when no-one is Holding the Agenda. If the Agenda isn't successfully held, a lot of very interesting ground can be covered, the client may get lots of insights and be thoroughly enjoying the process of the coaching, only to realise that there has been no significant progress towards the goal they had in mind at the start.

A coach who understands about Holding the Agenda within a conventional coaching context will have no problems at all including EFT in their toolset (it's one more way of moving towards the goal) or of knowing which Aspects to spend time on and which to leave as irrelevant.

Related sections:

6.2.12      Aspects ⇩

11.2        Tracking Notation ⇩

## 6.1.15 Accepting the Client without Judgement

*"Imagine someone who listens to you without judgment and allows you to show emotion - in fact accepts you without analysing you"* [2]

Acceptance of the client - of what they say, what they do, what they reveal about their past - is fundamental to the trust you are asking the client to place in you as a coach. The client cannot be expected to do deep change work with you and be totally honest with you about their motivations, fears and dreams unless the client knows that, in return, these most precious and rarely revealed parts of themselves won't be judged, rejected or otherwise hurt.

True acceptance of the client is about more than just keeping your mouth shut though. It is an energetic state in which not only does the client not **hear** any judgement coming from you, but they also don't **feel** any. It really isn't a skill you can fake. Clients (and people in general) are highly tuned to detect judgment coming from others, especially new acquaintances.

But acceptance also plays a fundamental part in EFT. The standard EFT setup involves the client asserting, in some form or another, that *"I deeply and completely accept myself"*. This self-acceptance serves to distinguish between the fundamental essence of the client (the "I" performing the EFT) and the problem the client (her "self") happens to have at the moment. Problems and emotions may come and go but the client's essence remains, and is always, acceptable.

It is said that a coach should never ask a client to do something that the coach hasn't already done or isn't fully prepared to do. It's all part of the "space holding" function of the coach. A coach can't "hold a space" for a client to move into if it's not a space the coach is fully familiar with and comfortable about inhabiting.

So if we are asking the client to accept themselves, the coach must "deeply and completely accept the client" **first!**

Many, many clients have trouble accepting themselves. I have lost count of the number of clients who have stopped halfway through the first setup statement and said *"I can't say that, because I don't accept myself"*. We do such clients a great service simply by modelling both self-acceptance (the coach accepts himself) and client-acceptance (the coach accepts the client).

Thus, coaching and EFT are completely in agreement on the importance of acceptance as the key to effective change.

Related sections:

6.1.13     Holding the Space ⇑

6.2.7      The Self-acceptance Statement ⇓

7.2.5      Modelling Self-acceptance ⇓

8.2.11     The Non-Judgement Pattern ⇓

## 6.1.16 Action and Learning

> *"Professional/personal coaching addresses the whole person - with an emphasis on producing action and uncovering learning that can lead to more fulfilment, more balance and a more effective process for living."* [2]

Although coaching is primarily about getting the client to action, good coaching is also about learning. It's the learning that transforms the client, empowers him and allows him to sustain change after the relationship has ended. Co-active coaching in particular emphasises the cycle of action and learning that is the basis for clients making progress towards their goals and altering their "way of being" in the process. In other words, learning from your actions changes who you are, which in turn changes your actions.

EFT is an incredible aid to learning - assisting insights and helping to make connections. But the practice of using EFT within the coaching, also acts to improve the client's focus and awareness on their thoughts and feelings. For instance, the client may have an action to perform as Homework. It would be good practice to not only have the client perform the action, but also to request that she notices her thoughts and feelings leading up to the action, during the action and afterwards - and to write these down and bring them to the next coaching session.

This information is useful even in conventional coaching, since it is the basis for the client's learning, particularly if the client failed in any way to perform the homework. But it's especially useful as information for the EFT Coach - because the thoughts and feelings will almost certainly identify beliefs, blocks and fears in relation to the homework task.

Although its usefulness is obvious if the client failed, it's also useful if the client succeeded but in some way did not feel good about what happened. Perhaps they went through a period of anxiety prior to the action, perhaps they felt as though "this isn't me" while they were doing it. Even though the client "pushed through their fear" to perform the action, it doesn't mean that they will do it again next time if they still have fear and unease around it still.

The key to successful and sustained action is internal congruency. The client must not only be able to **do** the action, but feel **no resistance** or negative feeling while they do it. Only when performing positive actions to achieve desired goals "feels like second nature" is the coach's job done.

As indicated above, deepening the learning can be achieved using conventional coaching methods. But adding EFT to the equation can vastly accelerate and ease the learning process, so that the "second nature" level of performance is achieved more quickly.

There's another way in which EFT really reinforces the "Action and Learning" cycle within coaching. If you are using EFT within coaching, the issues you apply EFT to will all in some way be related to obstacles to the client achieving their goals. So what's happening is this:

- The client needs to carry out certain actions on the way to achieving their goal.

- The client has various blocks, beliefs, fears etc which are preventing the client from taking action.

- The coach and client work on the blocks and beliefs one by one, using a combination of coaching tools and EFT to "unstick" the client and make action possible.

- The client goes back into his life and attempts to take one or more actions in furtherance of his goal.

- These attempts either succeed or they fail. If they succeed, he may succeed easily, or experience anxiety or difficulty on the way to achieving success.

Whatever the outcome of the attempted action, there is learning. Was the last Aspect we worked on with EFT the final piece of the puzzle that "unstuck" the client? Were there still blocks to the action occurring - and if so, what were they?

In other words, the test of the EFT (or any coaching) is the results obtained back in the client's life. Each time the client comes back, the client and the coach learn a little bit more about how this client works and what else needs to happen so that the client can achieve his goal.

The only difference with EFT is that as well as supporting this action/learning cycle between sessions, it allows cycles of action and learning to take place within sessions too, since a client can test his emotional reaction to the prospect of action over and over again within a session, after each round of EFT.

Related sections

8.1.2      Homework ⇩

8.1.2.3    Inquiries and Insights ⇩

8.1.11     Locking in the Learning ⇩

## 6.1.17 Gremlins

Gremlins are talked about a great deal among coaches and Richard D. Carson's book "Taming Your Gremlin"[10] is a coaching classic. But while the term "Gremlin" is a useful and fun shorthand for a particular sort of phenomenon in coaching, making it easy to talk about with clients, it's important for the EFT Coach to know what Gremlins really are.

In coaching terms, Gremlins are simply ingrained beliefs, usually so old that they are held unconsciously, and which determine the client's reactions to many aspects of their lives.

An example might be a belief which says *"I must be independent"*. A person can have a belief for so long that it takes on a life of its own - so it can rightly be named "My Independence Gremlin". This Gremlin might be triggered unconsciously whenever something happens to threaten the client's independence - such as someone telling him what to do, giving him unasked for advice, offering help, finding himself in someone's debt and so on.

Without being aware of the Gremlin, the client's experience may simply be one of feeling constantly irritated by the perceived interference of other people. Identifying the Gremlin is useful since it offers the client a different way to think about what's happening, and the possibility of different responses to events which "threaten" his independence. But knowing the Gremlin is there is not the same thing as being free of it.

In other disciplines, Gremlins are known by different names. In counselling or psychotherapy they can be known as "parts" (the "part" of the client that doesn't want to, fears to, or thinks they should). In NLP they may be thought of as meta-programs - persistent or dominant modes of thinking which are triggered at certain times or in relation to a specific subject. Gary Craig would call Gremlins the "writing on your walls" - the beliefs you inherited from people around you or derived from early experiences but which have remained unquestioned.

Contrary to popular belief, and thanks to EFT, clients do **not** have to be "stuck" with their Gremlin(s) for the rest of their lives. For one thing, people aren't born with them - they are acquired through various experiences which result in certain beliefs being internalised in order to provide protection from particular sorts of "dangers". Secondly, Gremlins do change over time, either maturing or being replaced by different Gremlins. Your "worst fear" when you were 12 is probably nothing like your "worst fear" now. So, Gremlins by their nature **are** mutable.

But the main thing to remember about all Gremlins, is that they are founded on fear. Their "function" is to protect the client from perceived danger. And the belief(s) the Gremlin is trying to uphold and protect is usually based on something that happened in the past and which "taught" the client to try and avoid happening again. Dealing with Gremlins' fears or beliefs is therefore simply to be treated as any other fear or belief.

There is another issue around Gremlins which EFT can help with. There is a danger of a coach effectively suppressing exploration of the client's feelings about a subject by labelling it as "the Gremlin" and refusing to talk to "it". From a client perspective (and I have experienced this as a coaching client) it can feel as though there are areas of the client's experience which are "out of bounds" and the client learns to edit what they say before they have even said it.

In my view this impoverishes the client-coach relationship. Gremlins may be real enough, but they are also part of the client and should be respected as such. In my opinion, refusing to talk to a Gremlin is effectively failing to coach the Whole client. In the section on "Parts" I show how to use EFT to deal with any "part" of the client, Gremlin or otherwise.

Thus, there is no section on "How to deal with Gremlins" specifically. The label "Gremlin" is actually superfluous to the coaching process. Even if you find the Gremlin concept useful to use with clients, the important thing is to listen to what the Gremlin/client is actually saying, identify the fear or belief being expressed and then work on that basis.

Related sections:

## 6.1.18  Values and Pseudo-values

*"Values are who we are. When we honour our values, there's a sense of internal 'rightness' that has nothing to do with morality."* [2]

Helping a client to connect with their values and use them as a guide in decision making, is one of the most powerful and lasting effects that coaching can do for a client. But although knowing their values and attempting to honour them in their lives might be a significant step forward in personal empowerment for many clients, there are some problems associated with them.

One of the problems is the possibility of "over-honouring a value". (i.e. honouring a value to such an extent that negative results start to occur or conflict with other values arises). If a value is characterised by "internal rightness" associated with honouring it, how can "over-honouring a value" even be possible? In fact this happens extremely commonly in coaching. In a profession where we are encouraging clients to find Balance between competing areas of their lives, finding Balance between two or more client values can be just as important a task in order to help the client find a solution that really works for them.

I believe that the idea of values in coaching can be taken one step further, to include the idea of "pseudo-values". Pseudo-values appear to operate like values on the surface but actually do not really belong to the client. These are values which can be inherited from parents, teachers or society, and which have fear as the underlying motivation.

For instance, suppose a client had a strict upbringing and it was drummed into them that they should always put others before themselves. This client may well hold a value called "Serving Others", or "Putting Others First", which by implication equates to "Putting Myself Last". Who is to say whether the value "Putting Others First" is held by the "true client" or whether that value is in fact a "pseudo-value"?

True values are those based on our core essence and are indeed Who We Really Are - or represent Who We Wish to Become.

But pseudo-values are more about Who We **Think** We Are - or Who We Think We **Ought** to Be.

Examples of pseudo-values might include the desire to be wealthy, the desire to be poor, the need to be loyal. It can't be judged in advance whether a particular value is a true value or a pseudo-value for a particular client. The test lies with the client themselves. What's driving this value? Where did it come from and what's at stake if it isn't honoured?

If what's at stake is the opinion of others or the client's image in the world, it's likely to be a pseudo-value. If what's at stake is the client's feeling of integrity with himself, regardless of the opinion of others, it's likely to be a true value.

Now, this can be confusing and unsettling territory, even for those with many years of self-development work behind them. Those used to examining themselves will be used to the idea of re-evaluating Who They Think They Are quite regularly, including questioning their values and beliefs along the way. For a new coaching client, it could just all be too confusing. It is very difficult to be told that the values you thought you had might actually not be real and that there is no real way of knowing in any case except by diligent noticing.

Luckily, EFT offers us a way to test the validity of a client's values, quite naturally and without either coach or client having to "judge" whether a value is a real one or a pseudo one. How to achieve this is covered below.

Even when values are true values, sometimes they can be in conflict. For instance, a client might have Intimacy as one of her values. She might also have Freedom. In some situations, these values may conflict. How to resolve such a conflict with EFT is also covered below.

EFT can also help identify and remove what's in the way of fully honouring a value. If a client feels there is a value that isn't being honoured in his life, there will usually be a reason for it - a belief, a block or a habit. How to address these is also covered extensively below.

Related sections:

6.1.6       Balance Coaching ⇧
9.4         Habits ⇩
9.5.6.2     Hand-me-down Beliefs ⇧
9.5.9       Testing Values ⇩

## 6.1.19  Most Coaching Happens Between Sessions

It is an observation of many coaches that what happens in between scheduled coaching appointments can be every bit as important to the client's progress, if not more so, than what happens in the 30-60 minutes when the coach and client were talking to each other. Coaching only has value if it has an impact on the client's life outside coaching. In co-active coaching especially, the client is expected to take action and continue learning in-between sessions.

EFT fully supports this paradigm. Since it was specifically designed to be an easy-to-learn self-help technique, it can easily be used by clients in between sessions to make further progress or generally to support themselves. Between-session use of EFT is common practice amongst practitioners using EFT in a therapy context. This contrasts with many therapies where the presence of the therapist is required before any progress can be made.

EFT allows progress to be continued in-between sessions in two ways:

- The client can do EFT by themselves either as planned homework or any time they want to if they meet a challenge.

- The client can test the effects of any EFT that happened within the coaching to see whether his responses to relevant triggers have been successfully altered.

Related sections:

8.1.2       Homework ⇩

## 6.1.20  Level 1, Level 2 and Level 3 listening

Most coaching training involves becoming aware of different types of listening awareness, although they are defined differently at different coaching schools. I use the CTI definitions as follows:

**Level 1** - focus on the self - the coach listening to their own internal dialogue (e.g. wondering if they are "doing OK", thinking about what to ask next or the last client call or even thinking about their own personal issues, possibly triggered by what the client has said).

**Level 2** - focus on the client - the coach listening exclusively to what the client is saying. The focus is on the client and the words and linguistic content of what is being said.

**Level 3** - focus on the entire environment, including the client. The coach is not only hearing what the client says, but is taking in the wider atmosphere and energy behind what's being said. It also includes background noises or anything else going on.

In general, the coach should be at Level 2 or at Level 3, most of the time. Being at Level 1 is to be avoided since the coach is not "with" the client at Level 1. Many of the self-management skills covered below are ways to get out of Level 1 or avoid going there in the first place. In brief, by dealing with their own "Level 1" issues with EFT before or during a session, a coach can enhance their ability to stay at Level 2 and 3.

Related sections:

7.1.2        Staying "Over There" with the Client ⇩


## 6.1.21 Bottomlining

Bottomlining is about the coach taking back charge of the session in order to keep focussed on the current goal. It's a way of getting clients to "cut to the chase" in their storytelling in order to get the focus back on what action they are going to take in their lives.

This skill is also important in EFT, since it is a common effect of EFT that the client starts to notice other issues - possibly related to the current issue or completely unrelated. It is the job of the practitioner to notice when a client has "switched Aspects" or even switched issues completely and to bring the client back on track and complete the original issue.

This often requires the practitioner to be somewhat abrupt. When a client starts relating some other issue it's necessary for the practitioner to say, for instance: *"That's a different issue. I want you to tune back into the issue we were just working on and tell me where you are with that."*

Another way that Bottomlining gets used is at the start of the session when the client appears to have many issues to work on. She may start telling you about some of them - how terrible they are, what they think is causing them and so on. While it is useful to listen to this for a while to get a general overview of what is on the client's mind, ultimately you cannot make progress until one issue is chosen and you start work. The same is true for coaching.

One of the fears about coaching becoming "therapy" is that the client ends up simply relating "what happened" and their associated thoughts about it all, resulting in no actual progress being taken towards the goal. The EFT practitioner would totally share in that fear, even for a use in a "therapy" application such as clearing a traumatic memory. With EFT, as with coaching, the practitioner needs to know just enough to understand what the client wants to achieve and something about the client's internal landscape (revealed by what language they use). After that, the emphasis is on action (applying EFT) and learning (what effect did the EFT have).

Related sections:

6.2.12        Aspects ⇧

## 6.1.22 Key Points

- Both coaching and EFT hold the client as fundamentally Creative, Resourceful and Whole, regardless of any current problems or goals. This can be expressed in a setup statement of the form: *"Even though I have this problem, I am Creative, Resourceful and Whole"*.

- Addressing a client's whole life includes their perceived past and their anticipated future. Both coaching and EFT work with the present. Coaching focuses on what the client needs to do today in order to achieve what they want in the future. EFT works and focuses exclusively on the client's current state whether the focus is on past, present or future.

- In both coaching and EFT, the agenda always comes from the client. In both, the client says what they want the outcome to be. In both, the client determines when the process is complete.

- In both coaching and EFT, success can only be achieved through an alliance between client and practitioner. Both coaching and EFT are co-operative ventures between client and coach/practitioner. EFT clients are fully empowered to use EFT for themselves at any time, just as coaching clients are fully empowered to take their learning, action and insights into their real lives.

- The idea of Fulfilment in coaching closely mirrors the unfolding of an EFT session or series of sessions. Although a client may start out with specific goals or problems to work on, the process of making progress acts to refine and redefine what the client understands he really wants and expands his idea of what is possible.

- The essence of Balance in coaching or life is relinquishing control. Since all control is based in fear, EFT can provide a key tool in reducing the need for control, increasing the client's ability to respond flexibly to new circumstances and achieve Balance.

- Coaching clients are encouraged to pay attention to not just their progress in the terms of results, but their Process in terms of who they are being and becoming. Process provides the learning and the insight that the client takes away with them after the coaching has ended. EFT also involves the client's conscious mind at every step of the way, allowing the client to observe fully their own Process.

- Both coaches and practitioners are trained to track and distinguish clients' Big Agendas and little agendas, in order to keep the session moving in the direction of the client's ultimate goal.

- Coachability depends both on the client and the coach. EFT expands the set of clients who can benefit from coaching without other emotional issues being a barrier, and it improves the ability of the coach to offer the benefits of coaching to clients who strongly desire to be coached but who do have significant emotional issues. I believe that clients who express a strong desire to be coached should be held as coachable until proven otherwise.

- Coaches, like EFT practitioners, use the client's own words and ideas as the basis for the process. The coach/practitioner's job is to elicit and follow, trusting that the client has the answers.

- The aim of coaching is to coach the "Real client", as opposed to his Gremlins or other fearful or doubtful parts of the client. But accurately identifying the "Real client" can be difficult and can depend on the coach's own judgement and beliefs. EFT offers a judgement-free way of testing which ideas are coming from the client's "Real self" and which are not.

- Although coaching content from the past may seem to risk doing "therapy", in fact it is perfectly valid to revisit the past as part of coaching - to learn and to reconnect with past resourceful states. EFT offers a way to accelerate any learning or releasing needed in connection with the past in order to assist progress towards a specific coaching goal.

- "Holding the space" is an essential coaching skill, involving setting and managing the atmosphere and environment in which the coaching takes place. As such it is very much an energy technique, and many of the self-management uses for EFT will assist the coach to "hold the space" effectively.

- It is the coach's job to ensure that the goal(s) agreed at the beginning of the relationship are not forgotten and remain the ultimate focus of attention and activity. A coach who understands about Holding the Agenda within a conventional coaching context will have no problems at all including EFT in their toolset (it's one more way of moving towards the goal) or of knowing which Aspects to spend time on.

- Acceptance of the client without judgement is fundamental to the trust you are asking a client to place in you as a coach. Similarly, EFT has self-acceptance at its heart. In general, coaches should never ask a client to do something they themselves would not do - which requires the EFT Coach to cultivate acceptance of the client. Thus, coaching and EFT are completely in agreement on the importance of client acceptance as the key to effective change. In addition, EFT as a self-management tool can enable coaches to cultivate the required acceptance of clients.

- Good coaching involves a cycle between Action (working towards a goal) and Learning (noticing results and "way of being"). EFT can be used to reinforce and accelerate this cycle. It can help to reveal insights into the client's reactions, and identify anxieties or blocks in the process of taking action. EFT therefore not only aids the process of learning, but releases any blocks identified along the way, leading back to more action.

- Gremlins are long-standing, often unconscious beliefs which determine client's reactions to events in their lives. In EFT terms, Gremlins are "the writing on your walls" - the belief system you inherited from people around you or derived from early experiences but which have remained unquestioned. Since Gremlins are usually based on some kind of fear - they exist to protect you from perceived danger - they can be released using EFT. EFT also allows a Gremlin to be accepted as part of the client and dealt with, instead of ignoring it and refusing to engage with it.

- Getting clients to connect with their values and begin honouring them fully in their lives is one of the keys to successful coaching. Unfortunately, some values can be pseudo-values - derived from family or peers or founded on fears or false beliefs. But trying to distinguish between them can involve judgement from the coach and confusion from the client. EFT offers us a way to test the validity of a client's values, quite naturally and without either coach or client having to "judge" whether it is a value or a pseudo-value.

- What happens in between scheduled coaching sessions can be every bit as important to the client's progress, if not more so, than what happens in the coaching session. In co-active coaching especially, the client is expected to take action and continue learning in-between sessions. EFT fully supports this paradigm since it can easily be used by clients in between sessions to make further progress or generally to support themselves.

- There are three different levels of listening: Level 1 (coach listening to his own internal dialogue), Level 2 (coach listening to the client), Level 3 (coach listening to the client plus the underlying energy and wider environment including background noise). The coach should generally remain at Level 2 or 3 during coaching. Level 1 is generally to be avoided and this can be assisted by using EFT as a self-management tool to deal with the coach's Level 1 issues.

- Coaches use "Bottomlining" to get the client focused on action and to move the coaching forward. It's used in particular to avoid lengthy storytelling and to "cut to the chase". A similar skill is needed in EFT in order to keep the work on track and focused on one issue at a time.

- In short, many of the assumptions and underlying principles and practices of coaching find their parallels within the practice of EFT. What this means is that combining the two methods should be possible since the two disciplines are highly compatible.

# 6.2  EFT Fundamentals

If you are unfamiliar with EFT this section serves as a primer in EFT terminology. If you already know EFT it serves as a way of noticing the parallels and relationship between EFT concepts and coaching concepts. If you have never used EFT before you are encouraged to try the basic EFT procedure for yourself using the instructions in section 12. This will familiarise you with the mechanics of the EFT method and will make what follows less abstract.

## 6.2.1  The Cause of Negative Emotions

*"The cause of ALL negative emotions is a disruption in the body's energy system"* [1]

To whatever degree you decide to use EFT within coaching, you need to understand this basic view of where negative emotions come from. In Energy Psychology generally (of which EFT is one particular technique) negative emotions are regarded as being ultimately caused by a disruption in the body's energy system.

This is a challenging concept if you regard your negative emotions as being caused by "my traumatic childhood" or "my unreasonable boss" or "my critical partner". But it is an extremely liberating concept if you want to find a way of not only being responsible for your own feelings, but having a practical and effective tool for releasing them.

It is entirely compatible with the coaching ethic of encouraging clients to take responsibility for their own lives and their own reality, to use a tool which assumes as a physiological fact, that negative emotions are the result of processes **within** the client, not outside.

EFT turns what was perhaps only a useful, life enhancing and self-empowering viewpoint, into a tangible and practical demonstration of that truth. As Gary Craig, originator of EFT, says repeatedly on his training tapes, *"It's all an inside job"*. Using EFT is the surest and quickest method I have seen of bringing the idea of self-created reality home to clients. It also enables coaches to more easily "walk their talk" by dealing with their own emotional issues effectively and to therefore model self-created reality for their clients.

So, although it is not necessary to really engage with this underlying assumption in order to successfully apply EFT, I personally find it satisfying to know that the tool I am using to assist my coaching rests on a principle which is so fundamentally affirmative of the idea of personal responsibility and self-empowerment - an idea which is so very much at the heart of coaching and its aims.

## 6.2.2  Working with the Client's Energy System

In EFT or other Meridian or Energy techniques, the focus of attention is the client's energy system. We are interested in seeing how it currently behaves (what the client says, does and feels) and we are interested in interacting with it in order to correct disruptions.

At first sight, this seems to put EFT and similar techniques firmly in the "therapy" camp. "Correcting disruptions" sounds like "fixing the client". However, even in conventional coaching, the client has behaviours and beliefs which aren't producing the results she wants - and so she seeks the help of a coach to help "correct" these behaviours and beliefs in the sense of choosing alternative behaviours and beliefs that will produce the desired outcomes. Making these changes aren't seen as "fixing" the client. The view is that the client's current behaviours and beliefs are "symptoms" and that underneath them all is the "real client" - the one who is Creative, Resourceful and Whole and doesn't need fixing.

If you regard EFT as changing the client's energy system to respond in new and more useful ways (as defined by the client), then coaching and EFT are doing very similar things - just in different ways. In EFT and in coaching, the client is saying *"I no longer want to have this response to this situation and I want to learn a new one that gets me closer to being, doing or having what I really want- and I want assistance in making that change"*.

But more significantly, it's important to understand that all coaching (like all interactions with all people for any purpose) involves making changes to the client's energy system. Of course, creating a relationship between two people (coach and client) in order to achieve what one person could not achieve alone, is energy work. But this isn't all the accidental kind which happens just by virtue of conversing and spending time with each other. Many or even most of coaching's conventional tools work because they are effective ways of manipulating the client's energy system.

- A visualisation exercise which puts the client in touch with their Future Self or makes the achievement of a goal tangible, is energy work.
- Asking the client *"What does your Future Self have to say?"* is energy work.
- Working with the client's Time Line and manipulating its shape and appearance to make goals easier to achieve, is energy work.
- Unsticking the client by getting them to listen to different music, wear different colours or take a new route into work, is energy work.
- Creating a plan of action where none exists, is energy work.
- Playing with the client's choice of association and dissociation at different times, is energy work.

And so on and so forth. Any coaching technique which alters the relationship of the client to himself or to his goal has altered the client's energy system. If the client goes away feeling different about any aspect of himself or his life, it is the change in his energy system that he is feeling.

What we are able to do with EFT is to work on the energy system very directly - and because it is so direct, it is also very fast. But don't let the directness or the speed of the work distract you into thinking that EFT is doing something that coaching doesn't do. In my opinion, they are acting on the **same** thing, and for the **same** ends, just in different ways.

However, you do not need to understand or even accept the idea of an energy system for you to start using EFT successfully. What matters is the results, not the theory. By following the integration process suggested below you will achieve the necessary personal experience of EFT which is what really counts.

Related sections:

5.3.2       Fixing versus Changing ⇧
6.1.1       The Client is Creative, Resourceful and Whole ⇧
8.1.16      Accessing the Future Self ⇩
8.1.17      Working with Time Lines ⇩
8.1.18      Visualisations ⇩
9.3.7       Unsticking the Client ⇩
11.1        Practice Integration Process ⇩

## 6.2.3  Psychological Reversal

*"I find the concept of Psychological Reversal particularly poignant when applied to people who have tried many times to make positive shifts in their lives, and somehow always seem to end up back where they started."* [3]

The concept of Psychological Reversal is so central to EFT and the way it is applied that it is worth mentioning it specifically because knowing how to recognise and more importantly how to overcome it gives any coach an incredible tool to tear down clients' blocks to progress.

But what is Psychological Reversal? Does it really exist or is it just a construct to explain the behaviour of people who don't have enough willpower?

In one very important sense, you don't need to know exactly what it is or how it works - you simply need to be able to spot the signs that is it operating and know how to deal with it.

Psychological Reversal can be thought of as a particular form of energetic disruption that occurs in the body whenever it is exposed to physical or emotional stress. Examples of physical stress would include illness, infection, toxins, fatigue, excess heat or cold and so on. Examples of emotional stress would include trauma, grief and especially fear. These types of stresses can cause the electrical polarity of the body to "flip" - so that energy is running in the wrong direction within the body. (You don't need to remember or even accept this description for EFT to work for you).

One common effect of this disruption is that the conscious mind seems to "want" one thing, but the unconscious/body-mind "wants" another. This is experienced as one part of the person wanting one thing (e.g. to quit smoking, start exercising or start work on an important goal) and the other part wanting the opposite (e.g. to smoke more, to avoid exercise, to procrastinate).

Does this type of behaviour look like absolutely classic coaching material to you? Do not the majority of clients and client issues come down in the end to persuading the part of the client that is resisting their goals to come into line with the part that wants them (the part that hired you)?

I have to tell you that as a person who is (or was) extremely prone to Psychological Reversal on a broad range of issues, coming across this concept (and its solution) was like being given a whole new lease of life. It released me from feelings of inadequacy and guilt about how little I thought I had achieved compared to my potential. It released me from feelings of frustration about why I was never able to really follow through with projects that were my own, as opposed to other people's projects which had deadlines and obligations to force me to complete them. But above all it placed me at choice with respect to my own life.

Psychological Reversal (referred to generally as "Reversal") can come in many different guises according to the situation and the client's belief or experience around the issue. Here are some typical types of Reversal that you may come across. This list in no way presents all possible varieties of Reversal - the intention is only to provide a flavour what a Reversal is and how it manifests itself in client language. (More types are listed in Goal Reversals and Blocks as Reasons Why Not)

| Reversal type | Example client statement |
|---|---|
| Safety | "Losing this fear would be dangerous" |
| Identity | "I don't know who I'd be if I achieved this" |
| Possibility | "It's not possible for this to happen" |
| Ability | "I don't have what it takes to do this" |
| Deservability | "I don't deserve to get over this problem" |
| Social | "I'm scared what my family will think if I start doing this" |
| Ecology | "This would turn my whole life upside down" |

In short, Reversals are the client's beliefs about "why not" which operate at the same time as wanting a successful coaching outcome.

(There is also a particularly stubborn form of Reversal known as Massive Reversal or Global Reversal. What this means is that the client's Reversals are not only specific to particular issues or events, but that the client experiences Reversal on almost every area of their life, even the things they enjoy. If a client describes long-standing problems in every significant area of their life (e.g. every spoke on their Balance Wheel has a low score), and they exhibit blocks or procrastination about things they say they enjoy doing (e.g. putting off reading a new book, putting off meeting up with friends, putting off booking a holiday) then it's a reasonable bet that there is Massive Reversal at work. Dealing with Massive Reversal involves very persistent use of EFT and/or other physical energy techniques which I won't cover here but which you will learn about if you undertake a practitioner level training.)

When a coach understands Reversal they have a tool for "unsticking" their clients, even if they don't use the full EFT procedure. Even more profoundly, when a **client** knows what Reversal is and knows how to overcome it, they have a tool for unsticking **themselves** any time they choose to. Creating clients who can "unstick" themselves is possibly the best and most lasting form of coaching possible.

You will be glad to hear that dealing with Psychological Reversal comes automatically as part of the Standard EFT procedure (it happens at the beginning with the setup statement), so you can proceed with using EFT quite successfully without necessarily having to think explicitly about Psychological Reversal as a separate issue.

But since the process of identifying and clearing blocks is a core coaching function, we do go into this in much more detail below.

In addition, an understanding of the concept of Psychological Reversal has another very positive side-effect within a coaching context. It allows you to take a detached and non-judgemental view of clients who exhibit (for instance) stubbornness, laziness, fecklessness, slipperiness (you can never pin them down to making a definite commitment) or even argumentativeness (clients who are reversed about an issue will come up with all kinds of "reasons" why they can't do something).

When you understand these qualities to be a sign of Reversal, and Reversal to be a spontaneous energetic disruption that occurs out of the control of the client, it is extremely easy to stay detached and non-judgemental about your client. It enables you to stay focussed on the client's true self, and maintain a feeling of unconditional acceptance for your client. Any viewpoint which allows you as coach to consistently, easily and congruently maintain this level of non-judgement about your client, has got to be a worthwhile one to investigate.

Related sections:

| | |
|---|---|
| 6.2.6 | The Standard EFT Pattern ⇩ |
| 6.2.10 | Where There is Willpower, There are Blocks ⇩ |
| 9.1.5 | Goal Reversals ⇩ |
| 9.3.1 | An Energy View of Blocks ⇩ |
| 9.3.3 | Blocks as Reasons Why Not ⇩ |
| 9.3.7 | Unsticking the Client ⇩ |
| 9.3.8 | Parts ⇩ |

## 6.2.4 Emotions as Physiological Events

*"Unless we as coaches take the body seriously we are missing an incredibly large piece of the coaching puzzle. This is simply due to the fact that the body is the domain in which action occurs and it is by dealing with the body that we can move our clients to new actions."*

*Pater Hamill, Somatic Coach*

It's surprising how many people view emotions as purely mental events. And since thoughts can give rise to emotions and emotions can give rise to thoughts, it's understandable how people are able to focus on the purely mental effects of emotion. It is probably this view of the nature of emotions which explains the many intellectual and cognitive approaches to dealing with emotional problems (e.g. counselling, psychotherapy, cognitive-behavioural therapy).

But emotions are not just mental. They are physiological events too - the effects of different chemicals on mood and emotion are very well known, from naturally occurring chemicals such as adrenaline (fear) and endorphins (wellbeing) through to herbal substances such as St John's Wort (uplifting), and pharmaceuticals such as nitrous oxide (laughing gas), tranquilisers (calming) or even Viagra (arousing).

In my experience, the best forms of coaching are those which acknowledge and include the client's physiological state and experience as part of their emotional condition and use that information within the coaching to track progress and achieve an outcome (e.g. *"Where do you feel this in your body?"*, is a good question used in Process Coaching as a way of getting the client to really connect with their emotion and get ready to explore it).

For EFT, physiological experience is the central focus of attention since emotions are viewed as not only being experienced in the body, but as actually occurring there. That doesn't mean that the EFT practitioner isn't interested in what the client thinks - far from it - but cognition is viewed as a symptom of emotional state.

This view is not doctrine or dogma that you are required to believe. It's the result of observation of many hundreds of clients who have undergone EFT to relieve an unpleasant emotional state (for instance anger towards a parent, or extreme anxiety when thinking about past traumas) and finish up spontaneously expressing 180° **attitude** shifts towards the situation or the people involved (e.g. *"Well I guess my mother was doing the best she knew how at the time"* or *"I guess he thought he had to attack me - he must have been in a lot of pain at that point"*). These kinds of perspective shift are the kinds of changes that counsellors, psychotherapists and sometimes coaches may spend many sessions attempting to facilitate but which are commonplace when EFT is used.

If you are a coach who already appreciates the power of getting clients to tune into their body as a way of contacting and processing emotions, then you will find EFT a very natural extension to that approach.

If you are a coach who tends to work primarily at the mental level (either because you prefer it or because your clients prefer it), then this physiological emphasis may prove something of a "congruency challenge" for you. However, I urge you to try EFT anyway, applying it at the mental level directly. The sections below show how EFT can be effective while working with entirely mental phenomena such as beliefs and values.

Even though EFT is clearly a physiological process (involving tapping on the body), it is quite possible to conduct a successful EFT session in which both client and practitioner talk only about what the client is thinking, as the basis for setup phrases. Since clients' cognitions are seen as much as a symptom of their emotional state as physiological experience (e.g. feeling butterflies in the stomach, changes in breathing or tightness in the chest), then you can work as well with cognitive symptoms as you can with physiological ones.

Related sections:

6.1.7       Process Coaching ⇧

## 6.2.5   Rating Scales

Effective application of EFT involves using rating scales to asses the client's initial state and to track progress. There are two varieties of scale used:

- SUDs = Subjective Units of Distress - measures **emotional intensity**, or for physical issues, levels of pain, stiffness or other symptoms

- VOC = Validity of Cognition - measures the degree to which a client **believes** a particular idea.

Both scales are 0 to 10, where 0 equals no distress, or zero belief. A rating of 10 equals maximum distress or complete belief.

In what follows, I do not refer again to either SUD or VOC directly since I prefer to avoid this type of jargon (especially with clients). But if you are entering this area you will come across these terms.

What's important for the EFT Coach to understand, is the value of using rating scales when applying EFT. Using scales allows you and the client to track progress thoroughly. Without using a rating scale, you risk the "much better syndrome", whereby a round of EFT may significantly calm a client, but not completely clear the issue. If you are a coach working with a client on their various blocks or beliefs, not using a rating scale means it is possible to leave your client with several low level blocks or beliefs (say at a level of 3 or under). Even though this may be a significant improvement on where the client started, these low level issues can still prove to be a background or insidious problem later on.

Rating scales have other benefits though. Firstly, getting the rating from the client requires them to tune into themselves, and notice what's really going on inside, both physiologically, emotionally and cognitively. Any coaching practice which develops a client's awareness of themselves and their reactions is to be welcomed. A client who can tune in like this easily is much easier to coach, since they are going to find it easier to find the answers inside themselves that will form the basis for creating their own solutions.

Secondly, there is a certain quality of truth to numerical rating scales that transcends verbal descriptions. Sometimes the client finds it difficult to really describe what they are feeling in words, especially if the territory is new, or if the client in general finds it hard to talk much about their feelings. A client in this kind of situation can easily cop out and say *"I feel OK"* rather than continue struggling to find the right words. But with a numerical rating scale, the client has the option of saying, for example *"Well, I still feel it's about a 1, but I can't really put a label on what the feeling is"*.

Using numerical ratings opens up powerful ways of working with clients that can avoid linguistic problems around labelling mental and emotional states, as well as maintaining full detachment and non-judgement on the part of the coach.

## 6.2.6   The Standard EFT Pattern

Although this book is not intended to teach you EFT in any thorough way, it is worth simply presenting the form of the Standard EFT setup statement here. This is to allow newcomers to EFT to recognise when Standard EFT is being used and when a variation of it is being suggested. (See also the QuickStart section for basic instructions on applying EFT).

Although each application of EFT involves tapping on the same set of points for every issue and every person, each application of EFT is totally customised to the individual's problem and the exact way they feel about it right now. This is expressed in the Standard EFT setup statement which begins each sequence:

The basic format of the statement is:

> *"Even though I have this problem, I deeply and completely accept myself"*

However, "this problem" can be expressed more explicitly in the words that the client would use to describe the problem e.g.

*"Even though I really hate my job, I deeply and completely accept myself"*

*"Even though I'm stressed, I deeply and completely accept myself"*

We will see later on how the number of possibilities for expressing the problem in the setup sentence is practically infinite.

Please also note that although the default ending for the setup statement is *"I deeply and completely accept myself"*, this can also be varied in many ways. In particular it can be altered if the client has a problem saying they accept themselves (and many clients do), or they simply prefer different words.

For the full EFT procedure download Gary Craig's original EFT Manual[1] or my EFT QuickStart Manual[9]. Both are free.

Related sections:

6.1.15     Accepting the Client Without Judgement ⇑

6.2.7      The Self-acceptance Statement ⇓

12         EFT QuickStart ⇓

## 6.2.7   The Self-acceptance Statement

I discussed the importance of Accepting the Client above. EFT asks the client to accept themselves every time they use EFT (see the Standard EFT Pattern above).

This self-acceptance is crucial to the overcoming of Psychological Reversal and to developing a distinction between the "self" who has the problem and the indestructible, infinitely valuable "I" who is deciding to release it. However, this phrase does not have to be exactly "I deeply and completely accept myself". Other variations include:

*"I deeply and profoundly love and accept myself."*

*"I deeply and profoundly love myself."*

*"I'm OK with myself."*

*"I'm a good person."*

*"I'm OK"*

*"I'm a worthwhile human being."*

Ultimately what's important is that the phrase involves saying something unconditionally accepting or positive about the person saying it. It needs to be something that has no significant "Tailenders" to it. Some mild Tailenders may be acceptable - and often clients get more comfortable saying it as they go on - but if the client really has strong objections coming up in their mind when they say the standard acceptance phrase, then it's important to come up with an alternative that they can say more easily. Mirror tapping may also be a useful technique to help clients cultivate self-acceptance.

Related sections:

6.1.15     Accepting the Client without Judgement ⇑

6.2.3      Psychological Reversal ⇑

6.2.6      The Standard EFT Pattern ⇑

## 6.2.8   The Choices Technique

With one single variation on Standard EFT, Dr Pat Carrington turned EFT from a technique which could remove the negative into a technique which could install the positive. Since much of coaching involves client choices - about who they want to be, what qualities they want to have, what actions they want to take - the Choices pattern is a stalwart in what follows.

The standard format of a Choices statement [7] is:

> "Even though I have this problem, I choose to be/do/feel this"

The Choices Technique is used only after Standard EFT has been used to bring a client's intensity down to zero or at least a low level (2 or less). After the Standard EFT has brought down the client's feelings about the issue right now, the Choices Technique can be used to help the client "program" future reactions to a particular situation.

So for example, suppose a client has an issue with feeling nervous and tongue-tied in the presence of their boss at work. Standard EFT can be used to bring down the intensity of this feeling to zero or close to zero. But suppose the client wants more than to just "not feel nervous anymore" (a rather neutral state), but would additionally like to feel confident enough to speak up in front of him. Some suitable Choices statements might be:

> "Even though it's my boss, I choose to be calm and totally confident."

> "Even though it's my boss, I choose to think of just the right words to say."

> "Even though it's my boss, I choose to speak easily and freely."

Choices can be used to help trigger positive thoughts in certain circumstances, such as:

> "Even though he makes me feel small, I choose to remember that I'm very good at my job and deserve respect"

It can be used to help useful memories come to the surface, e.g.

> "Even though I can't remember when this started, I choose to allow and notice any useful memories about this to come to me."

It can be used to bring the subconscious on board for problem solving:

> "Even though I can't see a way through this situation right now, I choose to find a creative and fun solution to the problem".

Choices can be set as homework or can be used as a Structure to help develop a new "way of being" or positive habit. These and other applications are covered specifically in what follows.

Those who want to use Choices in their work (either coaches or EFT practitioners) are encouraged to obtain Dr Pat Carrington's Choices Manual[7] and to subscribe to her email support list.

## 6.2.9  SLOW EFT

SLOW EFT was developed by Silvia Hartmann and is described fully in [4] and on Gary Craig's website at: (http://www.emofree.com/articles/sloweft.htm). I describe it very briefly here since I refer to it elsewhere as a useful variation of EFT in particular circumstances.

SLOW EFT (aka S-L-O-W EFT) is EFT done very slowly. The setup stage is identical ("Even though..."). The principle difference is that each EFT point gets tapped for a long time - perhaps 30 seconds or even a few minutes (although the speed of tapping is the same). The length of time spent on each point is up to the user - whatever feels right - and the cycle can be repeated as many times as the user wishes.

This pattern tends to be especially effective for allowing thoughts, images, memories, insights and so on to come to the surface and be noticed. It is especially useful for issues which are very big, vague or general such as "money", or "career". (Issues like this make it hard to choose just one specific aspect).

The thoughts or memories that are generated then provide material for doing more targeted standard EFT if desired i.e. they give clues about good places to start working. It can assist with a range of coaching applications, such as Homework Inquiries, Fulfilment Clarification, Finding the Learning, Ecology Testing and others.

Related sections:

| | | |
|---|---|---|
| 6.2.6 | The Standard EFT Pattern | ⇧ |
| 8.1.2.3 | Inquiries and Insights | ⇩ |
| 8.1.6 | Fulfilment Clarification | ⇩ |
| 8.2.6 | Finding the Learning | ⇩ |
| 8.2.8 | Ecology Testing | ⇩ |

## 6.2.10  Where There is Willpower, There are Blocks

*"For almost everyone in society, 'having a lot of willpower' to run roughshod over one's personal inclinations, emotions, bodies, intuitions, fears and uncertainties, is some kind of perverse badge of honour. For EFTers on the other hand, willpower is a diagnostic tool to tell you when you're still not done with a presenting issue; if you still have to use it, no matter how slightly, the problem has not yet been entirely resolved."* [3]

The title of this section could well be a motto for the EFT Coach.

Willpower, usually thought of as a positive force in achieving goals, is viewed quite differently by EFT practitioners.

Willpower is evidence of incongruence within the client. It shows that the client has a part of themselves which does not want the stated goal, but wants something else instead. A client with no objections and no "competing forces" to carrying out an action to achieve a goal, does not need Willpower - she simply does it.

Most clients will assume they will need to exert lots of willpower in order to achieve their goals. They assume it because most of our society assumes that anything worthwhile must involve "hard work", "discipline" and so forth.

Unfortunately, this is often a self-fulfilling prophecy. If most people are Psychologically Reversed about many of their goals in life (because most people aren't actually living the lives they really want to live), then this will have been their experience: it **was** hard work, and it **did** take discipline - so they must be right about needing willpower.

But as an EFT Coach you will be alert to the presence and symptoms of Psychological Reversal and how to address it. A client who talks about needing "willpower" is simply telling you they have a Reversal. The same goes for any other form of words which imply willpower such as "trying", "making myself", "pulling my finger out", "getting my act together" and so on. You may need to delve around to find out exactly what the Reversal - or block - is actually about, but basically the client has told you exactly what they need to get them "unstuck" and into action.

Related sections:

6.2.3      Psychological Reversal ⇧

9.3.7      Unsticking the Client ⇩

## 6.2.11 Persistence

Despite what you may have seen or read about EFT, not all EFT results in "one minute wonders", even though it can. Some issues and some people seem to need persistent and relatively prolonged application of EFT (over days or weeks) before results are seen. Gary Craig himself emphasises the need to be persistent in many cases - and his training videos and other people's case histories contain many examples of people who decided to be extremely persistent and eventually got results.

Clients come to coaches usually because they have attempted or intended to make changes in their lives before now, but haven't succeeded. They have tried "quick fixes", buying products or systems they hope will help them change, but it hasn't worked. Coaching understands - and needs the client to understand - that to make significant and sustained changes will require regular and persistent focus of attention on all aspects of the client's life that relates to their as yet unaccomplished goal.

An EFT practitioner who applies one round of EFT to a client without fully clearing a client's issue, would no more claim that *"EFT has failed"* or *"This client isn't EFT-able"*, than a coach would get to the end of one session, see the client still hasn't achieved her goal and announce that *"the coaching failed"* or *"the client isn't coachable"*.

In fact, coaching and EFT are remarkably similar in this respect. You can get "spot-coaching" for a very specific and bounded issue and achieve wonderful results for that issue - only to find that for your larger goal, there are other issues that you also want to get coaching on before all your obstacles are dealt with - or that there are other areas of your life which still need attention.

EFT operates in a very similar way. While a client should be able to get noticeable relief on a **specific** issue within a session, it may be that it is a very small and limited aspect of their more "global" problem such as "Procrastination", or "Stress", or "Problems with relationships".

Where the client's issue is a global one like these examples, then persistence with EFT **and** coaching in a longer term relationship is especially useful and compatible. With the discovery of each new aspect of the global issue comes a new opportunity for learning and one less impediment to action.

## 6.2.12 Aspects

Usually, clients have many issues that are on their mind - just as they have many different parts of their lives to which they want to pay attention.

And for each issue, there may be many Aspects, all of which contribute to the overall issue. The concept of Aspects is central to how EFT needs to be applied so that the issue is cleared thoroughly and completely.

There are two different types of Aspect to be aware of: Simultaneous and Sequential.

The classic illustration of an issue with Simultaneous Aspects is a phobia - let's take "flying" as an example. When a client is "afraid of flying", that is their overall issue. But underlying that overall fear are usually multiple elements of the flying experience, each of which has the power to trigger intensity **all by itself**.

So for flying, possible contributing Simultaneous Aspects might include: being up high, being over water, turbulence, flying at night, takeoff, landing, mechanical failure, being in a confined space, the sound of the engine, not being in control of what's happening, seeing the view, not seeing the view, contracting disease in aircraft etc etc.

The best example of an issue with Sequential Aspects is a traumatic memory - let's take "when my car crashed" as an example. Although the overall experience was traumatic, there were probably several mini-events within the client's memory, each of which may cause intensity when they are thought about.

So the Sequential Aspects of "when my car crashed" might include: realising the car was sliding out of control, seeing the trees ahead of us, thinking another car might come round the corner, hearing someone in the car screaming, the moment of actually hitting the tree, the quietness immediately afterward, seeing someone injured, hearing police sirens etc etc.

What Aspects apply to each client are completely individual and finding them out requires close questioning and listening to the client's language.

The different Aspects which contribute to the overall issue can be likened to a forest containing many trees (to use Gary Craig's analogy), with each tree representing something which has the power to trigger a negative emotion in the client. Clearing the overall issue (the whole forest), requires applying EFT to each Aspect in turn (chopping down each tree one at a time).

Not knowing about Aspects can be one of the easiest pitfalls in using EFT, since one might attempt to apply EFT to "my fear of flying", not get much if any change, and give up, thinking that EFT didn't work. The job of the EFT Coach therefore is to pay close attention to what clients say about their issues and to notice whether there are multiple Aspects around the central issue and to ensure they are each addressed.

Learning how to identify and work through Aspects in an orderly manner with clients is covered both on Gary's training videos and on the practitioner training.

## 6.2.13 Clients are Responsible for their Own Wellbeing

Whether in a workshop situation, using EFT alone or under the guidance of a practitioner, all EFT users and clients are required and encouraged to take responsibility for their own wellbeing. This means they have the right to say No to any particular direction for the session. It also means not putting themselves in any emotional or physical situation that will cause them pain or distress. It means communicating with the practitioner - or with themselves - about the areas they are willing and unwilling to explore right now.

This is totally in keeping with the spirit of co-active coaching and the Principle of Client Responsibility. The coach does not "do coaching **to** the client" - client and coach do coaching together. Ultimately, the client is in control. Adding EFT to the mix of tools and techniques doesn't change that.

Related sections

5.4.6     Principle of Client Responsibility ⇧

## 6.2.14 EFT Doesn't Erase Memories or Knowledge

EFT removes negative emotions - and nothing else! It doesn't make you "forget" a single detail of any memory - it simply allows you to recall the details without experiencing distress or any "emotional charge" while doing so. And it doesn't take away any positive feelings you may have towards people, places or objects.

This is very important to understand when thinking about the function of learning in coaching. Some clients might fear that if someone's memories or knowledge can be erased by EFT then this might interfere with the process of learning that is so vital and so rewarding in coaching - but this does not occur. EFT removes "energetic disruptions", not information or memories.

This means that any resourceful states from the past which the client may wish to access (e.g. a Peak Experience) will remain intact. The only "exception" to this may possibly be emotional states which the client decides to label as resourceful but which are actually founded on negative emotions - for instance using Anger as a motivation to stand up to an oppressor.

I have experienced clients who used Anger in this way and were consequently reluctant to "give up" their Anger using EFT for fear of having no drive or resources to deal with a situation (Anger had become their "strategy" in that situation). Be assured (as I assured my clients) that there is always something better (e.g. a sense of personal power) which can become a new strategy and without experiencing the unpleasant effects of Anger. I show how to do this using EFT below.

This is a nice example where coaching and EFT are very compatible. Simply removing emotional states which clients are using in resourceful ways, is not in itself very constructive. In fact, in my experience, clients tend not to let go of such emotions which are serving them in this way unless there is an alternative available. Working out what that alternative might be is a coaching conversation. Good coaching skills can therefore be of immense assistance in the successful application of EFT, not simply the reverse.

Related sections:

8.1.1.2    Retrieving and Cleansing Resourceful States ⇩
8.1.1.3    Anchoring Resourceful States ⇩
8.1.1.4    Negative Emotions as Resources ⇩
8.1.11    Locking in the Learning ⇩
8.1.12    Peak Experiences ⇩


## 6.2.15 Tailenders

"Tailender" is a term coined by Gary Craig to describe the negative thoughts, feelings or objections that can arise in response to a positive affirmation (in the absence of EFT).

So for instance, one might decide to increase one's wealth by affirming daily *"I am truly wealthy with all the money I could ever want or need"* (or something similar).

If you say this to yourself and then find yourself thinking things like:

>    *"Yeah right, in your dreams…"*

>    *"Nice goal, but it's not actually true is it?"*

>    *"And then all my friends would come sponging money off me"*

all these are examples of "Tailenders".

Tailenders have the power to totally wipe out the benefit of a positive affirmation. It's like saying "No" or "Cancel" to the affirmation before it has even had time to have an effect on your energy system or your thought processes.

Tailenders can also sabotage clients' best intentions and commitments to action. Luckily, if they can be identified they can also be eliminated using EFT, thus preventing this type of self-sabotage.

Gary goes into great detail on this subject in his trainings, and especially how to deal with them using EFT - but I merely mention it here as Tailenders will be referred to later on in the book, particularly around the subject of commitment.

Related sections:

9.3.9    Blocks to Commitment ⇩


## 6.2.16 Key Points

- EFT views the cause of all negative emotions as a disruption in the body's energy system. This view is compatible with the coaching concept of client's creating their own reality and is ultimately empowering.

- EFT works directly at the level of the client's energy system. Many conventional coaching techniques can also be viewed as affecting the client's energy system, in less explicit ways. In my opinion, both coaching and EFT are acting on the client's energy system, and for the same ends, just in different ways.

- Psychological Reversal can be thought of as a particular form of energetic disruption which often manifests as the conscious mind seeming to "want" one thing, but the unconscious/body-mind "wanting" another. Psychological Reversal is at the heart of many coaching conversations - persuading the part of the client that is resisting their goals to come into line with the part that wants them (the part that hired you). When a coach understands Reversal they have a tool for "unsticking" their clients.

- EFT views emotions as physiological events - not just experienced in the body, but occurring there. Mental aspects of emotion (such as what the client believes or says) are viewed as symptoms of the physiological state. Cognitive shifts tend to occur spontaneously as the result of EFT. However, EFT can still be effectively applied to the client's cognitive state (e.g. blocks or beliefs) as symptoms to work with.

- EFT uses 0 to 10 rating scales to measure and track progress in clients. Using rating scales avoids the "much better syndrome" which can result in lots of low level issues remaining unresolved. Getting in the habit of using rating scales also gets the client used to tuning into themselves and noticing their emotional and physiological state - a great benefit in coaching generally. It is also helpful in avoiding the problem of labelling emotions - progress can still be made even if the client can't find a description for how he feels.

- The Standard EFT pattern uses the setup statement: *"Even though I have this problem I deeply and completely accept myself"*. This pattern can be varied and several variations are used in this book.

- The acceptance phrase of the Standard EFT pattern (*"I deeply and completely accept myself"*) is particularly important in the overcoming of Psychological Reversal and in developing a distinction between the "self" who has the problem and the indestructible, infinitely valuable "I" who is deciding to release it. If the client really has strong objections to saying the standard acceptance phrase, then it's important to come up with an alternative that they can say more easily

- The Choices Technique is used when the rating for an issue is zero or very low (2 or less). It allows the client to install a positive Choice for a "way of being" in a future situation. The basic format is: "Even though I have this problem, I choose to be/do this".

- SLOW EFT is EFT done very slowly, with each point being tapped for a long time - perhaps several minutes. It tends to be especially effective for bringing thoughts, images, memories and insights to the surface and is useful for issues which are very big, vague or general such as "money", or "career".

- Willpower is evidence of a block, or Psychological Reversal. If willpower is needed, this means there is a part of the client that is resisting the desired goal for some reason - which is the definition of Psychological Reversal.

- Not all EFT results in "one minute wonders", even though it often does. Some issues and some people seem to need persistent and relatively prolonged application of EFT (over days or weeks) before results are seen. Where the client's issue/goal is a global one (e.g. "improving relationships" or "reducing stress") then persistence with EFT **and** coaching in a longer term relationship is especially useful and compatible.

- Aspects are all the different things that may contribute to an overall issue being addressed with EFT. Clearing the overall issue, requires applying EFT to each Aspect in turn.

- EFT clients are required and encouraged to take responsibility for their own wellbeing. This includes communicating with the practitioner about the areas they are willing and unwilling to explore right now. This is totally in keeping with the spirit of co-active coaching and the Principle of Client Responsibility. Ultimately, the client is in control.

- EFT removes negative emotions - and nothing else! It doesn't make you "forget" a single detail of any memory - it simply allows you to recall the details without experiencing distress or any "emotional charge" while doing so. And it doesn't take away any positive feelings you may have towards people, places or objects.

- Tailenders are the negative thoughts, feelings or objections that arise in response to a positive affirmation (in the absence of EFT). Tailenders have the power to totally wipe out the benefit of a positive affirmation and can sabotage clients' best intentions and commitments. Identifying, "catching" and eliminating Tailenders with EFT can be useful in preventing this type of self-sabotage.

# 7 EFT for the Coach

Even if you never use EFT with a client, there are many ways that EFT can help you to be a better coach. In this section we look at some common practices and skills of the coach and look at how EFT can help to strengthen these skills or improve on areas you'd like to be better at. In fact this is a good place to start experiencing EFT - by using it on yourself first.

You may notice that many of these skills relate closely to what has been said about fundamentals earlier. In the fundamentals section, the focus was on explaining the fundamental and showing how it is expressed in both coaching and EFT. In this chapter, we focus on how you can use EFT to assist or improve specific coaching skills, with specific suggestions for setup statements.

## 7.1 Self-management Skills

Self-management is a key skill and requirement for coaches and this involves many specific skills and attitudes. But all self-management skills are essentially emotion-management. And EFT is perfect tool for quickly achieving and maintaining the emotional state you want, before, during and after a coaching session.

### 7.1.1 Holding the Client's Agenda

#### 7.1.1.1 The Clients Agenda versus Your Own Agenda

Assuming that you agreed an agenda with your client and barring any memory problems on your part, the main thing which can get in the way of successfully "holding the client's agenda" is having your own agenda pop up during coaching and allowing that to influence the coaching.

This can happen if the client happens to be talking about something that also affects you, or which you have previously experienced or which you have a fear about - or in any way triggers your own concerns.

Since the object of coaching is to help a client discover their own solutions, Holding the Client's Agenda in such situations involves putting your own agenda aside and not imposing your fears, experiences or knowledge onto the client. This can be hard if the client is talking about an area where you have direct knowledge, personal experience or strong opinions.

Where this happens **during** a session, you can tap yourself while continuing to coach. Assuming it is a phone session, this will not be noticed by the client. In this situation, you do not use the setup statement or say anything to yourself while you tap - this would take you immediately to Level 1. The ideal is to remain focused on what the client is saying while performing only the physical EFT procedure. This may seem like "not doing it properly", but in fact it is what the client is saying which is the trigger for your agenda making an appearance - so focusing on it fully while you tap will have the effect of releasing the thoughts, opinions or concerns being triggered by what they are saying. By continuing to tap you maintain yourself in a neutral emotional state and you remove or reduce the "emotional charge" around what the client is saying.

In this neutral state, maintaining focus on the clients Agenda becomes much easier, allowing you to help the client find a solution uncontaminated by your own opinions.

Of course, all coaches are obliged to tell a client whenever they are on territory where they feel they cannot be neutral and successfully Hold the Client's Agenda because their own agenda is simply too important. If after tapping in the way suggested above you strongly feel that your own agenda cannot be neutralised or put aside, then you still have this obligation.

If you have forewarning that an upcoming session will involve territory that will make it hard for you to keep your agenda to one side, then you have the opportunity to apply EFT prior to the session. To do this thoroughly, make a list of all the Aspects of the issue that are concerning to you or which you feel may trigger your own agenda.

Then construct Standard EFT setup statements for each one and do at least one round of EFT on each Aspect. For example:

> "Even though I'm afraid my agenda will intrude on this coaching, ..."
>
> "Even though I have strong views about X,..."
>
> "Even though talking about Y really makes me mad,,..."
>
> "Even though I'm not sure I can avoid speaking my mind,..."
>
> etc.

Then check in with yourself about the forthcoming session. Do you feel differently? Does your agenda still feel like it might be a problem or do you feel that you can "park" it for the duration of the coaching?

If it feels less troublesome then finish off with a Choices round as follows:

> "Even though I know I have my own agenda on this issue, I choose to be a professional coach and Hold my Client's Agenda".

Even having done this, it is still probably a good idea to continue tapping yourself during the session as needed as a failsafe - or at least as a reminder to yourself of your intention to park your own agenda.

If your agenda still feels like a problem after all of this, then your existing coaching obligations come into play and you need to clear with your client at the start of the session and agree between you how to proceed. Your client depends on you to be neutral and to act in his best interests. He will trust you more to do this if you are honest about the times when you do experience conflict. In extreme cases of agenda conflict, you may even need to refer the client to another coach.

Related sections:

6.1.20    Level 1, Level 2 and Level 3 Listening ⇧

6.2.6     The Standard EFT Pattern ⇧

6.2.8     The Choices Technique ⇧

6.2.12    Aspects ⇧

## 7.1.1.2    The Problem of Shifting Aspects

A specific additional difficulty around "holding the client's agenda" within EFT Coaching arises from the know phenomenon within EFT of "shifting aspects". This occurs when the specific problem being worked on goes away or reduces significantly, but the client starts talking about something else.

For instance, suppose you are working with a client on their fear of filling in forms. Let's say one aspect of this fear for them is *"not knowing what all the terms mean"*, that it starts at an 8 and after a round of EFT falls to a 3.

Then your client says:

> *"Well, it's not so much that I don't know what they mean, it's just that I think they're so pompous and stupid it irritates me."*

You need to be able to distinguish whether what the client says is a new aspect of the issue being worked on, or about a new issue altogether. In this case, it appears to be another aspect of the issue - i.e. it does relate to how the client feels about filling in forms.

But suppose the client instead says:

> *"And all this paper! It makes me so mad thinking about how many trees get cut down every year."*

Is this aspect about form-filling? Or is it about the client's concerns about the environment? It's probably safe to say in this example that even if we could clear the client's anger about environmental issues, the client would still have a fear of filling in forms. And since it is the form-filling that is needed to achieve the client's goals, we can legitimately put the environmental concerns to one side.

That may have been a fairly black and white decision, but what about a less clear-cut example? Suppose the client says:

> *"Why do big corporations have to have so many forms anyway - I hate all that bureaucracy".*

Is this aspect about form-filling? Or is it about the client's annoyance with big corporations?

In other words, if you were to spend time doing EFT on the client's feelings about big corporations, would you be contributing to their ability to fill out forms and thus achieve their goal? It depends.

If they are applying for a job at a big corporation, you might decide that it **is** relevant - because their feeling about big corporations might be part of what's blocking them from filling in the form.

But if they are applying for a place at university, or filling in their tax return, then it may well **not** be relevant.

If the new aspects coming up are part of the root cause of the problem then it is legitimate to follow the trail and apply EFT to these new aspects.

If the new aspects coming up are about a completely different issue which has been bubbling under the surface waiting for the even bigger issue to get dealt with first, then it may not be appropriate to do EFT for that issue within the coaching context.

Ultimately, you have to make a judgement, based on relevance to the client's overall coaching goals (their "agenda"). But you can and should always check in with your client about what **they** think is relevant.

Related sections:

6.2.12    Aspects ⇧

## 7.1.2   Staying "Over There" with a Client

*"If you have a client who is very disturbed, crying, shaking, the last thing you want to do is go there and be there too - an utterly resourceless state that does neither of you any good whatsoever."* [3]

In addition to tapping along with clients when they are doing EFT, phone coaching also offers the opportunity to do tapping on yourself during the session. This is particularly useful if the coach feels himself become distressed or otherwise emotionally involved with what the client is saying. In these situations the coach's focus is immediately compromised from Level 2 (the client) or Level 3 (the client plus environment) focus, back to Level 1 (yourself).

If you are becoming aware of your own distress, then you are not maintaining focus on the client and you are certainly not "holding the space" as well as you could. However, simply ignoring or suppressing your own feelings means cutting yourself off from the totality of what's happening in the coaching and also involves reducing rapport (if you emotionally "retreat" from the interaction, this will have a negative effect on rapport). So how can you stay in rapport, maintain your emotional connection with client, and yet not have those emotions distract you from the client?

The simplest method is simply to tap yourself as the client talks and while you maintain focus on them. This will have the effect of dissolving your emotional response to them, allowing you to maintain a neutral attitude. Note that this does not mean that you should never allow yourself to respond emotionally to a client - your human response as a coach is a necessary part of the overall relationship. What you don't want though is to become **so** distressed or involved that you stop being a professional coach.

Having recourse to EFT at such moments is a way to

- Prevent the client's issue becoming your issue (see Avoiding Burnout).
- Maintain your professional composure and release you from Level 1 focus.
- Still allow you to maintain energetic rapport and focus on what the client is saying.

It's also possible, even likely, that tapping yourself while tuned into the client, will have some positive effect for the client also. However, this should not be your aim or your focus, since you want the client to be taking responsibility for their own progress as much as possible (Principle of Client Responsibility).

Having established the principle of client choice around use of EFT (Principle of Informed Permission), some might worry whether unintentional proxy tapping is a contravention of this principle. I believe not, provided that whenever you tap yourself it is **for yourself** and to help **you** manage your own emotional state as coach. In terms of any possible unintended benefits to the client, I compare this to the effect of normal coaching practice in "holding the space" for clients.

"Holding the space" is an energetic technique, involving the intention of the coach to create and maintain a safe, supportive space for the duration of the coaching. Many coaches attest to the power of this technique to facilitate coaching. However I have never seen anyone worry whether this practice contravenes a client's freewill or choice. And it has never been suggested that the client's permission needs to be first obtained. It is simply viewed as something that the coach does in order to create a good coaching atmosphere and to control his own emotional state in service of the coaching.

We should not be afraid as coaches of having an impact on the client. It's what they have come to us for. It's not the impact of imposing our ideas or opinions though - it's the impact of allowing and encouraging the client to be Who They Really Are and to expand into that in our presence. And it's this type of individual impact that coaches have on their clients simply by holding and radiating "good energy" that makes clients want to come back for more, or recommend them to others.

Related sections:

## 7.1.3   Clearing your Limiting Beliefs about what's Possible for a Client

To be a congruent coach, you **must** be able to believe in the validity of the client's goals and believe that the client can achieve them. If you have doubts, so will they. As a coach it is your job to hold the energetic space for you and your client to inhabit - and the space must be big enough to include the achievement of their goal. If you doubt they can achieve it, then you cannot congruently hold the space big enough for them.

I well remember two instances as a client when my own enthusiasm for a goal or a dream was dashed to pieces by a coach who wanted me to reign in my goals because they thought I was being unrealistic. If a client tells you they want to achieve a specific goal and you want to reign them in because you don't think it's feasible for them, then it's a good idea to examine and release this limitation in yourself.

Ask yourself: *"Why don't I think this goal is feasible for this client?"* and be very honest about your answers. Write down everything that comes back as an answer, no matter how ridiculous or how ashamed you may be of the answer. Nobody else will see your answers to this question - but your client will surely feel your lack of faith in their goal.

Once you have written down all your answers, construct opening statements around each one and do at least one round of EFT for each. Preferably, take a rating for how true each one seems to you and keep doing EFT (including any aspects that arrive) until it stops feeling like an obstacle to you believing in the client's goal.

Here are some suggested setups that illustrate the kinds of issues that might come up:

> *"Even though I don't believe this client can do this…"*

> *"Even though I would be terrified to have this goal myself,…"*

> *"Even though I think this is the wrong goal for him,…"*

> *"Even though I once failed at this myself,…"*

> *"Even though I'd be jealous if he achieved this goal,…"*

> *"Even though I think this goal is shallow and pointless,…"*

> *"Even though I can't see how to help him achieve this goal so I wish he'd pick an easier one,…"*

Ultimately, if you have done all the above and you still cannot seriously believe in the viability of the client's goal, you have an obligation to refer your client elsewhere. You cannot Champion your client - believe in them and be with them 100% - if you fundamentally doubt the validity of the goal you have been hired to help the client achieve. If you don't believe in a client's goal, there are two possible outcomes. Either the client will reign in their ambitions to match what you believe is possible for them - in which case you have been responsible for their underperforming. Or the client will go ahead regardless and achieve the goal despite your doubts - in which case you should be paying them.

Related sections

8.1.13    Championing ⇩

## 7.1.4   Clearing your Prejudices about Clients

We owe it to ourselves and our clients to be very careful only to work with clients who we feel a genuine "buzz" about, and who we "click" with. But often, any negative reactions to prospective clients are not about who the client really is, but about our reactions to them.

Before deciding that you can't work with a particular client, it's worthwhile using EFT on your thoughts and feelings about them to see if there isn't something which can be cleared. You may clear it and still feel that you wouldn't be the right coach for this client. But you may also find that with those issues cleared, you can see the client in a new light - and their goals seem suddenly that more interesting and exciting to you.

Please note I am not suggesting that you ignore your instincts and intuitions about prospective clients. Many coaches report getting an intuition about who and who not to work with. You certainly should pay attention to these intuitions and not try to override them without good reason. But it can be difficult sometimes to distinguish between a prejudice programmed by an incident so long ago you can't even remember it, and an intuition based on what sort of client is good for you. If there is a good reason to not work with a client, doing EFT on your feelings won't take that away - it may even help you clarify why that's the right decision.

Actually, using EFT this way - to "test" your feelings about a client - is a good example of how to use EFT with a client to test their own feelings about different issues (e.g. goals or values) - so it's a good one to try, if only for the experience. In this use of EFT, your intuition and instinct will have the final say, whatever the results of the EFT. You are not trying to "correct" or "fix" your feelings about the client - because you simply don't know whether it's a prejudice or a valid intuition at the start. Only by doing the EFT will you get a chance to notice whether your feelings alter and perhaps deduce afterwards whether any negative emotions were at work.

The method is as for most of these applications. Ask yourself *"Why don't I want to work with this client?"*. If you don't know why, do EFT on *"Even though I don't know why I don't want to work with this client,…"* and pay close attention to what ideas, thoughts or images come up.

Write down all the reasons you can think of (however ridiculous or embarrassing) and do EFT on each one, e.g.

> *"Even though they have a voice that puts me off,…"*

> *"Even though I just get a funny vibe,…"*

> *"Even though I'm not sure they're really committed to coaching,…"*

> *"Even though I don't like coaching men/women,…"*

> *"Even though I've never coached someone like this before,…"*

As above, if you still don't want to work with a client after doing EFT, then don't. Choosing your clients is your right and being sure that a client is right for you is also your obligation. The only difference this approach makes is ensuring the decision is based on positive choice, not negative prejudice.

Related sections:

9.1.2    Validating Goals ⇩

9.5.9    Testing Values ⇩

## 7.1.5 Dealing with your Own Performance Issues

*"...each person...has their own path, are in charge of their own destiny - but at the end of the day, many therapists are thoroughly unhappy when they don't get 'the results'. ... Taking the time to sit down after the client has left and to engage in just 5 minutes of 'basic therapists maintenance' as I call it, can make a lot of difference to your work and to your levels of energy and enjoyment."* [3]

Coaches can be equally subject to the pressure to "get results" with clients as therapists are - and for the very best of motives. But this type of pressure leads to the exact opposite state of mind and being that is necessary for good coaching.

It's hard to stay tuned into the client if you keep thinking *"How am I doing?"*. It's hard to create and hold a relaxed, expanded and safe space for your client if in the back of your mind you are feeling tense, energetically constricted because of your fear and feeling threatened at the prospect of failing as a coach. And it's hard to express real flair, intuition and insight within a coaching session if you are judging and editing everything you say, for fear it may be "wrong". But perhaps most important of all, it's hard to model congruence and integrity as a "way of being" to your client if you don't feel congruent and in integrity about sitting there and being their coach!

Assuming you have undertaken a good formal coaching training, then you **do** know as many tools and techniques as you need to move the coaching forward. I will also assume that if you have done a good coaching training then you have probably had at least one experience of when your coaching went well. And even by some small chance you don't think you had that experience on your training, then you will certainly have had good coaching modelled for you by the course leaders. In other words, your mind and energy system **knows what good coaching is and how to do it.**

If you are feeling lacking in confidence around your coaching, it is because you have beliefs or other negative emotions either around coaching in particular, or around performance, winning or success in general.

It is well worth your time doing as much EFT as you need to on these issues. When you have removed all the memories, beliefs and feelings that make you feel incongruent about being a good coach, then there will be nothing in the way of you simply being one!

As with many of these self-management suggestions, this is one way to obtain first-hand experience of working with your own belief system using EFT, so that you know how it feels when you decide to do similar work with a client.

Related sections:

9.5.2     Clearing Limiting Beliefs ⇩

## 7.1.6 Reinforcing Good Coaching

It's a classic coaching technique to make sure that clients who start to make progress, however small, receive explicit and fulsome congratulations from their coach. Receiving praise and recognition of success is a way to energetically "embed" the experience as a positive one within their system.

We will show later on how to use EFT to reinforce client's good feelings - but here I want to suggest that you use the same method to reinforce your **own** successes as a coach.

If you have general doubts about your abilities, then having one good coaching session can all too quickly be wiped out by negative thoughts such as *"Well, that was a one-off"*, or *"Well, the client made it really easy for me today"*, or *"Well, it happened to be on a subject area I know something about."*

By tapping while you are still feeling good about your performance (i.e. straight after the coaching session), you inoculate yourself against any thoughts like this that come long as "objections" to feeling good about yourself (a type of Tailender). As well as doing it straight after (and I would suggest tapping for a good few rounds straight away), also be vigilant if negative or judgmental thoughts come up later on, over the next few days. A good format to use would be:

> *"Even though I had that thought, I deeply and completely accept myself and I choose to remember how it felt after that coaching session"*

Or use the Celebration Pattern described below.

Related sections:

6.2.15     Tailenders ⇑
8.2.10.2   The Celebration Pattern ⇓


## 7.1.7   Avoiding Burnout

> *"It is powerful and energizing to be in the presence of personal change. It can be exhausting too - another sign of the emotional impact of being present in such a deep way in client's lives"* [2]

Even when coaching is going well, it's sometimes hard to maintain a healthy degree of detachment from the client and their issues. It's natural - and required - for the coach to care deeply about the client and the client's goals. But spending time and emotional energy outside the coaching thinking (worrying, mulling, planning, call it what you will) about the client is not required and adds nothing to the client's experience or progress - all it does is use up emotional energy that you need for your own life and goals, and which you need to have available for your next coaching session. And if you have a full practice, perhaps speaking to many clients a day, the result can often be exhaustion. Although this is common and perhaps natural, it is not necessary.

There are at least three ways to use EFT to prevent this:

**Tap while you coach.** Even if the client isn't doing EFT (and assuming you are on the phone), you can tap yourself at any point during the session where you feel concern or you can feel the client's issues "sticking" to you. (See also: Staying "Over There" with the Client)

**Tap after you coach.** At the end of each session you can use EFT to "clear" any lingering thoughts or worries about the client (e.g. what happened in the coaching, wondering how they will do with their homework, worrying about whether their unstable home life will get in the way of their career goals, etc.)

**Tap when you catch yourself thinking about your clients.** If you find yourself thinking about a client in any way that you sense is unproductive or exhausting to you, use EFT right then, in order to release the worry.  If you can't release the worry because you can't identify the root cause of it, then you can use the Choices format to "park" it (See also Principle of Client Responsibility).

> *"Even though I keep thinking about this client/Even though I'm worried about this client, I choose to park this until our next session".*

Related sections:

5.4.6      Principle of Client Responsibility ⇑
6.2.8      The Choices Technique ⇑
7.1.2      Staying "Over There" with the Client ⇑

## 7.1.8   Maintaining Detachment about Using EFT

When you have a "killer tool" like EFT in your coaching armoury, it can be incredibly frustrating when you have a client with a clear emotional block or who is in clear distress, but they don't give permission to use EFT.

When using EFT in a therapy context, it's understood by both client and practitioner that the reason the client is there is to apply EFT to their problem. In that situation, if a client decides that they don't want to use EFT, then the session is effectively over.

But in coaching, this is not the case. A client who withdraws permission to use EFT - for a specific issue, or at a particular time, or even for a long period of time - is still your client and you are still in a coaching relationship with them. You must find another route to take - choose a different coaching tool. (Of course, if you use EFT as a central tool for your coaching, and a client refuses to use EFT at all, for any issue - i.e. they have a fundamental objection to using it - then you may have to choose between coaching them using conventional methods or referring them to a different coach who works in a way the client prefers).

Being able to accept the client's decision without frustration or judgement can be a particular challenge, especially if you know that EFT could help this client and in very short order. But accept it you must. And you can use EFT on yourself to help you deal with any frustration.

> *"Even though the client won't use EFT on this issue,…"*

> *"Even though he is afraid to use EFT for this, I choose to remember the client has the right to change at his own pace."*

Using the Non-Judgement pattern may also be helpful as a way of emphasising that the client's choice to not use EFT is not necessarily a problem. For instance:

> *"She doesn't want to use EFT and I deeply and completely accept myself."*

You can also bring in the Both Of Us pattern to emphasise positive acceptance of the client as well as yourself:

> *"He doesn't want to use EFT here and I deeply and completely accept both of us."*

By maintaining your detachment about the use of EFT, you strengthen your clients' trust in you to respect their needs and wishes. It also reinforces the nature of the relationship as a coaching relationship rather than a therapeutic one (it's coaching with EFT, not EFT with coaching). And it also reinforces your credibility as a coach - that you have strong enough coaching skills to continue a productive relationship in the absence of EFT.

Related sections:

| | |
|---|---|
| 5.4.1 | Principle of Informed Permission ⇧ |
| 8.2.11 | The Non-Judgement Pattern ⇩ |
| 8.2.13 | The Both Of Us Pattern ⇩ |

## 7.1.9   Avoiding Faint Heartedness

> *"Coaching is not for the faint hearted."* [2]

Coaching requires courage on many levels. It involves speaking clearly and confidently, voicing your intuitions, interrupting the client when they are getting off track and asking them direct questions regarding their behaviour.

Many of these behaviours could be seen as rude, intrusive or over-bearing in normal conversation - and so it can sometimes require a bit of practice to get comfortable with exercising this level of assertiveness with a client.

What you probably know intellectually is that coaching with this kind of courage is a service to the client - it moves them forwards and is efficient in terms of time. But knowing it intellectually doesn't make it easy to overcome all sorts of emotional programming that says *"You mustn't contradict"*, *"You mustn't interrupt"*, *"You must be polite"* and all the rest. Pushing past this sort of programming to say or ask the things that need to be said or asked in a coaching relationship is hard work - unless you can use EFT to release your fears around "breaking" these conventions.

Using EFT for this purpose can be done as a "bulk session" - writing down all the ways you would like to be more courageous or assertive in your coaching and doing a round of EFT on each one.

Perhaps more thorough however is to do it over time and in response to specific instances that arise in your coaching. As with all EFT, results are usually much better when the client is focussed on an actual memory or incident involving the issue. If you have a session with a client in which you find yourself wanting to voice an intuition or ask a hard question and finding this difficult, then straight after the session is the best time to do EFT on that feeling - whether or not you managed to say what you wanted to say. By focussing in on the details of what actually happened with that particular client, you will most successfully "tune in" to the actual feelings and thoughts that were operating at the time, and therefore you are more likely to clear them.

Here are some example setups for the sorts of issues that may be operating in this area:

> *"Even though I find interrupting difficult, I deeply and completely accept myself."*

> *"Even though I can never seem to shut this client up, ..."*

> *"Even though I could feel the frustration rising inside me, ..."*

> *"Even though I went straight into Level 1 and lost all my power, ..."*

> *"Even though I get this ache in my back before I manage to interrupt, ...."*

> *"Even though I'm scared to say what I really think in case that's imposing my opinion,..."*

> *"Even though she seemed to ignore me when I interrupted,..."*

At a minimum, if you have a session where you experience any reluctance to speak out, you can apply EFT afterwards purely on the feeling associated with that until it is zero e.g. any feelings of embarrassment, heart-pounding, sweating, throat tightening - or whatever symptoms you notice. Clearing the symptoms may or may not clear the underlying issue, but it will begin to shift them. Your object then is to notice how you react in future similar situations and repeat the EFT based on what happens then. You are likely to fully clear any anxiety around this over time if done diligently.

## 7.1.10 Dropping the Need to Look Good

Even if you take great pride in your ability as a coach, the need to "look good" to your clients is a disservice to them. The second you put your image before your real self, you are moving out of authenticity. Staying in authenticity improves your ability to coach from the heart, using your intuition and maintaining Level 3 listening. It also models authenticity to your client - a key quality they will benefit from learning if they are to go forward and create their life the way they want it.

Moving out of authenticity - by worrying how you look to your client - takes you straight into Level 1, for a start. It also blocks skills such as intuition which are based on being connected with your true self. And it signals (unconsciously) to the client that they need to maintain their self-image too - which makes your job as coach much harder since your client is most likely to start moving towards their goals when they can connect with their true desires regardless of the opinion of others.

In other words, you cannot expect to bring forth your client's Real Self if you can't do the same for yourself.

You can use EFT to help drop this need to "look good". You can do this in a general way as follows:

*"Even though I'm worried about looking good with clients, I deeply..."*

What may be more powerful is to list all the specific ways in which you are concerned about looking good. As ever, the more specific you can be the more targeted and effective will be the EFT. Some examples might be:

*"Even though I want to come over as confident,..."*

*"Even though I hope they don't realise how new I am to all of this,..."*

*"Even though I'm worried what they think about my fees,..."*

*"Even though I think they're judging me,..."*

*"Even though I think I should have printed all this out professionally,..."*

As mentioned above, the best way to get specific on these issues is to notice any particular image-conscious thoughts you find yourself having during coaching and to write them down and apply EFT specifically to those thoughts after the session.

You may be surprised at how many of these you have when you start noticing. But working through them as they arise will reduce the overall level of them over time, and will then allow you to be the authentic coach that you can be.

Related sections

6.1.11    Coaching the Real Client ⇧

6.1.20    Level 1, Level 2 and Level 3 Listening ⇧

7.2.3    Intuition ⇩


# 7.1.11 Coaching Outside your Comfort Zone

Usually the coach's job as a guide involves encouraging the client to go into areas they either wouldn't have thought of going themselves, or if they would have thought of it, would have been too scared to go by themselves.

There's another tricky situation that occurs when the client is all too eager to head off in a direction, but the **coach** is reluctant. This can occur when the client wants to talk about something that triggers very negative feelings in the coach, reminding them of something they find hard to look at in their own lives. The risk is that the coach will see the scary subject coming, will head the client off at the pass and find a related or different topic to focus on instead, thereby totally missing the opportunity to serve the client.

EFT can help you resolve or reduce your fears around coaching a particular topic. There are two approaches to this:

**During the session:** If it occurs during the session, your best recourse is simply to start tapping. Since you will still be mostly focussed on the client, you will not be expecting to fully clear the emotional charge around the subject or find and clear all the aspects that relate to it. What you are aiming to do is to take the edge off, and release you long enough so that your will to focus on the client and go where they need to go can get back in charge of the coaching. By reducing the fear even somewhat, you make it easier to go where the client is going - and by keeping tapping, to make that not only bearable but to receive many insights along the way. However, you do need to ensure this remains the client's process, not yours.

**Between sessions:** If you have been alerted to a piece of territory that you feel unwilling to coach, it's a good idea to try and deal with it outside the coaching environment when you will have the time to really explore its roots and aspects and clear them. If it's a really tough one, find a fellow coach and/or practitioner to guide you through it. If you notice an issue like this and then find yourself putting off dealing with it, this is a sure sign that you need outside help to make sure it doesn't hang around and pop up in further coaching sessions.

If you are going to use EFT to deal with it by yourself, and assuming it's a reasonably large issue for you (large enough to make you do anything to avoid going near it within a coaching session), you probably need to do some pre-work on it first before diving in to the usual procedure of finding aspects etc. This is the same sort of pre-work an EFT practitioner would do with a client who was fearful about beginning work on the main issue.

First of all you need a measure to know when you have done enough pre-work to allow you to proceed with dealing with the main issue. Ask yourself:

*"On a scale of 0 to 10, how willing do I feel to work directly on this issue?"*

As well as getting a number, scan your body for any physical signs of anxiety or tension.

If you get a 5 or less then you have significant pre-work to do. If you get between 6 and 8, some pre-work will probably be useful. If you get a 9 or a 10, then you have little resistance to working on the issue. It's probably unlikely that you will have a 9 or 10 at this stage or else you probably would not have experienced the resistance to dealing with it during the coaching. If you do get a 9 or 10, **and** you experienced strong resistance to coaching that issue, you need to look at what exactly was scary in the session for you and adjust what you want to work on.

Pre-work setups should be based on how you feel about having the issue, how you feel about not being able to go there with clients or with yourself, reasons why it's scary for you to go there, and so on. These will be specific to you, but here are some suggestions:

*"Even though I don't really want to look at this issue yet...."*

*"Even though I think I have to look at this issue because of my coaching..."*

*"Even though part of me wants to deal with this and part of me wants to run a mile..."*

*"Even though I hate myself for feeling like this about this issue..."*

*"Even though I think I'm a coward for not dealing with this..."*

*"Even though I feel bad about letting my clients down on this issue..."*

You will know you have dealt with all the "fears of the fear" when you find yourself naturally wanting to get on and work on the issue itself. Doing the pre-work may lead naturally on to working on the fear directly, or you may feel like taking a break and coming back to it. Both are fine. Sometimes the energy builds up momentum which it feels good to "ride" and get straight into working on the issue. Sometimes the effect of the pre-work requires a bit of time for neurological rewiring to take place before the system is ready to make more progress. Both are natural outcomes of this type of work and neither is better or worse.

What's important is to be as gentle with yourself as you would be with a client and go where the energy leads. If you have done a fair amount of pre-work and get the urge to take a break, this doesn't mean you are "giving up" or "failing". It means either that you have done a lot of releasing and the system needs a break to consolidate, or that there is fear of finally getting close to dealing with the issue - or both. If the latter occurs, this means that even doing the pre-work is triggering significant anxiety.

The answer to this is to backtrack and dissociate even further to a safe distance and work from there. For instance:

*"Even though even this pre-work is scaring me...."*

*"Even though the slightest reference to this issue is really freaking me out..."*

and so forth.

If this doesn't start to clear the fears, even after a break, then you almost certainly need to get help from another practitioner to help you work on this. In the extreme case, if you are ultimately unable to bring yourself to work on a particular area with your client, then you need to refer your client to another coach who can.


## 7.1.12 Controlling Your Own Gremlin

*"First notice. Make sure you record it well in your mind. What was the Gremlins' criticism or observation, precisely?"* [2]

It's not just clients who have Gremlins - coaches have them too. (By the way, I treat Gremlins as special types of belief - but if you think of particular beliefs as Gremlins then it's fine to continue using this term). Working on your own Gremlin using EFT is an excellent thing to do as a precursor to working with a client on theirs.

The classic "method" of controlling or managing a Gremlin lies in noticing and observing the Gremlin at work. It's a classic technique that removes you from being "in" the thought (*"I am thinking this thought about myself"*) to being removed from it (*"I am watching a part of me say something to me"*).

Learning to detach from the Gremlin (or any belief) puts you back at choice. You can decide whether to dismiss what it is saying (*"Oh that's just my Gremlin"*) or to accept it as truth (*"Well maybe I really am a terrible coach! Maybe I should arrange some practice or do another course."*). Without EFT, this process of noticing and detachment is usually slow. And even if it is successful, the Gremlin is still there.

But the process of noticing is still useful even if you want to use EFT to actually get rid of the Gremlin.

As with all EFT, the key is being able to connect with the problem, identify all the aspects and get specific about the issue. In EFT generally, the more specific you can be the more likely it is that the EFT will reduce the emotion or belief. By noticing precisely what words the Gremlin used and what it is actually criticising you for, you can then use those words directly in your EFT setup statements to combat it.

Be aware that the specific thing that the Gremlin said to you today, may not be all there is to the Gremlin. There may be bigger underlying themes of which today's criticism was merely one aspect or one possibility. But by cutting down each specific criticism as it pops up, you gradually limit the Gremlin's options for getting at you. Having identified a Gremlin, there are two ways to clear it

The most thorough way is to dig around and find the fundamental belief or fear that's behind it. This can be interesting and give you many insights along the way. It can also be hard work. Sometimes the driving fear is so old that you may not be able to access it consciously or even articulate it in language. And sometimes, if the Gremlin is active, it can be hard for you to get the perspective or detachment you need to really understand the underlying belief or fear.

A longer way is to deal with each aspect of the Gremlin as it appears, one at a time. This can be a thorough method if done diligently over time, for each thought or action you notice coming from the Gremlin. In one way this method can be seen as equally good if not better than finding the fundamental belief straightaway, since working on each actual thought from the Gremlin keeps the EFT focused on very specific aspects and the emotions connected with them (as opposed to an intellectual exercise that might be rather abstract and unemotional, and therefore not very strongly tuned in to the emotional content of the Gremlin).

In the end, choose the method that seems to flow most easily for you and which feels intuitively better.

"Gremlins" can often speak the truth - or refer to the truth even while they are making you feel bad.

> *"Self-management is also about knowing when it wasn't the Gremlin - when you really are in over your head"* [2]

EFT can help you with that knowing. EFT never taps away the truth about a situation. If your "Gremlin" has been saying *"You really should get more practice with this, that was terrible"*, even if it is true and you do need more practice, you still want to get rid of the bad feeling you got when you heard it. If it's true that you do need more practice, this will come into sharp focus for you as a result of the tapping. But by taking away the negative emotions that happened when you heard it (shame, guilt, feeling useless etc), you allow the positive energy needed to correct the problem to come into play and help you arrange more practice.

This is a great way to turn criticism around so that not only are you more likely to take positive action to correct the problem, but you can also feel genuinely grateful to the person who criticised you, even if it was yourself.

Related sections:

9.5.2      Clearing Limiting Beliefs ⇩

## 7.1.13 Key Points

- EFT can be used to clear your mind of distracting thoughts before a coaching session to ensure you are fully focussed on your client during the session.

- EFT can help you "Hold the Client's Agenda" by helping you put your own agenda aside while coaching. EFT can be used during the session by simply tapping while continuing to focus on the client. Or it can be used prior to a session by applying it to all the aspects of the situation that are problematic.

- EFT can help you "stay over there" with your client at times when you find yourself becoming distressed or otherwise emotionally involved with a client and the inclination is to detach. Since this usually happens unexpectedly during the coaching, the best solution is simply to tap yourself while maintaining focus on the client.

- To be a congruent coach, you **must** be able to believe in the validity of the client's goals and believe that the client can achieve them. EFT can help you clear any of your own issues which may be undermining your ability to fully believe in the client's goal.

- EFT may be used to clear any prejudices you may have about particular prospective clients. It can be used to "test" whether your dislike of a client is based on negative prejudice or correct intuition about whether a client is right for you.

- EFT can be used to deal with your worries about your own performance as a coach. Assuming you have received professional coach training, it's likely that if you lack confidence about your coaching it is because you have beliefs or other negative emotions either around coaching in particular, or around performance, winning or success in general. It is well worth your time doing as much EFT as you need to on these issues.

- EFT can be used to positively reinforce the occasions when your coaching goes well. By tapping while you are still feeling good about your performance (i.e. straight after the coaching session), you inoculate yourself against any thoughts like this that come along as "objections" to feeling good about yourself.

- Even when coaching is going well, it's sometimes hard to maintain a healthy degree of detachment from the client and their issues and eventually this can lead to exhaustion and burnout. Using EFT during and between session whenever thoughts or worries about clients arise, helps to stop client issues "sticking" to you and helps to maintain your energy levels.

- Not all clients want to use EFT - and maintaining detachment about whether it is used can be difficult. You can use EFT on yourself to help you deal with any frustration. By maintaining your detachment about the use of EFT, you strengthen your clients' trust in you to respect their needs and wishes.

- Coaching requires courage to speak clearly and confidently, voice your intuitions, interrupt the client when they are getting off track and ask them direct questions. EFT can be used to deal with the social conventions and fears that can make this uncomfortable.

- The need to "look good" to your clients is a disservice to them. The second you put your image before your real self, you are moving out of authenticity. You can use EFT to help drop this need to "look good". Working through any image-conscious thoughts you have as they arise will reduce the overall level of them over time, and will then allow you to be the authentic coach that you can be.

- EFT can help you resolve or reduce your fears around coaching outside your comfort zone. If necessary you may need to do some pre-work on the fear of addressing the issue or even seek out a practitioner to help you work through the issue.

- It's not just clients who have Gremlins (negative self-beliefs) - coaches have them too. Working on your own Gremlin using EFT is an excellent thing to do as a precursor to working with a client on theirs. Gremlins can sometimes speak the truth - using EFT is a great way to turn criticism around so that you are more likely to take positive action to correct the problem.

- Many of these self-management techniques may be useful in improving your confidence and performance as a coach, even if you do not use EFT with your clients.

# 7.2  Coaching Skills

This section looks at many common coaching skills and looks at how compatible EFT is with each one and how EFT can be used to enhance or demonstrate that skill.

## 7.2.1  Listening Without Judgement

When you are familiar with EFT (or any other energy technique), something spontaneously occurs to the way you look at other people and think about what they say and do. When you come from the viewpoint that "all negative emotions are a disruption of the energy system", it becomes almost impossible to hold a negative judgement about anyone. When you know that the appropriate adjustments to a person's energy system would reveal only a beautiful, loving, forgiving soul, it becomes extremely easy to distinguish between the "true person" and the particular energetic disruptions that are displaying themselves at this moment.

Even when I am not using EFT with someone, I find that the training in EFT is strongly affecting how I think about - or judge - what someone is saying and what it means. With this viewpoint, "listening without judgement" becomes completely natural and logical. Instead of noticing how objectionable someone's views are, or what terrible decisions they've made in their life, instead you start to notice the disruptions in the energy system. Then you become curious about what might have triggered them and what might have caused them - which leads us to another key coaching skill.

Related sections:

6.2.1      The Cause of Negative Emotions ⇧

## 7.2.2  Curiosity

It is a coach's curiosity which demonstrates to the client that the coach cares passionately about them and their goals. It is a coach's curiosity which drives forward the coaching dialogue. And it is the coach's curiosity which shines the light on the client's issues so that the client can see them more clearly or from a different viewpoint.

As already indicated, viewing the client as an energy system tends to excite curiosity quite naturally. The types of question that accompany an EFT session also happen to be the sorts of questions which generate insights from the client and deepen the client's understanding about how they function. For instance: What triggers this reaction in my client? Does this always happen or only at home, at work or with certain people? How does it really feel to be in this state? What other thoughts, images or bodily sensations accompany this state?

Adding EFT to your coaching toolbox therefore augments the level of curiosity about what makes your client tick and the exact nature of their experience.

## 7.2.3  Intuition

*"The natural tendency is to hold back at first, to analyze the intuition, to make sure it's viable....The most powerful moment is the first. Fear and timidity, hesitation, will pass it by."* [2]

You can use EFT to improve not only your own intuition as a coach, but also that of your clients if that is relevant to their goals. Feeling the intuitions about clients in the course of a coaching session is the ultimate in being "tuned in" to your client. It's also an incredibly useful skill in a profession that perhaps spends a maximum of 30-60 minutes with someone once a week or less.

There is a limited amount of information you can really know about your client in that time, especially at the start of the relationship (although pre-intake questionnaires and intake sessions themselves can give you the basics). So the more "information" you can access through alternative channels the better. Now, I am not talking about "woo-woo channelling" here (although I have met coaches who use that method quite explicitly as part of their technique). Here I am referring only to the down-to-earth type of coaching that can be taught in most coaching schools.

But it is a fact that there is far more information coming at us than we are able to pay attention to consciously and make available for processing. All the rest is perceived unconsciously, and, for the most part, stays unconscious. But it is possible to open our ability to access information that exists in the unconscious, and specifically attune our systems to make available information that we have picked up which is relevant and useful to our (or our clients') goals.

So, we can unconsciously pick up information from a client's voice, or their manner of dress, or something they mentioned back in the intake session. Or we can use information we've picked up over a lifetime experience of meeting different people and being in different situations, so that when we have a client in front of us, something they say or do somehow triggers a memory pattern from long ago. Suddenly we have images, words, music or sensations that we now suddenly and for "no reason" strongly associate with the client and which seem to be presenting themselves as important and relevant to the situation.

A recent example I saw of this type of memory-based intuition concerned a fireman who decided, based on his strong intuition, to pull his men out of a burning building even though there was no overt sign of danger at the time he did so.

At the time, his men couldn't understand why he had pulled them out, since they couldn't see any problem - and the fireman could not explain his feeling in any other terms than having a strong sense of unease. A few minutes after all his men had left the building safely, the entire building exploded and collapsed. Later analysis of the fire revealed that there were three specific oddities which usually precede the occurrence of "backdraft" - a highly dangerous event which leads to intense and sudden explosion. Although the fireman did not consciously notice the three oddities at the time (one of them was the fact that the fire was silent, rather than making the crackling sound of a normal fire), he had been around enough other fires in the past, for his unconscious mind to notice that this fire was different - the patterns didn't match.

I believe we operate like this much more of the time than we realise.

We already know that EFT can be used for bringing to consciousness memories from long ago which are relevant to our problem today. In fact this often happens spontaneously even when the client has no idea that there is a memory relevant to their issue when they start. If intuition depends even partially on the availability of information from past memories, then EFT has the power to increase our intuition profoundly. This means we can use EFT to increase intuition generally:

> *"Even though I don't think I'm very intuitive, I choose to be more intuitive every day"*

It also means we can also get more specific about what we want to be intuitive **about**, and specifically invite the memories that are relevant to the chosen situation:

> *"Even though I'm not getting any intuition about this client, I choose to access any memories or past information that would assist my intuition".*

It's one thing to have an intuition about something - it's another thing to act on it. Many people, myself included, often experience a strong intuition about something, only to realise later on why the intuition was valid (just like the fireman). Why don't we act on our intuitions? Probably because we don't fully trust them. And are not trust and self-doubt emotionally based issues which can be addressed with EFT? This means that it is possible to use EFT to reduce your own resistance to listening to your own intuition. Each person's doubts or distrust of their intuition will take a slightly different form - so use opening statements that reflect your own specific feelings about it. Some examples might be:

> *"Even though I don't trust my own intuitions, I deeply..."*

> *"Even though I feel my intuitions aren't good enough on their own, I deeply..."*

> *"Even though I'd rather wait and see if my intuitions are correct before believing them,..."*

> *etc*

Then, even if you learn to trust your intuition, there may be other things holding you back from using them within your coaching. This relates to fear of voicing your intuition, fear of being wrong, or looking foolish. This also is an EFT-able fear. Again, the fear will be specific to each coach, but here are some possibilities:

> *"Even though I'm afraid of telling someone else my intuition,..."*

*"Even though I trust my intuition I don't think anyone else will,..."*

*"Even though I'm afraid my client will think I'm not a serious coach if I start going all woo-woo,..."*

*etc*

In my experience as a coaching client, it has always been the intuitive abilities of a coach which have made the difference between an OK coach and a really impactful one. A coach who sticks only to the observable facts may be effective in getting you moving, but it can feel a bit like going through the motions. A coach who is expressing their intuitions with me - even if they are wrong sometimes - is the coach who most effectively makes me feel that I am being truly empathised with and listened to. Intuition is often the ingredient that makes a client feel "They really get me". Holding back on your intuition is holding back on your coaching and therefore your client.

Related sections:

9.2.1     Clearing Fears ⇩


## 7.2.4   Building Rapport

It's probably true to say that without rapport, effective coaching cannot occur. While rapport is important in any inter-personal interaction where someone cares about the outcome (whether it be physical therapy, counselling, business relationships, being on a date or negotiating with the taxman), coaching is perhaps one of the few types of interchange where almost nothing can occur without rapport.

There are many techniques for establishing rapport with clients - including mirroring posture, breathing and language. But there is one factor which underlies all of these - and that is the emotional and attentional state of the coach to start with.

In EFT terms, rapport means aligning and maximising connection between your energy system and that of the client. If you are focused on your client - as you will be at least to some extent if you are talking to them - then there is already a degree of connection of the type that happens spontaneously whenever two people talk to each other. But the degree to which the two energy systems really align and merge is dependent on (a) the level of focus and (b) the degree of distracting energetic activity in one or both parties.

This is a rather complicated way of simply saying that if one of the parties is feeling distracted by an negative emotion they are currently experiencing (worried about getting back to the office on time, upset about the row they had with someone earlier, or even being put off by something about the person such as their dress, manner of speech or content of what they are saying), then the likelihood of rapport with **anyone** they talk to will be reduced.

So, apart from all your existing rapport-building techniques, one of the most effective things you can do as a coach to build rapport with a client, is to bring yourself into a state of minimum emotional distraction. When your energy system is feeling calm and balanced, this creates a kind of "blank slate" which can then easily respond and fall into alignment with whatever emotions or issues are coming from the client. And using EFT to create this balanced state is something you can do before the session even begins. This is as much a self-management skill as it is a coaching skill.

Applying EFT to your current thoughts can help reduce the emotional charge. Even if the issue isn't fully cleared (and it does not need to be), you can reduce it enough that it isn't demanding your attention when the coaching begins.

To use EFT to clear your mind of distractions before a session, first tune into what the dominant thought(s) or subject is and then write it/them down. Next, construct an opening statement based on what you've written and do enough rounds of EFT on each one so that it no longer feels like a big deal and your mind starts naturally thinking about other things. (Losing interest in your issue is one of the best tests there is that EFT has removed the emotional charge from the subject.)

Examples might be:

*"Even though I'm still thinking about the last client, I deeply and completely…"*

*"Even though I'm worried about my child, I deeply…"*

*"Even though I keep thinking about my medical exam next week, I deeply…"*

*"Even though I'm excited about my date tonight, I deeply…"*

*"Even though I'm absorbed in my book project, I deeply…"*

Note that what is distracting you may not be in itself a negative thought (e.g. being excited about something, or being absorbed in a project). And doing EFT won't reduce those positive feelings. But **thinking** about them right now, is a problem for you and that is what we are targeting the EFT at.

After doing the Standard EFT, you can also use a Choices round in order to help set your positive intention for the next session:

*"Even though I'm still thinking about the last client, I choose to let all that go and be totally focussed on my next client."*

*"Even though I'm excited about my date tonight, I choose to fully focus on my client."*

*"Even though I'm totally absorbed in my book project, I choose to fully focus on my client"*

Apart from clearing your head of distractions, you can use EFT to address the issue of rapport more directly. This can be done by applying EFT while you hold an image of the client in your mind. If you have difficulty establishing rapport with a specific client or with all clients, use the Standard form of EFT to deal with any reversal about that:

*"Even though I find it difficult to have rapport with this client, I deeply and completely accept myself."*

*"Even though I find it difficult to have rapport with clients, I deeply and completely accept myself."*

and then use "Rapport" as the reminder phrase.

If you don't perceive building rapport as a particular problem, but simply want to get to a rapport state more quickly, then use a Choices statement such as

*"I choose to establish rapport easily and quickly"*

*"I choose to build rapport"*

*"I choose to have excellent rapport with Jill"*

Pay close attention to any "objections" or worries you have about building rapport that come up while you do this. If anything specific does come up, do EFT on that to reduce it.

I'm going to assume that if you are a coach you have had some level of formal training in rapport skills and that you know in theory and practice what rapport feels like and what techniques you can adopt to induce rapport.

If you have had this kind of training and yet still feel a lack of confidence about being able to build rapport, then I would strongly recommend using EFT to address this issue. Knowing fully and completely that you can and will build rapport in a reliable way with almost any client who comes your way will surely turbocharge not only your coaching sessions (because a client who experiences rapport is going to trust you more quickly and get down to the real stuff more readily), but also improve your ability to present yourself as a coach to prospective clients and get them enrolled.

If you never use EFT with a single client and only use EFT to address your confidence issues around rapport it will be perhaps the single most useful thing you will have done improve your coaching. So we will spend a little time here suggesting how to do this with yourself.

Firstly, think about how you feel about your rapport building skills and notice what thoughts or feelings come up. Do not edit your thoughts or dismiss any of them as trivial or not relevant. It can be the **most** trivial thought about an issue which has the power to totally undermine your confidence and your skills in an area. You are looking not just for emotions (fear, doubt, anxiety), but also your beliefs about rapport.

Here are a few possible examples which may or may not apply to you, but which should give you a feel for the type of issues you should be looking for and writing down.

> *"I'm OK face to face but it's impossible to really have good rapport on the phone"*

> *"I think rapport depends on the client"*

> *"I can only get rapport when I really like the client"*

> *"I know mirroring works but I feel it's manipulative"*

> *"I don't think I should be trying to build rapport - it should just come naturally"*

> *"Only the top coaches can build that type of rapport"*

> *"Rapport is a black art that I don't think I'll ever crack"*

> *"If I use rapport techniques the client's going to notice and find it artificial"*

> *"I can't pay attention to what a client is saying as well as their rapport signals"*

> *"I'm a visual person - I'm no good at doing the voice rapport thing."*

> *etc*

Mark each belief or feeling out of 10, where 10 indicates you feel the feeling strongly or you believe the statement totally. For each item you have listed, do EFT at least 3 times and take a new rating.

Although this could be a time-consuming process consider it an investment in yourself as a coach. Compare it with the amount of time (and money) you would consider worthwhile spending to go on a "Rapport skills for coaches" seminar.

Having worked on your general level of emotional distraction and your fears and beliefs about your rapport skills generally, what do you do if you come across a specific client with whom you find it hard to build rapport? In EFT terms, what this means is that there is an Aspect of your issue with rapport that has not yet been addressed - i.e. something about this particular client which is creating an emotional distraction in you or triggering a belief about your ability to build rapport with someone like this.

To address this problem you need to do EFT on the rapport issue while holding an image of the client in your mind. If there is an Aspect of the client which you know or suspect is making rapport difficult for you (e.g. their gender, their age, their background, their voice), then focus on this Aspect directly. Construct setup statements that reflect these aspects or how you feeling about the client. Examples might be:

> *"Even though I find rapport with men/women much harder, I deeply,..."*

> *"Even though I just can't seem to feel comfortable with this client,..."*

> *"Even though I feel this particular client is difficult,..."*

*"Even though I'm at a loss how to build rapport with this client,..."*

*"Even though I just don't seem to connect with this person,..."*

*"Even though I feel I don't even want to have rapport with this person,..."*

Honesty is required here. Assuming you have reasonable rapport skills with most of your clients, if you meet a client who you just can't create rapport with, it could mean you need to do more work on your rapport, or it could mean this client isn't right for you. Using EFT as suggested here will help you work out which it is.

Related sections:

6.2.6      The Standard EFT Pattern ⇧

6.2.8      The Choices Technique ⇧

6.2.12    Aspects ⇧


## 7.2.5   Modelling Self-acceptance

In the section on "Accepting the Client without Judgement", we noted how important it was that if we are to ask the client to accept themselves, then we as coaches must first accept them. It's also critical however that the coach models **self**-acceptance to the client - that is, the coach accepts herself.

I urge you as a matter of basic self-development to test your own "level of truth" for the statement:

*"I deeply and completely accept myself".*

Say this out loud to yourself and pay close attention to what thoughts or feelings come up in response. Rate how strongly you agree with the statement, 0-10, where 0 means you don't believe it at all, and 10 means you believe it completely.

If you get less than a 5, then you must address this fast - your non-acceptance of yourself will be felt energetically by your clients.

If you got a 6 or 7, you would still benefit from working on this, but your clients probably aren't going to notice anything particularly negative as this is still a reasonably good score for the average person.

If you got an 8 or 9, you are doing pretty well compared to a lot of people - even people with good self-esteem will usually be able to find some aspect of themselves they don't feel totally positive about - but you would still be doing yourself and your clients a favour by rooting out the remaining 1 or 2 points, finding out what they are about, and dealing with them.

If you got a 10, you are either exceptionally well developed as a person, having a very good day, or deluding yourself.

Remember that deep and complete acceptance of yourself is independent of any particular problem or flaw you may be aware of in yourself. Giving yourself a 10 is not contingent on being unable to think of anything about yourself that you'd like to improve. The sort of acceptance we are aiming for here - in yourself and in your client - is **unconditional acceptance**. It's about your fundamental worth as a human being.

I am labouring this point for a reason - and not just because it's important for you to do this work and be able to model self-acceptance for your client. It's important for you to experience directly how it **feels** to go inside yourself and see to what degree you accept yourself, and to understand experientially the distinction between unconditional acceptance and acceptance based on external judgement about how you look, what you do, what you said, how you feel, what you think, and so on.

If you are going to work on self-acceptance issues with clients - and if you work with EFT it is bound to come up pretty frequently because its basic structure invites it - you need to have been there yourself.

When a client says to you *"But how can I accept myself when I can't even manage to do my homework/pay my bills/forgive my father/be a good mother?"*, you need to **know** how that feels and you need to know what their conflict is really about (conditional versus unconditional acceptance).

But even if these questions never come up in client session as an explicit issue, you still need to be able to model your own self-acceptance. Clients want to be assured - explicitly or implicitly - that the person they have hired to be their coach is a little bit further along the road of self-development than they are. And although coaches shouldn't really be "gurus" for their clients, the fact is that clients do look at their coaches lives and make judgements about whether their coach has got their own act together around the issue that they have come to coaching for. Developing self-acceptance in yourself as a coach is core to every other self-development issue your client could possibly bring to you.

Related sections:

6.1.15     Accepting the Client without Judgement ⇧

## 7.2.6   Allowing Silence

If listening is a cornerstone of coaching, then allowing silence to happen is a necessary precursor. If you've asked the client a particularly searching or powerful question, it can take the client time to really search inside for an answer. In fact, silence is a good sign that you are not about to get the client's superficial, pre-rehearsed responses or reasons on a subject, but that new work is being done. The client is thinking about something she hasn't thought about before, or considering it from a new perspective, or making new connections between ideas.

Silence is also required in EFT, and for very similar reasons. After each round of EFT, you will ask the client to say how they feel now about the issue you just tapped on. After each round, the client is required to tune into the issue once again, and notice closely what response that produces in their emotional, mental or physical state. They need to examine their new state of being. They are not the same person they were a minute ago and they cannot depend on things being the same as they were then - they have to look afresh. They can only do this if they are not being distracted by what you're saying or what they are themselves saying.

However, silence is also uncomfortable, at least in normal social interactions with people you don't know well. Add to that the perceived pressure of "being in charge" as a coach, and it can become even harder to simply shut up and let the client's process go on without prompting, rephrasing or even suggesting options.

The need to fill the silence is based on fear. If this is something you find difficult you will know all too well the feeling of rising anxiety that can precede the urge to speak.

If you know this is a problem for you generally, then the usual method applies. List all the thoughts, beliefs or fears you have around silence and use them to construct setup statements. Examples might be:

*"Even though I think I must say something or else the client will think <X>, I deeply..."*

*"Even though silence just makes me feel I've lost control of the coaching,..."*

*"Even though I dislike silence because I just want to get onto the answer,..."*

*"Even though silence feels like the coaching has stopped,..."*

*"Even though I never know how long to allow the silence to continue,..."*

*"Even though I think silence on the phone is a problem because I can't see the client and I don't know what's happening, ..."*

*"Even though I think silence means the client needs help, ..."*

*etc*

As well as or instead of this method, you can use EFT during the session when the silence occurs and as soon as you feel any anxiety about it. Since the client isn't speaking you can easily tap or massage a few of the EFT points without in any way disrupting the client's process or your own attention on what's happening.

Reducing your anxiety "on the spot" like this allows you to focus away from your anxiety and onto the real energy of the silence. What kind of silence is it? Is it thoughtful silence? Or stunned silence? Is it confused or is it peaceful? In the silence, and having released any anxiety about the silence itself, you have the perfect space in which to exercise and listen to any intuitions that may be occurring.

Usually only the most intimate of relationships allow extended silence to occur without causing discomfort to either party. By cultivating the possibility of comfortable silence between yourself and a client, you not only respect the space they need to be in their process without distraction, you also have a most profound way of really "being with" your client. Implicitly you are expressing the level of intimacy which is allowed between you. And assuming that the client is willing, this can help to accelerate the process of entering into the really important issues with you.

## 7.2.7   So much to remember!

One of the challenges of coaching is to be applying multiple skills simultaneously and unconsciously.

For instance, the coach may know she needs to main listening at levels 2 and 3. She also wants to check that rapport is being established, exercise curiosity, maintain non-judgement, hold the client's agenda, hold the coaching space, listen to her intuition...

Phew! To start with it all seems like a lot of stuff to think about.  But it's actually worse than that. To do all these things effectively, you need to **not** think about them, but simply **do** them - because if you are focused on how you're doing and running through a checklist of all the above skills, then you are already failing to do several of these things.

Of course the usual way to learn a multi-faceted skill is lots and lots of practice. Practice allows you to perform skills unconsciously so that your conscious attention can be put to some other use - like adding in the next skill, or preferably just being totally focused on the client.

There are many examples of EFT successfully aiding and accelerating motor-skill and mental-skill acquisition - from sports performance, learning to drive (a classic multi-faceted skill), learning a new musical instrument, studying for exams and many, many more. We can combine this with visualisation, an established coaching technique for mentally rehearsing a skill before actually putting it into action.

So here is how you could use EFT-assisted visualisation to help you acquire and combine multiple coaching skills much more quickly.

**Step 1:** Apply EFT - at least 3 rounds - to each individual coaching skill that you want to improve. Use either the Standard pattern or the Non-Judgement pattern depending on how you feel about each one. For instance:

*"Even though I have trouble trusting my intuition, ..."*

*"I want to stay at Level 2 and Level 3 listening, ..."*

*"Even though maintaining non-judgement is often hard for me,..."*

**Step 2:** Apply EFT to your ability to perform all skills simultaneously covering as many aspects of why this is a problem for you, as you can.

*"Even though this is too much to remember,..."*

*"Even though I think I'll never manage all of it,..."*

*"Even though I can't imagine being able to do all this unconsciously,..."*

*"Even though I think you have to have years of practice before you can do all this,..."*

**Step 3:** Build up a visualisation for yourself, including sounds and feelings as you wish, which somehow contains all the skills you want to learn. Start with one skill and visualise yourself performing it excellently, while tapping 3 full rounds. Add in one skill at a time, doing 3 rounds of EFT for each one. It's important that the basic scene does not change or flip from one perspective to another. You are creating a single scene that when you bring it to mind will encapsulate **all** the skills you want to perform simultaneously. Add in each skill one by one until all the skills you want are somehow represented in the scene.

**Step 4:** At the beginning of each coaching session or practice session, bring the whole scene to mind. If it's not crystal clear, tap to bring it into the level of focus and clarity that feels solid to you. Even if you happen to focus on one particular skill in the image, you know and your unconscious knows that all the other skills are there too. By focusing on any one, you implicitly trigger all of them.

This technique can be used with clients too.

If you are thinking "But that could take hours!" compare the time with what you would be willing to spend at a "Skill improvement for coaches" seminar. (I made the same point above regarding rapport enhancement). Just as EFT can become a self-empowerment tool for your clients, it can become one for you too.

Related sections:

6.2.6      The Standard EFT Pattern ⇧

6.1.20     Level 1, Level 2 and Level 3 Listening ⇧

7.2.4      Building Rapport ⇧

8.1.18     Visualisations ⇩

8.2.11     The Non-Judgement Pattern ⇩

## 7.2.8   Key Points

- The central assumption of EFT - that all negative emotions are a disruption of the energy system - allows the EFT Coach to view clients (and people in general) in a much less judgemental way. This viewpoint invites detachment from the particular behaviour of the person and encourages compassion for the underlying person whose energy system has been disrupted.

- The questions that an EFT practitioner needs to ask in order to conduct a thorough EFT session are highly curious questions. Adding EFT to your coaching toolbox therefore augments the level of curiosity about what makes your client tick and the exact nature of their experience.

- You can use EFT to improve your own intuition as a coach and to reduce your fears around voicing your intuitions in the service of the client. Much of what we experience as intuition is in fact allowing unconscious memories to come into play in our conscious minds. So the ability of EFT to bring unconscious memories to the surface can be used to enhance this natural process.

- It's probably true to say that without rapport, effective coaching cannot occur. In EFT terms, rapport means aligning and maximising connection between your energy system and that of the client. You can use EFT to assist rapport in two ways. Firstly, by minimising your own emotional distractions before a session so you can fully focus on the client. Secondly, by applying EFT to any doubts or difficulties you have around specific aspects of establishing rapport.

- It's vitally important to be able to model self-acceptance for your clients, even if it doesn't come up as an explicit issue in client sessions. You are encouraged to test the degree to which you agree with the statement *"I deeply and completely accept myself"* and if it is less than a 9, to address it as a matter or urgency.

- Allowing silence within coaching and within EFT-assisted coaching is important - because clients need to space to go inside themselves and assess who they are now following a round of EFT (or even a powerful coaching exercise or question). You can deal with any fear or anxiety around allowing silence using EFT.

- There is significant evidence that EFT can accelerate learning for new skills (e.g. driving, playing musical instruments and learning new academic subjects). You can help accelerate and integrate the learning and practice of multiple coaching skills using a combination of visualisation and EFT.

# 8 EFT for the Client

This chapter covers the use of EFT to assist or augment your existing coaching tools and techniques that you use with a client. In some cases, EFT offers completely new tools.

This chapter is primarily a "how to" guide. It assumes familiarity with all the coaching and EFT fundamentals and principles presented above and moves onto the specifics of different ways to use EFT within the coaching process.

This chapter is split between ways to use EFT to assist or enhance tools and techniques that are already used by conventional coaches; and new uses for EFT in a coaching context.

## 8.1 Enhancements to Existing Coaching Techniques

This section covers tools which are already used within coaching and shows how EFT can be used to enhance them.

If you are a coach thinking about how to add EFT to your toolset, this section should make sense to you. But if you are an EFT practitioner thinking about moving into coaching, then you may be wondering whether you need to learn these coaching techniques or whether you can simply start work identifying blocks, beliefs and goals and start tapping.

Choosing a specific coaching technique to address a client issue with EFT is simply a way in to the client's mental and emotional world. They are ways to begin a dialogue with the client, providing a kind of larger structure of narrative and often helping to define when the session is complete, since coaching exercises all have a defining outcome which can be worked towards. Having a coaching exercise to structure the use of EFT, very usefully defines the boundaries of which issues are relevant to delve into. This avoids the problem that can occur in "straight" EFT sessions where it's possible to be led down a very interesting but frighteningly infinite set of interconnecting issues. Using EFT within a structured coaching exercise helps to avoid this problem, and allows both coach and client to achieve resolution within a session.

### 8.1.1 Resourceful States

EFT can be used, like NLP, within a coaching context to access, anchor and consciously trigger resourceful states within the client.

This is achieved by a combination of "straight" EFT to remove negative states, and the Choices method, which installs or anchors positive options.

Resourceful states are states of mind which allow a client to make positive progress. Resourceful states may be very general, such as "feeling positive", "feeling happy" of "feeling relaxed". Or they can be very specific, referring to specific tasks or previous experiences, for example "having my writing head on", or "that graduation feeling of I can't fail".

There are at least two ways to use EFT to access resourceful states:

## 8.1.1.1    Creating Resourceful States

If there is no previous experience to refer to, it is necessary to create the desired resourceful state from scratch, perhaps using bits and pieces of knowledge about the client's values.

The first step is to get the client to tune in to what a resourceful state would look like, if they could achieve it. This step may involve reference to a role model who seems to exhibit the desired state, or to the client's own Future Self. Or it could be elicited using the "Who Do You Need to Be?" tool. The client probably won't be feeling the state yet - but they can start to describe it in terms of what it would empower them to do and what sort of action they would expect someone in that state to carry out.

The second step involves accessing how it feels to be in the state - and this is usually the hard part, depending a great deal on the client's ability to "sentise" the state and/or the coach's ability to guide them to do so. With a client who finds connecting with their own bodily sensation difficult or unusual, this step tends to stop short at being an intellectual exercise. Even though a purely intellectual imagination or visualisation of the new state will have some positive effect, we know as coaches and as EFT practitioners that there is really no substitute for really connecting with how the state feels.

It is therefore at this step that EFT can be useful. At the same time that the client is imagining and visualising the actions they would carry out in their new resourceful state, ask the client to tap. This allows any negative feelings connected with the action to be released and allowed to move within the body. It also, of course, helps to dispel any resistance to the new state, any worries or doubts about it, and even any doubts about the wider process they are undergoing.

As well as general tapping, EFT can be used to address any specific Tailenders that the client has around getting into state. For instance:

>  *"Even though I'm not really feeling this state very much,..."*

>  *"Even though I can't stay in this state for very long,..."*

>  *"Even though I think I should be feeling different,..."*

>  *"Even though I'm not convinced this is going to work,..."*

The feeling of being in the resourceful state may be freely augmented by including any other images, sounds, words, movements which the client associates with the state or which help the client inhabit the state.

Related sections:

6.2.15      Tailenders ⇧

8.1.14      Who Do You Need To Be? ⇩

8.1.16      Accessing the Future Self ⇩

## 8.1.1.2    Retrieving and Cleansing Resourceful States

Getting clients to access Peak Experiences from their own past is a classic coaching technique for getting clients to tune back into times when their values were being expressed, they felt fulfilled or otherwise had the energy and resources to achieve what they wanted. These Peak Experiences provide useful reference points for the coach.

Any time the client is feeling unresourceful about a goal, the coach can refer back to the state the client was in during the Peak Experience, and ask the client to view the current situation from the viewpoint of how they felt during the Peak Experience.

But when a Peak Experience is a long way back in the client's past, the memory of it can become overlaid with negative memories, beliefs or feelings. For example, suppose a client's Peak Experience involves how they felt when they got their degree at age 21.

Even though they regard this as a Peak Experience, the feelings that are brought up when they think about it, may not produce anything like a Peak Experience feeling right now. The memory of that achievement may trigger other less positive memories or feelings such as;

*"Yeah, but that was 15 years ago - and what have I achieved since then?"*

*"Yes, but later I realised that it wasn't even my goal and I'd wasted those 3 years when I really should have done something else"*

*"I remember straight after that happened my grandmother died."*

These "Tailenders" to the Peak Experience can be dealt with using EFT. By cleaning up the Tailenders, this increases the power of that memory to produce only positive and resourceful feelings.

If the Tailenders are hard to identify, or too many, or would take too much time to work through (and this would be a matter of judgement by the coach and the client), EFT can still be helpful in "cleansing" the memory by simply focussing on the memory directly and tapping - possibly using SLOW EFT. Cleansing a Peak Experience can make excellent homework for the client - and is likely to be pleasant work too - since it involves focussing on something which the client has already identified as one of their most positive memories.

Related sections:

6.2.9      SLOW EFT ⇧

6.2.15    Tailenders ⇧

8.1.12    Peak Experiences ⇩

### 8.1.1.3   Anchoring Resourceful States

Once a resourceful state has been created or cleansed, it is ready for use. The object is not only for the client to experience the resourceful state in a session with you, but to be able to remember and bring it into play when it is needed after the session and in response to a specific situation.

For example, you might work with a client on the resourceful state called "The confidence to speak up for myself".

For this state to be an effective resource for the client, he needs to be able to enter the state at specific times, such as when talking to his boss, negotiating with a partner or making family arrangements. (Usually, the application will be already known and may have been what triggered the resource work in the first place.)

In NLP terms this requires the state to be "anchored", so that it is triggered automatically in the required situation. NLP has its own particular methods for creating these anchors, but it is possible to do it using EFT also.

The basic structure of an EFT or Choices setup statement, effectively anchors the first part of the setup (*"Even though I have this problem"*) to the second part of the setup (*"I deeply and completely accept myself"* or *"I choose...."*).

The anchoring works partly by repetition (just like learning a song or a nursery rhyme - hearing the first half of a line immediately brings to mind the second part), and partly due to the physical tapping. Tapping while repeating a particular phrase makes the phrase a physical event. Recalling the phrase then involves the body recalling, and recreating the physiological state associated with it.

So here's what needs to happen to make anchoring with EFT work:

**Step 1:** Create or retrieve the resourceful state and connect to it using EFT - by getting rid of anything that's preventing the client experiencing that state (see above). Give the state an explicit and appropriate label, such as "Speaking up with confidence".

**Step 2:** While still in the resourceful state, repeat an appropriate Choices statement. The first part states the situation the client wants to deal with using the resourceful state (*"Even though I'm talking to my boss..."*). The second part says what resourceful state the client wants to be triggered in that situation (*"...I choose to speak up with confidence."*). The Choice needs to explicitly use the label for the state that was chosen earlier. The subconscious mind is very literal and will regard, for instance, "feeling confident" as a different thing to "speaking up with confidence".

**Step 3:** Repeat the Choices statement and do a full round of EFT several times (at least three). Set the repetition of the Choices statement as homework for the client to do once or more a day for several days. Pat Carrington recommends writing the statement down - or having the client write it down - on a piece of card and keeping it by the client's bed or in the client's wallet so that it will be seen frequently. The repetition is an important part of the anchoring process.

You can test whether the anchoring has occurred by asking the client to visualise or recall the relevant situation (e.g. speaking to the boss) and seeing what reactions occur.

However, as with all EFT, you and the client do not know whether the anchoring has worked until the client has to deal with the situation in real life. An ongoing coaching relationship allows the client to test the anchoring back in real life (either it happens spontaneously or it may be deliberately engineered as a homework exercise) and for any tweaks to be made.

Related sections:

6.2.8        The Choices Technique ⇧


## 8.1.1.4   Negative Emotions as Resources

When a client has developed a particular emotional response as a normal way of dealing with things, this emotional response can end up looking like it is the client's resourceful state for dealing with the situation. For example:

- When a client habitually responds to perceived injustice with anger prior to setting to and seeking justice.

- When a client habitually responds to work deadlines with stress.

In these cases, the client might want to be coached on finding alternative responses to these triggers. EFT would of course be a perfect tool for taking down the negative emotion around a typical trigger situation (an injustice or a work deadline).

I have experienced multiple clients who - perhaps when their anger or stress has dropped to a manageable level (say a 2) - feel they **need** their negative emotion in order to act successfully in the situation. Such clients will quite simply tell you that they don't **want** the remaining anger or stress taken away thank you very much.

In other words, the client has formed an energetic relation to the anger or the stress - it is no longer simply an emotion. It has become strongly linked to the client's resources of "dealing with injustice" or "meeting deadlines". To remove the emotional response altogether feels like a threat to the ability of the client to access these resources and to cope at all.

When this happens, we are firmly in the realm of coaching - finding new ways for the client to be and looking for new strategies for the client to try.

Using a "Who Do You Need to Be" approach is one way of working with the client to come up with a new solution or response to the problematic situation. You could also use the Perspective technique, simple Idea Generation, asking the Future Self or even a homework Inquiry. Once the client has chosen an alternative "way of being" as a response, you can then use the techniques above to connect the client with the state, and to anchor it firmly as the new response.

With the new response firmly anchored, the client can now fully release the negative emotion previously being used as a resource. You may even find that it has released anyway.

Related sections:

| | | |
|---|---|---|
| 8.1.2.3 | Inquiries and Insights ⇩ | |
| 8.1.3 | Perspectives ⇩ | |
| 8.1.10 | Idea Generation ⇩ | |
| 8.1.14 | Who Do You Need to Be? ⇩ | |
| 8.1.16 | Accessing the Future Self ⇩ | |

## 8.1.2   Homework

Since EFT was originally designed to be an easy-to-learn self-help technique, it is highly suitable as a homework exercise. The applications for use as homework are as infinite as the applications of EFT itself - but here are a few specific applications for you to adapt.

Related sections:

| | |
|---|---|
| 6.1.19 | Most Coaching Happens Between Sessions ⇧ |

### 8.1.2.1   Pure EFT

EFT can be a good form of homework, especially for an issue which seems to need persistent application. This would apply to any issue where there seems to be a strong emotional block to the issue clearing and it is desirable to "loosen" the resistance over time, or where the issue involves an ongoing aspect of the client's life.

As with all homework, setting EFT as homework must be done with full client agreement. The client can accept, reject or make a counter-offer. Remember it is always the client's choice how they choose to move through their issues or blocks and if they decide to "be with" their issue a while longer, think about it or simply try something else, that should be respected.

If it is used as homework, it is useful to be very specific. For instance, rather than say "Do some EFT on this issue", agree with the client exactly:

- What setup statement(s) to use (they can change this of course, but they must have a default to work with).

- The frequency and timing of the EFT sequence(s) - so they know when they have done it or not. For example - 3 rounds in the morning and 3 rounds in the evening for 3 days in a row. (Part of coaching is getting clients used to setting and definitively achieving goals - so they get used to the feeling that occurs with achievement).

- Any particular circumstances which should trigger use of EFT (e.g. just before or just after particular relevant circumstances).

- Any particular action required to accompany the EFT - for example writing down any aspects or other insights that occur during the EFT, tracking intensity ratings, noticing any differences in feeling or behaviour afterwards, and so on, as appropriate to the application. Whether this type of additional noticing and recording is appropriate is down to the judgement of the coach: for some applications you simply want the client to benefit from the effects of doing the EFT; for other applications it is also useful to develop the client's ability to tune into and notice their own feelings and behaviour.

This specificity should also be constructed in agreement with the client so that they are clear about why the chosen wording, frequency and timing have been selected - and again they have the option to accept, reject or make a counter-offer with respect to all these aspects, to ensure that the homework is achievable within their life circumstances.

You need to exercise caution and judgement as an EFT Coach regarding how much EFT to set as homework.

Some clients (often the perfectionists) will try to be extra ambitious about how many times they intend to do EFT and what issues they will do it on. It's tempting for clients who are keen and who see how fast EFT can work, to think that they can whizz through whole chunks of their emotional landscape in an evening, not realising the proliferation of Aspects that can occur if specific and bounded issues are not defined and adhered to. While you don't want to curb the enthusiasm of clients like these, neither do you want to set them up for "failure" by setting excessive homework. It's a good idea in these cases to agree a minimum amount, and then allow the client free reign to do additional homework and to report that if they wish.

Ultimately, a client who successfully manages to clear just one small and highly specific issue on their own, is going to build up trust in EFT and in the coaching generally, much more quickly than a client who is ambitious, ends up getting lost in the process of trying to do too much at one time and concludes that EFT is difficult or doesn't work.

Related sections:

6.2.12     Aspects ⇧


## 8.1.2.2   EFT as Homework Support

As well as being homework in its own right, EFT can also be set as a support for other homework.

For instance, a client may have homework to make certain phone calls to people who can help them in a project, beginning a class in a new activity or getting down to work on a creative project they have been putting off for some time.

In these cases, where there is a suspected fear or block around the issue, the previous session will have looked at those blocks, worked through them (with or without EFT) and got the client to the point that they want to take action. Hopefully, the work within the session will have been sufficient to clear the block or resistance and the client will be ready, if not eager, to take action.

However, this won't always be the case - some hesitancy may still remain. Or the client may feel confident while in the session but then express doubts about whether they can carry this forward into the real situation. This is common and coaches vary in their approach to this. Some coaches simply leave the client to carry out the homework, trusting that if they are committed to doing it they will benefit from the experience of realising they can act despite their doubts. Indeed this can be a useful learning experience for clients - it certainly empowers them and emphasises that it is they, and not their coach, who is responsible for their progress. Other coaches might give the client some type of support structure to take with them - whether it is a "Structure" of some kind, or a keyword to trigger the resourceful state they experienced in the coaching session.

EFT can be used as just such a structure. A round or two just before taking the action, or afterwards can be enough to reassure or take away any nerves that may be present. In this context, even **not** doing EFT - but simply knowing they could - can be enough to give the client courage. For me, this is where the self-empowerment qualities of EFT marry up completely with the self-responsibility emphasis of coaching.

Related sections:

5.4.6      Principle of Client Responsibility ⇑

8.1.5      Structures ⇓


### 8.1.2.3   Inquiries and Insights

*"And to help clients stick with the question, there may be action attached to the Inquiry. …The key is to look at the Inquiry in a new way each time and to keep engaging it every day…for fresh perspectives."* [2]

Inquiries are questions where the answer may not be immediately clear and will typically take some time for the client to develop an answer. Inquiries are designed to expand the client's consciousness about an issue or about themselves. They depend for their success on clients taking the Inquiry with them into their life following the coaching session, and having the client achieve some insight into their condition as they go about their daily life.

Examples of Inquiries might be:

*"What has X cost you?"*

*"Who do you become when you are doing Y?"*

*"Where are you honouring your value of Z and where aren't you?"*

*"What would honouring your value of Z mean?"*

EFT (or SLOW EFT) can be a very helpful support to an Inquiry. Focusing on (repeating) the Inquiry, while tapping, can lead to an opening up of creativity and ideas around the issue. In this application it is useful to give the client two additional meridian points to work with: the third eye (in the middle of the forehead) and the crown of the head. These points are especially useful for alertness, creativity and insight.

Adding EFT to Inquiry homework is also very helpful in making what can be a rather nebulous and open-ended piece of homework, into something much more tangible. The danger with Inquiry homework is that the client doesn't think about it at all between the end of the session and the start of the next one. (And if the coach happens to forget the homework it may end up never being mentioned again). By including set times and frequency for doing EFT while focussing on the Inquiry, you make the homework more tangible for the client - **and** you also much increase the chances of actually getting the positive insights you were hoping for.

The tangibility of the homework can be strengthened further by asking the client to write down what thoughts or images arise - especially if SLOW EFT is used. These can be sent to the coach as evidence of the homework (if that seems appropriate and the client agrees). As well as frequently triggering excellent insights for the client at the time, the contents of the session can provide extremely useful material for the next coaching session.

One of the benefits of asking the client to write down what thoughts or images occur while tapping on the Inquiry, is that this releases the client from necessarily having to find "the answer" to the Inquiry. They may have thoughts or images which don't seem to connect to the Inquiry at all. By recording them and bringing them to the next coaching session, these thoughts can become material for the coaching and may reveal their relevance later on while talking to the coach.

It's possible that you are thinking: *"But I don't want my client to just spend 10 minutes a day doing EFT on this Inquiry in isolation to his real life - I want him to notice things in his real life that are relevant".*

Even though the Inquiry/EFT homework is done "in isolation", it is usual for the relevance to the client's real life to come through quite clearly in the images and thoughts that are provoked. And because the client **isn't** actually in his real life right then, there is actually a much greater chance of actually noticing it, writing it down and starting the process of thinking about what it means, finding a solution, or whatever is relevant.

But if you would like your client to be still working on the Inquiry in his real life as well, this can be requested as part of the homework - and it can be enhanced by using the Choices pattern:

> *"Even though I don't have the answer to this Inquiry, I choose to notice anything that happens over the next week that is relevant.".*

As well as helping the make the activity of the homework more tangible, using EFT as a support allows the client to detach from the question and the answers.

> *"The inquiry... is not an easy place for most clients to go. It's often challenging enough just to wrestle with the hard questions when they are on a coaching call with you - let alone keep wrestling when they are alone. But part of their becoming more resourceful includes learning to spend time with challenging questions."* [2]

Indeed, may clients find inquiries so challenging that they don't really know **how** to spend time with it - and therefore avoid it altogether or come up with a superficial response to it 5 minutes before the next session, just to have something to say.

By asking them to use EFT and simply note what answers, thoughts, images, feelings occur along the way, the client is released from feeling the need to "generate" answers. In so doing, the client learns that considering such questions need not be a fearful or difficult thing. Simply cultivating the ability of the client to ask and spend time with Inquiry type questions without fear, is in itself a huge step forward in self-development.

By the way it's very important that the client is actually interested in the Inquiry. All too often a coach gets to the end of a session, thinks about what homework to give and comes up with an Inquiry on the spur of the moment. Or the coaching reaches a certain place where the coach is champing at the bit to get the client to realise something about themselves, but like good coaches they hold back from imposing their agenda onto the client and instead come up with an Inquiry which they hope will lead to the answer they think the client is just a moment away from getting. It's important to check in with the client by saying *"Is this something you'd like to know the answer to?".* Again, it's about client avidity[4] and client co-activity. In an EFT/Inquiry situation, ensuring buy-in from the client is even more important:

Suppose you are working with a client on how they repeatedly sell themselves short with regard to their coaching goals. Let's assume that you know, based on what the client has said in many sessions, that the issue of self-worth is a major one for them.

You might then give them an Inquiry that asks: *"Where does your self-worth let you down in your life?"*

Now this looks like a perfectly well-formed Inquiry - it's open ended, demands the clients to notice different times and places where self-worth issues have let her down. And it **might** be a suitable Inquiry for this client.

But, what if the self-worth issue is so big for this client that even the thought of thinking hard about it brings up resistance? If it produces extreme anxiety, it's possible that the client won't spend **any** time on it, for fear of what might be unearthed.

Now, before you object: *"But the client is Creative, Resourceful and Whole! She can take it!"*, this isn't about whether a client can "take" the anxiety of dealing with a particular question. Of course she is and of course she can. The question is rather, **will** she spend time with it, or will she avoid it?

By checking in with the client you avoid having to make the judgement yourself. The client can respond to all homework suggestions, including Inquiries, with a Yes, a No, or with a counter-offer.

If you sense sufficient anxiety to the question and are receiving less than full commitment from your client, then you can use a classic EFT technique, which is to backtrack one step and address the anxiety of working on the problem before you work on the problem directly.

In this case you could reform the Inquiry as follows:

*"In what ways do you avoid really looking at the issue of self-worth?"*

*"In what ways do other people demonstrate their own self-worth or lack of it?"*

*"Who in your past modelled self-worth for you? And who didn't?"*

All of these examples allow the client to start looking at the issue of self-worth but from a dissociated viewpoint (Watching myself not deal with it, Watching other people do it, Remembering other people who did or didn't do it).

By offering these alternatives, you are offering the client safety, rather than being face-to-face with one of her most difficult issues for a whole week. More importantly, you get her buy in because one of them is likely to be a question she's genuinely interested in knowing the answer to. And because of both these things, she is likely to actually spend time on it. And if she is doing SLOW EFT in her chosen Inquiry regularly for a week, there **will** be progress either in the form of insights or in the actual improvement in her self-worth.

Related sections:

| | | |
|---|---|---|
| 6.1.1 | The Client is Creative, Resourceful and Whole ⇧ | |
| 6.1.4 | The Designed Alliance ⇧ | |
| 6.2.9 | SLOW EFT ⇧ | |

### 8.1.2.4   Mirror Tapping

Mirror tapping involves getting the client to look at themselves in a mirror, maintaining eye contact with themselves while they tap.

This is an especially good homework exercise for any issue involving self-acceptance, self-worth, identity or relationship with self, and would therefore be valuable in any Being-dominated coaching application such as Self-esteem coaching, Consciousness or Spiritual coaching.

Eye contact is well documented as a way of enhancing relationships between people. Holding eye contact with someone indicates acknowledgement or acceptance of the other; avoiding eye contact signals exclusion or non-availability for contact. The emotional response to eye contact is hard-wired and goes back millions of years in terms of evolutionary significance. Evolutionarily speaking, the brain has no way of distinguishing between what it feels when it has eye contact with another person and what it feels when it has eye contact with a mirror image of itself. Many personal or spiritual development programs include mirror exercises for just this reason..

But by tapping at the same time as looking in a mirror, the client will be not only releasing around the stated issue being tapped on, but also on any negative feelings or thoughts triggered by the act of looking at oneself.

A huge range of issues can be helped to release using mirror tapping, including appearance, ageing, guilt, or dislike of oneself for any reason.

The mirror technique is especially helpful if the client has basic self-acceptance issues, to the degree that they find it uncomfortable or even impossible to say the self-acceptance statement: *"I deeply and completely accept myself"*.

Where this occurs, the acceptance phrase can be freely adapted to use words that cause the client less problem, such as "I'm a good person", "I'm OK" and so on.

In a "therapy" situation one can be content for the client to use whatever acceptance phrase that results in the desired drop of intensity for the issue at hand - and it may be that the client leaves the session free of their fear of flying but still with their problem about self-acceptance intact. But in a coaching context, the coach is likely to be far more concerned about addressing the self-acceptance issue directly, since so much else derives from it in terms of values, beliefs, Life Purpose and working towards fulfilling goals.

Many coaching sessions could easily be spent on the issue of self-acceptance alone - the reasons for it, what the client thinks will make them feel more self-accepting, whether it's right or even desirable to achieve self-acceptance (you would be astonished at the number of completely logical and value-driven reasons that clients will find to justify why they shouldn't have self-acceptance as a goal!). Using mirror tapping bypasses all these conscious objections to the subject and allows the barriers to be released at an ecological rate, over time and under the complete control of the client. There are many variations on mirror tapping for the purposes of building self-acceptance.

Perhaps the simplest is to use no setup statement at all - simply holding eye contact while tapping through the normal EFT sequence. This variation avoids the client having to say he accepts himself in any form.

If the client has a problem looking in the mirror at himself, a second variation is to use a setup statement that addresses this reluctance directly:

> *"Even though I don't like looking at myself in the mirror,…"*

If the reluctance is extreme, to the point that the thought of it brings up distress, then do pre-work prior to working in front of the mirror. Find out what the client **is** comfortable doing and start there - perhaps standing in front of the mirror but not looking into it, perhaps looking in the mirror but looking at his own forehead rather than the eyes, or perhaps imagining himself looking in a mirror.

If the client's issue is around saying "I accept myself", then use a variation which addresses this. Obviously this requires creativity and co-active work with the client to come up with an acceptance phrase which is acceptable! Use whatever world view or self-view the client already has that can be drawn upon as a model for acceptance or which allows acceptance to be built up over time. Some possibilities might be:

> *"Even though I don't accept myself, I would like to accept myself."*

> *"Even though I don't accept myself, I choose to accept myself more and more."*

> *"Even though I don't accept myself generally, I accept myself right now for doing this."*

> *"Even though I don't accept myself, I know I am a well-meaning person."*

> *"Even though I can't imagine myself accepting myself, I'm open to finding reasons to accept myself."*

*"Even though I don't accept myself, I know God/Jesus loves me unconditionally."*

*"Even though I don't accept myself, my friends/family/partner/children seem to accept me."*

Related sections:

6.2.7      The Self-Acceptance Statement ⇧
10.4       Consciousness and Essence Coaching ⇩
10.14      Self-esteem Coaching ⇩
10.15      Spiritual Coaching ⇩

## 8.1.3   Perspectives

*"The hard part [is] finding new ways of looking at the world. The strain [is] actually inhabiting those different perspectives and getting inside the possibilities."* [2]

Perspectives is a particularly powerful conventional coaching technique which can create powerful shifts in client viewpoint and therefore the possibilities for action around an issue. Essentially it's a "way of being" technique. That is, it takes an issue or event which, in itself isn't going to change, or which the client wouldn't even want to change (e.g. "looking after my child", or "getting married next month", or "getting this project finished on time") but which is causing some sort of stress or problem. When the facts of the situation cannot be changed (or would not be changed even if the client had the choice), the only way to alter the client's experience of the situation is to alter the client's perspective on it. It is a very practical exercise in the client creating their own reality.

The Perspectives technique involves first generating ideas for alternative perspectives for an issue, starting with the client's existing perspective and then being as wild and creative as possible (e.g. what would the complete opposite of your current perspective look like? what perspective would John Wayne have on this issue? etc).

Once several perspectives have been generated (typically at least six), the client gets to "inhabit" each perspective to see how it "fits", how it feels and whether it "works" as a solution to the original problem. Finally, the client is guided to choose or synthesise the perspective that seems to fit best with his goals, values and general feeling.

But often the process of choosing a preferred perspective - or synthesising a new one out of features of different perspectives, can prove harder. It requires the client to "try on" each perspective and see how it really feels to think about his problem from that perspective: What feels good about being here? What feels bad? What's here that you didn't expect to be here? What actions are possible here that weren't before? This starts the process of the client noticing elements he wants and elements he doesn't want in the final solution.

But fully "inhabiting" perspectives that were generated a moment ago, can be hard work for clients (especially if one of them involves being Sylvester Stallone's leopard, for example).

And since the process of inhabiting is crucial for properly assessing the merits and demerits of each one, choosing one and then taking action based on it, anything that can make that process of inhabiting easier and more vivid is going to increase the quality of the final solution.

There are conventional coaching methods for helping clients to do this - such as getting them to stand or sit in different places or positions or asking them what they might choose to wear in each one, in order to create differentiation between alternative perspectives. In a face to face coaching session, the coach might even provide props, toys and other objects which the client can select to represent different perspectives and hold them or wear them to help take on the perspective more vividly. As with all types of visualisation, EFT can assist the process of inhabiting the perspective vividly.

But what's really important - and often difficult - is choosing one of the perspectives to adopt as the basis for a solution. If you have done a good job of creating several solutions, most of which have some attractive features for the client, choosing between them can be a hard job.

And here's where EFT can help. For each candidate perspective, ask the client to tap while they inhabit it until the good and bad aspects of it become very clear to them. You are asking a general question for each alternative:

> "How right does this perspective feel?"

Getting a 0-10 rating helps you to rank each perspective and see which one looks most promising.

If you don't get a clear winner doing this, (i.e. there is more than one perspective with equally high scores, or there are no really high scores, just lots of middling ones) then you and the client will need to create a new perspective out of elements the client liked in the candidate ones. At this stage in the process the client is usually fairly expanded in terms of coming up with new ideas and perspectives - so simply asking him to create a new perspective which contains specific elements may well be all that's needed for him to come up with one.

If it doesn't come easily, EFT can be used once again. Ask the client to create a blank canvas (or empty room or similar metaphor for "starting over"). Then ask him to put all the good elements identified previously (you need to list them one by one for the client) into the picture somehow. Make sure the client can clearly see (or hear or feel) the presence of each element. Now ask them to put a perspective around that - perhaps by inventing a story that involves all the elements, perhaps by choosing some clothing, some music or an animal that somehow sums up all those elements for them.

The purpose of this is to seek synthesis. If all these elements, or at least most of them, need to be part of the solution that's going to really work for this client, there needs to be some sort of connecting idea, principle or feeling that ties them all together. If one does not appear fairly quickly, ask them to tap while they focus again on the set of elements, perhaps mentioning each element as each point is tapped.

Having found a perspective which the client feels is good, the exercise can be consolidated with a Choices round. Supposing the perspective that the client chose was called "The Tiger perspective" (all perspectives need to be given titles as they are generated). Having discussed the perspective using this title, considered its good and bad points, inhabited it and so on, by now the words "Tiger perspective" is highly imbued with a raft of images and meanings and can now be used as a trigger word in a Choices statement.

The format links the original problem that the Perspective technique was aimed at, and the chosen Perspective.

> "Even though <original problem>, I choose the Tiger perspective"

or

> "Even though <original problem>, I choose to be the Tiger"

It's useful to select the words according to the title of the perspective to make the choice as powerful, positive and active as possible. As well as doing a Choices round a couple of times in the session, it's a good idea to set it as homework to ensure the choice of perspective is firmly embedded.

The final stage of the Perspectives technique is to take the chosen perspective into action with regard to the problem - and that involves making commitments. But the more strongly the chosen perspective has been inhabited and then embedded as a "resource", the more strongly the client can work from that perspective while carrying out any commitments or actions required.

Related sections:

## 8.1.4   The Compelling Way

*"This image of what we are drawn to do has the power to overcome the bonds of lethargy and fear."* [2]

"The Compelling Way" is a powerful coaching technique based on firm NLP principles. It involves creating as vivid and "compelling" a scene as possible of the client's goal - complete with as much sense details (sights, sounds, smells, feelings) as possible. The idea is not only to make the scene as desirable as possible so that the client feels drawn towards it, but to make it seem so real that it is almost as though the client has already achieved it. This creates and strengthens new neural pathways in the client's brain, which then assists the creation of the scene in external reality.

I have seen "straight" Compelling Way coaching achieve remarkable shifts in clients, resulting in significant and tangible acceleration in goal achievement. But sometimes, the process of compelling scene creation isn't so easy. Sometimes the client has difficulty really creating a vivid, fully sensory scene. And sometimes the client experiences a series of cognitive objections to the scene. These objections are the client's "Tailenders" for the goal in question, and can include all the reasons why she thinks she can't do it, all the fear she has about what might happen if she does do it, and so on. These, of course, are all blocks (in coaching terms) or Reversals (in EFT terms).

Of course we know we can use EFT to address any blocks which are found directly. But we can also use EFT directly on the scene creation task, without necessarily mentioning any of the blocks which are making things difficult. This involves using EFT in exactly the same way as for any other type of Visualisation task e.g.

*"Even though I can't seem to see myself in this scene..."*

*"Even though I can't seem to feel what this would feel like..."*

*"Even though it seems blurry and far away...."*

It is absolutely fine to switch between tapping for trying to get the image bigger or brighter, and tapping on the client's realisations about the task itself (e.g. that if she achieves this goal then she will be the centre of attention for a while, which she doesn't like the idea of), and then switch back to working on other aspects of the scene. Whatever comes up as the "problem" at a particular instant is the problem that needs to be worked on.

Related sections:

## 8.1.5   Structures

A "Structure" is an external object or physical action designed to reinforce learning, and remind clients of either an intention to action or a new "way of being" that was experienced within the coaching. For instance, a very basic Structure might be a post-it note to remind them to do something every day. But it's possible and desirable for chosen Structure to be much more creative. Spending time choosing a Structure that is effective, creative and fun, further reinforces the client's intention to act. However, being creative also makes it more likely that it will stand out and be noticed by the client (one more post-it note amongst several might not get much attention after a day or two).

In this section I present two ways that EFT can support the use of Structures: by accompanying the use of a physical Structure, and by using EFT itself as a Structure. Thirdly I present different ideas for applying EFT as a Structure depending on the type of issue involved.

### 8.1.5.1   Augmenting Physical Structures

A "Physical Structure" is any object or tangible physical action which is used as a reminder of an intention or commitment. For instance, wearing a wedding ring is a common Structure used by married people to signal their status to themselves and to others. Using Physical Structures in coaching is a way for the client to consciously create and benefit from reminders they have chosen themselves - as opposed to reacting unconsciously to the hundreds of Structures that are already operating in clients' lives every day. Choosing a Structure is way of breaking out of a client's conditioning. In EFT terms it's a way of altering or at least consciously adding to "the writing on their walls".

Choice of Structure is agreed between client and coach and can vary greatly depending on the preferred modalities of the client (visual, auditory etc) and the situation referred to by the Structure. Physical Structures are usually images or objects placed in a visible position which are significant to the situation, but they can also include anything that has strong significance for the client, such as playing a particular piece of music or wearing particular clothes or jewellery. The strongest structures are often those which the client has had to buy or make themselves - such as taking a photograph of a significant object or place, cutting out a picture of a desired object or printing out an inspiring passage or poem.

Sometimes the Structure involves making physical changes to the client's environment to support a new "way of being" or activity - such as reorganising their office, or redecorating with a colour that resonates with the new "way of being". Structures can also be auditory - for instance beginning the day listening to a particular piece of music, or using a particular alert sound on their computer as a reminder. There is literally no limit to the creativity that can be used to create Structures which are totally unique and powerful to the individual client.

So how can EFT augment these kinds of Structures?

When using EFT for therapeutic purposes it is often useful for the client to tap while focussing on a photograph of the person or issue involved [3]. The photograph serves to keep the client "tuned in" to the issue and so the repetition of reminder phrases can often be dropped.

This technique can also usefully be adapted to coaching, by getting the client to tap while looking at the chosen Structure. Done persistently over a period of time, perhaps as homework, this will slowly (or quickly!) reduce the negative feelings, doubts, uncertainties, fears or blocks that pertain to the specific goal or commitment represented by the Structure. Sometimes such tapping will produce specific insights or fears which can be worked on in the next coaching session or by the client on their own, as they prefer.

Structures can also be used as representations of goals. Using or creating external representations of the achieved goal can also be a useful alternative process for clients who really do have a hard time getting the full sensory experience of the achieved goal in their mind. All kinds of creative ways can be found to create in physical reality the types of objects or outcomes that realisation of a  goal would actually produce.

Here are some ideas for choice of Structures relating to a specific goal or intention:

- Where the goal is an exam or test - create and frame a certificate of achievement, or use an old exam paper.
- Where the goal involves a public appearance or community project - create a fake news cutting reporting the successful event and pin it to a notice board in the client's office.
- Where the goal relates to sales or business success - create fake orders and invoices for the amounts the client is seeking to achieve (not to be submitted to the tax man of course!).
- Where the goal relates to a sport - create a trophy, rosette or medal acknowledging success.
- If the goal relates to the writing of a book - create a front cover for the book and wrap it around another book and place it somewhere visible - or write a letter of acceptance by a publisher or agent including the amount of money required as an advance.
- If the goal involves many steps along the way (e.g. passing an exam, applying for a job and achieving a specific income) - create objects which represent the successful completion of all the major steps involved. It's hard for a client to really believe the end goal if they haven't first established belief in all the things they know to be a necessary precursors or milestones along the way.

Related sections:

6.2.8      The Choices Technique ⇧
6.2.15     Tailenders ⇧
8.1.4      The Compelling Way ⇧
9.3        Blocks ⇩

## 8.1.5.2   Using EFT as a Structure

EFT can be used as a Structure in its own right. Indeed, most of the applications of EFT presented elsewhere, especially where the client uses them outside the coaching session, can be thought of as Structures.

Like other structures, EFT can be individualised, using whatever words or references that help to trigger the client into the desired state of being.

The format is basically the Choices format (*"Even though…, I choose…"*). To make it an effective Structure the chosen statement needs to be repeated as homework. Initially I suggest two or three times a day for several days to a week. It is also often useful to create physical Structure to support the EFT, such as writing the statement on a piece of card which the client keeps in a prominent place such as by the bed, on their desk or in their wallet or bag.

It's very important not simply to hand out an EFT Structure and expect that to be sufficient to produce the desired change - although it may. Settling on a Structure statement should be the **final** stage after having addressed all the Tailenders, Reversals and blocks around an issue. A Structure should be a kind of "summation" and reminder of a conclusion and decision that has already been reached during the coaching.

The range of ways that EFT can be used as a Structure are manifold, but here are some suggestions based on broad categories of application.

## Structures for feelings (I feel...)

In this application, the intention is to reconnect with particular states of feeling that were contacted during the prior coaching exercise. This might include connecting with a chosen Resourceful State. The EFT statement should be based on the words that the client used during the exercise, although always in discussion with them to find out which words really "trigger" the desired state.

> *"Even though I have this challenge, I choose to feel positive and energised."*

## Structures for ways of being (I am...)

In this application, the intention is to trigger the new "way of being" that the client wants access to in the future. A "way of being" is about the client's identity rather than purely how they feel in that identity - it's about Who They Are or Who They Wish to Become.

> *"Even though I have this challenge, I choose to be empowered and courageous in this type of situation."*

> *"Even though I have this problem, I choose to be Creative and Resourceful in dealing with it."*

> *"Even though I often feel I am hopeless at this, I choose to remember I am Creative, Resourceful and Whole."*

## Structures for commitments (I will...)

Commitments are usually carried out in opposition to habits, ways of being and feelings that might prevent the commitment occurring - so much of the above is relevant here. But a Choices statement expressing a Commitment is much more definite about what physical action will occur. The basic format is:

> *"Even though I find it hard to go to the gym, I choose to go to the gym."*

But it's possible to be creative around this format to add in some "Compelling Way" or other element to make the chosen commitment more appealing.

> *"Even if I don't feel like going to the gym, I choose to enjoy going to the gym."*

> *"Even if I don't feel like going to the gym, I choose to enjoy the feeling I get afterwards."*

> *"Even if I don't feel like going to the gym, I choose to go and feel proud of myself."*

## Structures for goals (I desire...)

It's a good idea not to say "I want" in this format, since this reinforces the client's lack of something and can often signal a negativity within a goal - i.e. wanting to move away from something rather than towards something. "I desire" is a positive statement, not founded in lack or fear - it's a "move towards" word which has more chance of coming from the client's true self. "I desire" is also a form of words which instructs the mind to begin finding solutions and to start eliminating behaviours and choices which are inconsistent with the desire.

> *"Even though I'm in this job, I desire a job that is fulfilling and rewarding."*

> *"Even though I'm overweight, I desire to be fit and healthy."*

The beginning part of the statement needs to be firmly based in the client's actual current situation and should represent the emotion or state of being that they no longer want to have and yet are constantly reminded of, by their everyday circumstances. Once the whole statement has been anchored through tapping (preferably through regular repetition over several days or even weeks), then thinking of the current situation ("I'm overweight") will automatically trigger the mind to produce the second part of the statement ("I desire to be fit and healthy").

Related sections:

6.2.3      Psychological Reversal ⇧

6.2.8      The Choices Technique ⇧

6.2.15     Tailenders ⇧

8.1.1.3    Anchoring Resourceful States ⇧

8.1.4      The Compelling Way ⇧

9.3        Blocks ⇩

9.4        Habits ⇩


## 8.1.6   Fulfilment Clarification

If goals represent the "Doing" of what the client wants for themselves, Fulfilment represents the "Being" - what inspires them and what makes them feel good about their lives. In practice, working on goals and Fulfilment should happen together and with reference to each other. But since the two concepts exist separately within coaching I am treating them as separate entities here.

Just as EFT can be used to test client goal validity, EFT can complement Fulfilment coaching by testing the client's ideas about what Fulfilment means.

Everybody wants Fulfilment. But finding out what it means can be as hard as getting there. In particular the feeling of "being fulfilled" is confused with "having fulfilment". So people look for Fulfilment by acquiring things - possessions, income, qualifications, relationships and so on, only to have the **feeling** of Fulfilment remain out of reach or fade after a while.

Finding out what Fulfilment means for a particular client is important, because it will be the basis for goal setting, establishing values and measuring success. In conventional coaching it involves an extensive discussion to find out what the client really means by Fulfilment and what he expects it to look like or feel like when he gets it. Sometimes clients come to coaching especially to look at Fulfilment - and so for these clients it is especially important to get a strong grip on what this really means to the client.

EFT can be an incredibly useful tool to help clients access the truth about what Fulfilment means to them. I love this application because it's a particular example of how using EFT need be absolutely nothing to do with "therapy" or "raking over the past". The focus is 100% on understanding the client's value system and what they really want for themselves.

In this context, the objective is to generate insights and material for further study, not for removing any particular emotion. SLOW EFT is a particularly useful pattern of EFT here, but standard EFT can also be used.

The exact words to be used are down to the creativity of both client and coach (this is a great place for the client to be co-active and take this work in her own direction by experimenting), but here are some suggestions for uses of EFT for specific issues around Fulfilment. Essentially the task is to discuss with the client the concept of Fulfilment and for the coach to take note of any feelings about Fulfilment, and any blocks or Reversals that the client mentions specifically. These will vary, of course, according to each client, but could cover issues like not knowing what Fulfilment means, not knowing what it feels like, not feeling worthy of Fulfilment, not believing it's possible and so on. Here are some possible setup statements:

> "Even though I don't know what Fulfilment means for me yet...."

> "Even though I don't know how to recognise Fulfilment, I deeply and completely accept myself"

> "Even though I don't know what Fulfilment feels like, I choose to allow myself to feel Fulfilled."

> "Even though I don't allow myself to feel Fulfilled..."

> "Even though I don't deserve to feel Fulfilled...."

> "Even though I think I should feel Fulfilled with everything I have...."

> "Even though I have no idea what Fulfilment feels like..."

> "Even though I don't believe it's possible to be really Fulfilled in this lifetime..."

> "Even though I think Fulfilment is an illusion..."

Then use the word "Fulfilment" as the reminder phrase, (saying it several times on each point if using SLOW EFT). The client and coach pay close attention to whatever thoughts, words, images or sensations occur during this process, since these are likely to be relevant. Alternatively, it can be set as homework and the client can write down what happens. Some clients prefer doing this type of work alone as it's far more private and enables the client to really focus in on his own internal landscape.

A particular area in which EFT can aid the search for Fulfilment is testing what the client believes they **should** have in order to be fulfilled. Much of what clients (and the rest of us) believe we need to do or have to be fulfilled is the result of conditioning by society, religion, parents, teachers and peers.

Coaching serves the client when it helps the client distinguish between things the client really wants and the things they think they should have. It can save the client a lot of time spent wasted on goals that won't ever provide the Fulfilment he is seeking. And it can accelerate the client's understanding of his true essence - the part of him that has desires and dreams that are all his own and nothing to do with anyone else's expectations of him. This is discussed further under goals.

Related sections:

6.1.5    Fulfilment Coaching ⇧

6.2.3    Psychological Reversal ⇧

6.2.9    SLOW EFT ⇧

9.1.2    Validating Goals ⇩

9.3.3    Blocks as Reasons Why Not ⇩


## 8.1.7    Achieving Balance

As discussed under fundamentals, the purpose of Balance coaching is to develop behavioural flexibility - to allow the client to move freely between different parts of their lives and to make the changes necessary to achieve the Balance that brings them Fulfilment.

This means getting them "unstuck" from their current pattern of life and keeping them unstuck and moving fluidly. It was also noted that at the root of "stuckness" is a desire to control (keep things safe and predictable) and at the root of that is fear (of what will happen if control is lost). Since EFT can address both of these, it is also a useful tool in achieving Balance.

Whenever you come across a client who is resisting making changes in order to achieve Balance, an EFT Coaching line of enquiry would be to find out what the client is trying to control by staying where they are. Then, you can go further and find out what the client fears might happen if he **loses** that control. Whatever comes up as a fear can be addressed with EFT.

(Incidentally, clients are never going to drop their need for control completely - if they did you would probably have a great spiritual master on your hands! But you can shift them into wanting to have control over their emotional state instead.)

Another aspect of Balance that EFT can help with is improving the ability of the client to make choices - to stand up for the parts of her life that are important to her and say No sometimes. A client will never be able to achieve the Balance they seek if they constantly allow other people to determine where they should be, what they should be doing and for how long. Saying No to employers, to partners, to people trying to sell you something, to children, to in-laws who invite themselves for the weekend, etc, is hard for many people.

At the root of not being able to say No are issues such as:

- Fear of the reaction (*"I'll get sacked", "They'll leave me", "They'll make my life hell"*)

- Not feeling important enough for one's preferences to matter (*"I should put my children first", "I'm just one employee"*).

Often, the anticipated negative reactions of the people the client wants to say No to, are actually projections or a cover-up for the client's pseudo-values. For instance, being unable to say No to an employer may not really be about a fear of being sacked - but the client's need to fulfil his idea of himself as a hard-working, dedicated employee - he may be far more afraid of undermining his own sense of identity than what his employer will actually do.

Or, being unable to say No to the in-laws may be less about what the in-laws will think or say than the client's idea of herself as a good wife and homemaker - she may be far more afraid of appearing not to be able to "handle" unexpected guests and appearing disloyal to her husband than what the in-laws will actually do or say. And all these fears, limiting beliefs and pseudo-values are addressable with EFT.

Related sections:

6.1.5      Fulfilment Coaching ⇧
6.1.6      Balance Coaching ⇧
6.1.18    Values and Pseudo-values ⇧
8.2.14    The Yes/No Commitment Pattern ⇩
9.2.1      Clearing Fears ⇩
9.5.9.1   True Values, Limiting Beliefs ⇩

## 8.1.8   Supporting Process Coaching

A particular aspect of Process coaching is the act of simply being there with the client, in whatever mood or state she is in. Process coaching comes from the perspective that being with a client during the down times as well as the up times, allows the client to feel safe in expressing their emotions and even exploring them, rather than trying to suppress them, switch them off or fix them. This is a form of unconditional acceptance of the client, irrespective of their current emotional state, which an EFT practitioner will recognise.

EFT also offers the client a way to build confidence in working with their emotions - noticing them, feeling them and exploring them - but in a slightly different way - by offering them the assurance that these feelings can be released whenever the client chooses to do so.

It also explicitly asserts the acceptability of the client in having the emotions. Having EFT as a tool can, therefore, act as a kind of safety net within Process coaching. Even if it is not used - and it need not be used at all - having it there enables the client to know they she can safely explore all kinds of issues without the fear of being overwhelmed by what may arise emotionally. It also enables the coach to enter into Process coaching without fear, knowing that she has a tool capable of dealing with any emotion that might arise.

This is one very good reason why EFT should be introduced right at the beginning of the coaching relationship, so that it can be brought into play at times like this, or not. Trying to introduce the client to the basic procedure just when she is going through a particular emotional process will simply be an interruption.

Related sections:

6.1.7        Process Coaching ⇧

6.1.15      Accepting the Client Without Judgement ⇧

## 8.1.8.1    Valuing the Learning from Negative Emotions

It is a very fine line indeed that the EFT Coach walks during Process coaching. It is absolutely true that the client **can** derive huge learning from their negative emotions, if they are coached well. And so it is not always appropriate for the coach to respond to negative emotions with a suggestion to do EFT.

Process coaching usually occurs some way into the coaching relationship - after having set goals, made commitments and perhaps entered a period of struggle. If you have introduced EFT early on, then the client should be fairly familiar with EFT and what it can do by now. At all times the client has the choice whether to use EFT or not. But I incline to the view that for Process issues particularly, this choice must be expressed by the client, not suggested by the coach.

This is to avoid the coach prematurely ending the client's emotional state before the client has had the time he needs to get whatever value or learning from it that he can. Of course it is always the client's prerogative to end an emotional state anytime he wishes - but the desire must be expressed by him.

There comes a time for all Process coaching and all clients in negative mood states where the client says: *"Enough - I want to get on with my life"*, or *"You know - I think I've had all the learning I want from this state right now - staying in this state isn't moving me forward and I want to get out of it."*

When that turning point comes, EFT can be there in the wings to help, if it is requested. It can also be put aside indefinitely whenever the client says *"No, I want to stay with this feeling for a bit - I think there's something in here I can't quite grasp and I want to see how it unfolds"*.

It's my view that when **either** of these responses occur from an EFT Coaching client, you can be very proud indeed - you have created a client who is in total charge of their emotional life, taking conscious decisions about which emotions to allow and explore without fear and which emotions to clear as soon as possible because they are simply getting in the way of having a fulfilled life. There are few people on the planet with that sort of control over their inner life - but your client can be one of them.

### 8.1.8.2   The Coach's Response to Process

Having EFT as a coaching tool should not be used as a way for you to avoid feeling uncomfortable around your client's negative mood states.

But what if a client reaches for EFT the second they feel any kind of negative emotion? What if you, as their coach, feel they are trying to avoid "facing their feelings" and are "reaching for the aspirin" the moment they get so much as a grazed knee?

If so, that is your opinion - and if it causes you any frustration you need to check whether you have an agenda about how much or for how long your client **should** be with his negative emotions before it's "OK" to feel better.

Since the client by now will know how to apply EFT himself, you can actually no more control his use of it to feel better than you can control whether he responds to his negative emotions by going on a spending spree, booking a holiday, or going to the pub to get drunk, in order to cheer himself up. If your client wants to use EFT this way, he is using it the same way as thousands of self-help users of EFT around the world use it every day.

Before you can be a congruent EFT Coach, you may need to examine whether you can "be with" the idea that clients may zip through their Process emotions, material and learning in minutes or hours instead of days, weeks or even months. This won't necessarily happen, but it can. And you need to decide if you can "be with" the idea that clients can move so quickly through their Process that you as coach may not actually get to be there when it happens (e.g. if they have EFT homework). If you have a need to see it happening for it to feel like "proper Process coaching" then you have begun to need your clients to be a certain way for you to feel good as a coach.

If this causes you any kind of challenge, then use of EFT during the coaching as a self-management skill can help you stay back and allow the client's Process to unfold. You can also do EFT specifically on any issues after the session, for example:

> *"Even though I thought she seemed to be rushing through her emotions,..."*

> *"Even though it went so fast I didn't feel in control of what was happening,..."*

Ultimately, your decision to use or not use EFT in a Process context must be taken congruently. If you feel unsure about it or have any reservations, then don't. Possibly the best way to use it congruently is to work through some of your own emotions in a Process type of way so that you get to experience directly how using EFT can accelerate you through emotional states. When you get to experience how this feels and reassure yourself that you didn't "miss" anything by doing it that way, you will be in a position to use it congruently with clients.

Related sections:

| | |
|---|---|
| 5.3.4 | "Coaching should be about results, not about making clients feel better" ⇧ |
| 6.1.15 | Accepting the Client Without Judgement ⇧ |
| 8.1.2 | Homework ⇧ |
| 11 | Integrating EFT into your Coaching Practice ⇩ |

### 8.1.8.3   Managing the End of a Process Session

Since Process coaching can involve some significant emotional content (with or without EFT), clients can be in quite an emotional state at the end of the session.

Sometimes it is appropriate and entirely healthy for a client to stay in a particular state and work through it on their own. But I do not believe it is productive to leave clients in extreme or even moderate states of distress. Distress is rarely a resourceful state and therefore is not a state that you should want your client to be remaining in for any length of time if it is avoidable.

In my experience as a coaching client (of inexperienced or trainee coaches), there have been times when I have been left in a state of distress because "time was up" and the coach had no tools to quickly bring me into a less distressed and/or more resourceful state. In my opinion, at this point invoking the mantra that *"the client is Creative, Resourceful and Whole and therefore they can take it"* feels like an abdication of responsibility.

If you are any sort of good coach, your client will trust you enough to go into difficult and highly personal territory, because you are with them, supporting them and they don't feel alone while it happens. In my opinion, to allow this to happen on the premise that they are supported, and then to end the session and withdraw that support without ensuring the client is back into a reasonably secure space, is frankly, an abuse of trust. If the client knows that this can happen, they will be less willing to allow themselves to be vulnerable with you again. Not to mention the fact that a client should be looking forward to their coaching, not dreading it.

Some readers may be thinking *"But looking after a client's emotional state sounds like therapy to me"*. The distinction I would make here is between looking after the client's emotional state and paying attention to their state of **resourcefulness**.

As a coach I am only interested in a client's emotional state to the degree that it is affecting their ability to make progress towards their goals. If a client feels unsettled, or upset during coaching but they are telling me they can see a way through, or they know what to go and do next, I am content. If they are upset and saying they feel they don't know what to do next and can't see a way through, then I believe it's my job as coach to help bring about a more resourceful state before completing a session.

A suggested solution for ending an emotionally charged Process session, is to use a variation of the EFT setup that was suggested earlier:

>*"Even though I feel this way, I am Creative, Resourceful and Whole"*

or

>*"Even though I feel this way, I choose to remember I am Creative, Resourceful and Whole"*

One or two rounds of this pattern of EFT at the end of the session not only produces non-specific calming in the client (i.e. whatever issue caused the upset has not been directly addressed and remains there for future processing), but focuses the client on their own resourcefulness to deal with the situation.

I would then follow up immediately with some agreed actions and/or homework, paying close attention to whether I am hearing a resourceful state from the client in response.

If part of the client's problem at this point is worry about being overwhelmed emotionally after the session (e.g. if the agreed actions involve issues which they fear could cause distress), then of course setting some EFT as part of the homework would be appropriate.

Related sections:

6.1.1      The Client is Creative, Resourceful and Whole ⇧

8.1.1      Resourceful States ⇧

8.1.2      Homework ⇧

## 8.1.9   Metaphor

> *"...metaphors...are the language of the unconscious mind. ... EFT can be used most creatively and most successfully to change metaphors, to move them along, and to discover their relevance and meaning."* [3]

Remembering that all coaching should be following the client's lead, there are times when the client will spontaneously hand you a metaphor on a plate (if you pardon the metaphor).

They will say things like

> *"I feeling like I'm floating around in a fog."*

> *"My life is a complete roller coaster at the moment."*

> *"Working on this project is like wading through treacle."*

> *"I just feel terrible when I'm with my boss - like she's the ugly sister and I'm just some Cinderella having to be at her beck and call."*

Metaphors encapsulate for their user, not just the physics of the situation, but very much what is going on energetically.

Having a metaphor to work with can let you, as coach, find out more about the Aspects and Reversals that may be operating on the problem - but without directly needing to ask the client analytical questions such as *"What are your blocks here?"* which can be hard to answer.

Having found out the Aspects and Reversals in metaphorical terms, EFT setups can be constructed using those terms, without having to analyse what the terms really mean. The client, or at least his unconscious, knows **exactly** what they mean, because they came from the client in the first place.

How to use EFT in this way is best explained through examples. When you are presented with a metaphor you can do the following:

**Look for fears:**

> *What don't you like about the fog / the roller coaster / the treacle / being Cinderella?"*

The answers give you an idea of the client's core fears - which usually are fears that are more significant than just the current issue. Again, this is a much easier question to answer than *"What are the things you fear most in life?"* which might invite resistance, either because the client doesn't know or doesn't want to look at their core fears in such a blunt way (and who could blame them), or because the client won't see why they need to tell you their core fears in order to help them finish their project, handle their boss, etc.

But by asking about the metaphor they have just given you, the relevance issue is dealt with automatically, as is the level of resistance to talking about their feelings. You can then apply EFT to the answers that come back: e.g.

> *"Even though the fog makes me feel isolated and alone and no-one can hear me cry for help..."*

> *"Even though the roller coaster makes me feel out of control and powerless..."*

> *"Even though I think that if I really fall in the treacle I'll drown and never get out..."*

> *"Even though being Cinderella makes me feel I'll always be poor and lonely..."*

**Look for Psychological Reversals:**

You can also ask:

> *"Is there anything nice about the fog / the roller coaster / the treacle / being Cinderella?"*

The answers give you an idea about what the client may be getting (unconsciously) from the situation. This is much easier for the client to answer than the question *"What are you getting out of having this problem?"* which often invites resistance or at least confusion.

You can then apply EFT to whatever the answer is: e.g.

> *"Even though it's kind of comforting being enveloped by the fog…"*
>
> *"Even though the roller coaster gives me a feeling of excitement in my life…"*
>
> *"Even though I like being able to focus on the treacle and not the goal…"*
>
> *"Even though if I'm Cinderella I can believe that someone might come and rescue me…"*

**Look for solutions within the metaphor:**

But as well as looking for Reversals and fears implied by the metaphor, we can also use EFT to work on the metaphor directly, as a way to get rid of blocks or to find solutions to the problem itself.

By solving the problem as expressed by the metaphor we can start to solve the real problem it refers to, since energetically the metaphor **is** the problem in the client's world.

How the metaphor could or should be changed for the better, should always come from the client, as usual. But you can elicit their ideas by asking:

> *"If you could alter the fog / the roller coaster / the treacle / the Cinderella picture to make things the way you'd like, what would you do?"*

Notice that asking a client to creatively alter a metaphor is a much easier process than asking them to come up with a solution to their problem. It really does involve different parts of the brain and in so doing helps to bypass the areas which will probably also come up with "reasons why not" at the same time. Also, by staying at the level of the metaphor which is a representation of the client's energy in relation to the problem, we are helping the client to work on their energy around the problem, as well as the problem itself.

Again, we can then apply EFT to whatever answers come back from the client:

> *"Even though I wish I could just breathe on the fog, warm it up and make it disappear…"*
>
> *"Even though I'd like to have a personal brake pedal which I could use any time I wanted it to stop…"*
>
> *"Even though I'd like to become a treacle bird that could just fly straight over the treacle…"*
>
> *"Even though I'd really like to turn out to be the Fairy Godmother all along and just zap myself right out of there…"*

You may want the client to come up with several possibilities and then choose the one that feels best. ("Best" is defined as the easiest to imagine and bring about in their imagination and most effective at solving the problem.)

Having found an energetic "solution" to the problem presented in the metaphor, you need to translate back into the client's real life, so that the learning that took place in the metaphor world can be consciously processed and embedded. (By the way, it is quite possible that ideas will come up spontaneously while doing the EFT in the previous stage.) As always, this process is begun by asking the client a question about it:

> "So in your real life, what would happen if you decided to blow away the fog? (Try doing that now - what do you see?)"

> "So what could you do to create a personal brake pedal in your real life? (Let's generate some ideas for a few ways that you could create one)"

> "So how could you become the Treacle Bird while you finish this project? (What structures could we use to help remind you to be the Treacle Bird? Let's think about some)"

> "So how would the Fairy Godmother deal with your boss? (What would she feel about her? What would she say?)"

In other words, using the client's own metaphor - and then using EFT on how the client thinks about the metaphor, allows coach and client to work at levels of creativity (and safety) which totally transcend the original metaphor and also totally bypass the client's normal system of resistance and objections to finding solutions to their problems.

By the way, be prepared for the eventuality that the solution created this way may not be the total answer to the client's issue. In all coaching, the client may need to try out and refine several different strategies before finding one that really sorts out the problem. The same goes for solutions created using metaphors. The metaphor the client gave you to start with was just one of many that she could have used to describe the problem and how it feels. It was significant that of all the metaphors possible, that one was chosen at the particular point in time - and so was important to work with. Another point in time, and another energetic state, might produce a different metaphor and therefore a different solution to try.

But even with this caveat, I believe metaphor work - assisted by EFT - offers about the easiest, most playful and most fun way to do extremely deep work with a client and but without having to ask overtly scary questions.

Also notice that never at any point in the entire process do we look at **why** the client chose that particular metaphor. Nor do we ask whether there are any memories associated with fog, roller coasters, treacle or Cinderella that might give us clues about what the metaphor signals to the client or might indicate why the client is responding to their current situation with this metaphor.

Delving into the significance of the metaphor and events from the client's past that helped form them, is an approach that might be taken in a therapeutic EFT session. And while this option may be open to you if you find the client presenting the same metaphor to you over and over for different issues, it's important to realise that deep and significant coaching work can be done by focussing only on how the metaphor feels **now**, and how the client would like to manipulate the metaphor in the future.

Related sections:

6.2.3      Psychological Reversal ⇧

6.2.12     Aspects ⇧

8.1.5      Structures ⇧

8.1.10     Idea Generation ⇩

## 8.1.10 Idea Generation

Whenever Idea Generation is required in coaching (e.g. in Perspectives work, or in generating a list of possible solutions to a problem), combining use of metaphor with EFT can make the difference between run-of-the-mill ideas and truly inspired ones.

As discussed above, using metaphor takes us directly into the energetic world of the client, bypassing a certain amount of rationalisation and analytical thinking. By heading straight for the world of Metaphor and then working with it using EFT, we are getting directly to the client's energetic relationship with the problem and allowing solutions to be found which are energetically "correct" for the client.

In the Idea Generation situation, it is the coach who initiates the metaphors, not the client, but still in the form of a question:

*"If there was one animal that could just deal with the problem straightaway, what animal might that be? (Tell me what it is about that animal that allows them to deal with it)"*

*"If there was a famous person from history who could just deal with the problem straightaway, who would that be? (What qualities do they have that let them deal with it?)"*

*"If the solution to this was a particular colour, pattern or shape, what would it look like?"*

*"If there was a piece of music to accompany you while you easily solved this problem, what music would you choose?*

These types of question do two things. Firstly, and obviously, they elicit ideas and feelings about the problem that start to indicate energetically what a solution to the problem might incorporate.

But secondly, it gets the client away from actually thinking about the problem directly - and so triggering all his fears, doubts and general stuckness around it. It is pretty difficult to maintain the thought *"This is a really hard problem and I can't see a way out"* when you are trying to remember your favourite characters from history, or visualise a rainbow of colours to choose from. And being separated from the stuck energy of the problem is the best way of generating a solution that is not limited by that stuckness.

EFT can help this process in two important ways. Firstly, it can help when the client can't think of anything in response to your question. EFT can be used to get the ideas flowing:

*"Even though I can't think of anyone/anything…."*.

You can then use a relevant reminder phrases while they tap to further stimulate their ideas: e.g. "Animal". (By the way, EFT shouldn't be used to labour a line of enquiry that just isn't "landing" with a client. If they don't resonate with animals, they might resonate with the music idea instead. But this use of EFT to get ideas flowing can be used when the client likes the idea of finding an animal but can't quite come up with one right now.)

Secondly, it can help when the client is overwhelmed by options in response to your question. EFT can help the client focus in and pick the one that resonates best - or perhaps even amalgamate options to create a new ideal one.

*"Even though I have all these options…"*.

Then use reminder phrases to help the client focus in on the most useful option: *"All these options, one perfect option, the ideal option, the best option, most creative option, choosing an option, the strongest option, the most vivid option…"* etc

Having generated ideas for several solutions, if the preferred solution appears to involve a metaphor generated this way, then the process of turning that metaphor into a real world solution is as described above.

Related sections:

## 8.1.11 Locking in the Learning

As presented in the Fundamentals section, coaching is as much about the client learning as it is about action. But coaches don't only take the client through a process in which they learn. They make sure the client **knows** that they have learned and **what** they have learned. Unconscious learning can be missed or dismissed by the client. It can make them think that the coach did it, rather than them realising that not only did **they** do it themselves, but they can do it again, because they now have learning they can use in the future.

EFT also emphasises (by its essential nature) conscious client understanding of the process and the outcome. I contrast this with other forms of "therapy" or healing (e.g. Reiki, massage, or even sometimes NLP) in which the practitioner performs an intervention and the client ends up feeling different, but they don't know how or why it happened. EFT can therefore be a great support in ensuring that client learning is conscious and fully "locked in".

Bringing learning into conscious awareness can be greatly assisted by using EFT. This can be done either during a session with the coach listening and feeding back to the client (which can further help the client gain conscious awareness), or as homework if the client prefers to do this in his own time.

SLOW EFT can be particularly appropriate for this application. The client simply focuses on the relevant event (e.g. the outcome of a previous homework action) and taps on each EFT point for a while and notices what thoughts arise. Repeating the reminder phrase "learning" may also be helpful but not absolutely necessary.

Once the learning is in consciousness, it's useful to "lock it in", especially if it is learning that the client recognises as being potentially useful to draw upon in future situations. Having identified the learning, a suitable format for locking it in is a Choices statement:

> *"Even if this situation occurs again, I choose to remember that..."*

Here's an example of a coaching dialogue in which EFT is used in these ways.

> *Coach: "So how did last week's homework go?"*

> *Client: "Well, I made an appointment with my boss and we talked about the situation."*

> *Coach: "That's great. What was the outcome?"*

> *Client: "Well, not so great really - he said he was snowed under by the budget preparation thing at the moment and didn't really have time to think about it right now."*

> *Coach: "OK, so did he actually say No?"*

> *Client: "No, it was neither Yes or No - just that he was busy and now wasn't a good time."*

> *Coach: "OK - so what's next?"*

> *Client: "Well, I feel a bit disheartened to be honest. I'm probably going to have to get my courage up to talk to him again another time."*

> *Coach: "OK - so what did you learn?"*

*Client: "That I wasted my time?"*

*Coach: "Did you?"*

*Client: "I don't know - I guess I'm pleased I managed to get to speak to him. This time last week that seemed like a really big deal."*

*Coach: "Yes, that's true. Shall we use some EFT to see what other learning there might be around this?"*

*Client: "Sure - if I'm going to see him again that would be useful."*

*Coach/Client: "Even though I'm not sure what the learning is from this, I deeply and completely accept myself......Learning...Learning......."*

*Client: "You know what? I learned that my boss is willing to talk to me even if he's not able to give me the answer I want right now."*

*Coach: "Great - and what else?"*

*Client: "And that he has his own stuff going on. Saying Yes or No to me isn't the only thing on his mind and - well, it's not personal is it? - I mean he's just doing his job the best way he knows how."*

*Coach: "That's great. Do you think knowing all that will make it easier to talk to him next time?"*

*Client: "Totally"*

*Coach: "OK, well, let's lock that in with some EFT so it's there next time you talk to him."*

*Client: "OK - sounds good."*

*Coach/Client: "Even though I still need to get my boss's permission, I choose to remember that talking to him is no big deal really, and anyway his response isn't personal."*

This example shows how even an apparent "failure" can, if handled skillfully by a coach, result in some superb learning for the client which then positively assists in the client's future actions. EFT further enhances this process by firstly helping to reduce the initial negative reaction to the event (*"I wasted my time"*) allowing a more positive interpretation of the event to come forward (*"My boss was willing to talk to me"*). Secondly it offers a way to "lock in" what was learned explicitly, anchoring a future event (*"talking to my boss again"*) to the lessons learned.

Although the above dialogue is entirely fictitious, the sort of cognitive shifts that are represented there are to be seen repeatedly on Gary Craig's training CD's and are the commonplace experience of EFT practitioners.

Related sections:

6.1.16    Action and Learning ⇧

6.2.8     The Choices Technique ⇧

6.2.9     SLOW EFT ⇧

8.1.1.3   Anchoring Resourceful States ⇧

## 8.1.12 Peak Experiences

Eliciting a client's "Peak Experiences" is a good way of learning about your client's value system. Peak Experience work can be used as a general "getting to know you" exercise in the first couple of sessions, since it can be done without reference to any specific goal or event and it is usually a fun experience for the client. Peak Experience can also be used in a more focused way to elicit an experience that is relevant to a specific issue (e.g. if the client has a work goal, remembering a time when she was extremely successful in a work context can produce many insights that can be used in the current situation.)

The value in recalling a Peak Experience is two-fold. Firstly it reconnects the client with a positive state they may not have experienced for some time, and this may form the basis of a Resourceful State that can be used in the future.

Secondly, it can reveal insights and conscious awareness in the client. Some of these insights can involve revealing the clients values - but others are possible, such as understanding behaviour patterns, making connections with other significant life events or decisions.

Using EFT while focussing on a Peak Experience can be useful in fully eliciting the memories around an event and in noticing any insights or connections that may be relevant to the current situation.

There are two ways of using EFT to enhance Peak Experience work.

It can be used informally - by simply getting the client to tap while they talk. In terms of dialogue flow, the coaching dialogue is exactly as it would be without the EFT. If tapping through the whole sequence is distracting to the client, he can instead tap on just a few points or just one point. The best points to use for this application are the Third Eye point (middle of the forehead), the Eyebrow point and the Side of Eye point. Also useful is the Crown point (on the top of the head). If the client is clearly managing to connect with the experience and tell you all about it and you can hear insights and connections being made, then this is probably all you need in the way of EFT assistance.

But it can also be used more formally if you sense that the client is not connecting with the experience fully - or is even having trouble identifying an appropriate memory.

> *"Even though I can't find a relevant Peak Experience,..."*
>
> *"Even though I can't remember that much about it, ..."*
>
> *"Even though it just seems so distant and nothing to do with me any more,..."*

Although the aim is for the client to reconnect with a positive experience, this should not be forced beyond what occurs naturally with the help of EFT. If a client cannot connect with a particular memory to make the Peak Experience exercise work, even with the help of EFT, then it is not to be. There may be another memory that is more relevant. Or there may be some other very good reason why the client does not wish to explore that particular memory. The client always gets to choose which Peak Experiences to explore and which to avoid, even if EFT is available to help.

Related sections:

8.1.1      Resourceful States ⇧

9.5.9      Testing Values ⇩

## 8.1.13 Championing

Championing involves explicitly and enthusiastically expressing your belief in the client and her abilities. For example: *"I know you can do this - you have all the energy and all the skills to do it".*

In Championing, the client gets to experience one person (perhaps the only one currently in their lives) who fully believes in the client and totally supports them in achieving what they want. It's also where you convey how big you hold the client - allowing and encouraging them to step into that bigness.

Championing can be included very effectively when constructing a Choices statement. Remember that constructing Choices statements is ideally done co-actively, the client needs to end up with a statement she can believe in 100%, and represents what she really wants around an issue. But the coach has a role too - not simply making sure the client doesn't include any negative or counterproductive phrasing, but also to help the client expand her idea of what's possible and what this Choice could really mean.

For instance, suppose a client is constructing a Choice regarding their future responses to a particular colleague. (The past anger etc has been diffused with standard EFT, but the client knows she will have to deal with that colleague again and wants to avoid building up new anger).

A perfectly adequate Choice statement might be:

> *"Even though this colleague is sometimes difficult, I choose to remain calm in his presence."*

But if you bring in the idea of Championing, you can raise the power of the Choices statement to a whole new level. You can help the client generate much bigger ideas about herself by first championing:

> *"I know you are an incredibly powerful and compassionate person..."*

And then questioning:

> *"...so what's the most powerful and compassionate response to this colleague, that you could imagine?"*

This invites a whole new level of Choice to be created:

> *"Even though this colleague is sometimes difficult, I choose to remain in my power and find creative ways to find and nourish the Oneness between us".*

Or

> *"Even though this colleague is sometimes difficult, I choose to feel unconditional acceptance and to extend unlimited compassion to him."*

As with Championing within coaching, it must be based on what's actually true about the client, and which the client will also recognise as true. You can't Champion someone on the basis of their courage if you haven't actually seen the client display much courage so far, or if the client hasn't somehow taken on courage as a value or acknowledged it in herself at least to some degree. Championing based on qualities the client doesn't have or doesn't associate with herself will create "Tailenders" for any Choice that tries to tap into them - i.e. little voices that pop up and say *"But you're not"* or *"But that's not possible for you."*

By using Championing to help clients create powerful Choices for themselves, they are effectively learning how to Champion themselves - ultimately a far more powerful and long-lasting method than relying on the coach to do so.

Related sections:

6.2.8      The Choices Technique ⇧

6.2.15     Tailenders ⇧

## 8.1.14  Who Do You Need to Be?

Often, in order for the client to Do something different, they also need to Be something different. The best coaching models (in my opinion) address both Doing and Being as part of the client's development. Addressing the Being of an action can make the difference between a one-off action carried out with willpower and courage, and sustained consistent action over time carried out as a natural expression of the client's expanded self. And so a common technique is to ask the client *"Who do you need to be in order to achieve this?"*

This question asks the client to examine Who They Think They Are, and compare it with Who They Need to Become in order to be "the sort of person who does this".

Although the question is intended to find out what qualities the client needs to adopt and express in order to carry out a particular action, sometimes you do get more literal answers, such as *"I'd have to be Superman"*, or *"I'd have to be Boadicea"*. But then it's quite easy to elicit the perceived qualities of the people the clients have chosen as role models for Being and use these qualities as the basis for what follows.

EFT - particularly the Choices pattern - allows clients to choose who they want to be - what qualities they want to express in particular circumstances and to loosen or eliminate any emotional blocks to achieving them.

The format of the setup statement is based on the type of circumstance relevant to the new desired "way of being", and the chosen quality or type of action that the client would like to experience or have triggered when that happens:

> *"Even though <insert circumstance>, I choose to be <insert quality>.*

So, for instance:

> *"Even though my boss is being unreasonable again, I choose to be calm and professional"*

> *"Even though I sometimes feel down, I choose to be creative and positive about whatever is happening"*

> *"Even though I sometimes doubt I'll ever achieve this, I choose to be focussed and persistent."*

If the person has chosen a particular person or character to model themselves on (a legitimate tool within coaching), the EFT can be carried out while focussing on the person while they tap (perhaps literally focusing on a photo or image of the person). Note that if this is done, the client is not "tapping in" the positive qualities of the other person. What they are doing is tapping away any blocks to the client exhibiting those qualities.

Please note: I strongly believe that people do not acquire desires to Do or Be without also being given the capability to express that Doing or Being in **some** form. If a person truly resonates with the qualities they admire in another person, object or place, this must mean that that quality resides within the person to some degree and can therefore be developed, unleashed and expressed. So, a person who admires an Olympic athlete may not become an Olympic athlete themselves, but they can start to express the qualities of physical fitness, discipline, drive and focus in terms that are relevant to their own lives.

Sometimes, Who the Client Needs to Be is Herself. That is, take a "way of being" she uses quite naturally in one area of her life and develop that "way of being" in another area of her life. For instance, a client may feel totally confident and be highly admired and successful in her working life; but feel ill at ease or very shy socially. Conventional coaching methods might find ways of transferring the "way of being" at work to the client's "way of being" socially. In a way this is simply playing with Resourceful States.

But in EFT terms, what is happening here? Why does a person behave confidently in one area but not in another? Because there are different Aspects operating in the two situations. By eliciting the Aspects in the two different areas of life, the EFT Coach can help the client identify the aspects which are different between the two and target EFT on the problematic ones.

It's also useful to use the confidence in the work arena as the basis for a Choices statement. This allows the client to tap directly into the feeling of confidence that he is already familiar with and apply it to the new arena (once any significant Aspects have been dealt with).

> *"Even though this is a social situation, I choose to feel the same way I feel at work."*

> *"Even though I'm at a party with strangers, I choose to feel the same way as being in a work meeting with strangers."*

The outcome of the Who Do You Need To Be exercise can be further supported by the Doing and Being Pattern, a variation on the Choices Technique.

Related sections:

| | |
|---|---|
| 6.2.8 | The Choices Technique ⇧ |
| 6.2.12 | Aspects ⇧ |
| 8.1.1 | Resourceful States ⇧ |
| 8.2.12 | The Doing and Being Pattern ⇧ |


## 8.1.15 What are you Tolerating?

"What are you Tolerating" is a classic coaching tool aimed at uncovering the part of a client's life which need changing.

"Tolerations" are in fact a form of block to progress. They are they things which the client has "got used to" in their life because they don't think they have the power to change them or which don't cause quite enough pain that they demand to be dealt with.

Although none of these things may look big or important by themselves, among these tolerations are some of the things that the client will probably need to say No to, in order to say Yes to their goals.

If there are any beliefs or other emotional attachments keeping these things in place, then it makes it harder to say No to them and therefore harder to achieve the overall goal.

Things which are being tolerated in life are usually being tolerated for a reason - often in the form of a belief (about what should be tolerated) or a fear (of the alternative). In either case, EFT can address whatever it is that keeps the client tolerating it.

Related sections:

| | |
|---|---|
| 8.2.14 | The Yes/No Commitment Pattern ⇧ |
| 9.2.1 | Clearing Fears ⇩ |
| 9.5.2 | Clearing Limiting Beliefs ⇩ |

## 8.1.16 Accessing the Future Self

Contacting or creating a vision of the client's Future Self often occurs in the early sessions of coaching, using a guided visualisation. Just like values, the client's Future Self can become a point of reference for future decisions and future coaching.

For instance, when a client is stuck over a decision that has to be made, or some other problem in the client's life, the coach can simply ask *"What does your Future Self have to say about this?"*

At it's most superficial level it gets the client to view his current situation from a detached viewpoint, as though it were all over and done with years ago, unencumbered by the issues and fears that appear to be so important right at this moment. It's a way of cutting through the present trivia and getting the client focussed on what's really important to him and what he really wants.

However, the Future Self can work on an even deeper level. Sometimes the client's vision of his Future Self is so vivid and present, it really seems to take on a life of its own. When this happens, clients can almost "channel" what the Future Self has to say, with little or no conscious thought.

But sometimes, the client is so completely stuck in whatever is going on, that when asked *"What would your Future Self say?"*, they just get a complete blank. Either they have trouble even visualising the Future Self, or there is too much emotional chatter going on for that particular part of the client to be able to come through at this time. It is at these times that the client probably most wants to get the guidance of the Future Self - but it seems to be blocked.

EFT can be applied directly to this block, possibly without even directly addressing what the client is emotionally hooked into. For instance:

> *"Even though I can't access my Future Self at the moment…"*

> *"Even though I feel totally blank when I think about my Future Self…"*

> *"Even though I can't even see my Future Self…"*

> *"Even though I can't hear what my Future Self is saying…"*

For all these setups (or any other you might use to reflect the nature of the block), use the reminder phrase "Future Self". Or if the Future Self has a specific name, use the name as the reminder phrase.

It's important to get the client to report whatever thoughts, ideas or feelings come up during the tapping. Sometimes it will be a clue to what the block is about and what needs to be tapped on next. Sometimes it may be images or words which the client will recognise as having come from the Future Self. (It isn't important to determine whether they did or didn't, since the Future Self is already a part of the client, and so it all comes from the client in the end - but sometimes the client will experience the appearance of some words or images and really feel *"that wasn't me - I didn't make that up"*.)

Sometimes the client can so successfully access words or images from the Future Self that what appears is not easy to interpret. I have experienced hearing my Future Self say something that feels immensely profound and relevant to the current problem, but also have the feeling of not fully grasping its full meaning. Although somewhat frustrating, it does help convince me (or a client) that it was not "made up".

EFT can be applied to what the Future Self provided - words, images, sounds or feelings - in much the same way that EFT can be used to help get insights into dreams[3]. For instance:

> *"Even though I don't fully understand how this applies to the problem…"*

> *"Even though I want to know what this means,…"*

EFT can also be applied as though it were the Future Self doing the tapping, in order to come up with ideas or resources for the client:

*"I am my Future Self. Even though I haven't given <client> any ideas on this yet..."*

*"I am my Future Self. Even though I don't know what advice to give for the best yet..."*

*"I am my Future Self. Even though <client> has this problem, I deeply and completely accept <client>..."*

These can be complex mental manoeuvres for some clients and are not to be forced if the client doesn't take to it fairly naturally. As with all exercises and techniques, it's best to remain client-led at all times. As a client becomes acquainted with different tools and variations, and if you have a good co-active relationship established, you will find your client making their own suggestions for variations. In fact, you should not be surprised if you and a client end up creating whole new patterns or applications in the course of the coaching. EFT and its cousins are infinitely adaptable to different situations, and as humans we love to make and adapt tools to our immediate purposes.

In presenting ways that you might use EFT with the Future Self concept I do not mean to say "this how it must be done". It serves simply to inspire you with the possibilities.

Related sections:

8.1.18    Visualisations ⇩

## 8.1.17 Working with Time Lines

Time Lines are a specific NLP technique which can be used to help a client see how their internal representation of their past, present and future actually looks. Having discovered how it looks (what's visible, what's out of sight, what clear, what's fuzzy, what's on the Time Line and what's off it), it can then be adjusted according to the preferences of the client in order (for instance) to make desired events more achievable or, in a therapeutic setting, to heal past events.

Using EFT to enhance work on a client's past Time Line, for the purposes of healing past events is well described in Advanced Patterns of EFT[4].

However, I am going to focus here on using Time Lines for coaching purposes - and primarily for looking at the future and how the client represents that to themselves.

The reasoning behind using Time Lines as a coaching tool at all is this: that the client's mind is giving him a representation of his future which is congruent with his current beliefs about it. In other words, if a client is having trouble imagining or visualising the future there is likely to be some emotional reason or belief behind this.

So for instance, someone who believes *"There's no point making plans more than a year ahead because everything will have changed by then"*, will have trouble seeing anything past the point that marks one year away.  Someone who strongly believes in "living in the now" may have trouble with any sort of future representation at all. A person who strongly believes that they aren't going to live past 60 because that's when their mother/father died, might have a complete blank after age 60 on their Time Line. In contrast, someone who believes strongly in life after death may have no trouble seeing a Time Line that runs over hundreds of years.

So a client's Time Line representation is a window into the client's belief system around time and especially (in a coaching context) his beliefs about the future. We will see later in the book how EFT can be used to directly alter and redesign a client's belief system. Here we work on the client's belief system indirectly by using EFT to redesign the client's Time Line. By "correcting" features of the Time Line in a way chosen by the client, we are indirectly addressing the client's underlying beliefs that chose the original representation.

Related sections:

9.5        Beliefs ⇩


### 8.1.17.1  Eliciting the Time Line

Before you can start redesigning the Time Line - or even using it to understand the client's belief system around time - you need to elicit their existing representation.

The most common ways for people to represent their Time Line are:

- Left to Right (past on the left, present in the centre, future to the right)
- Back to Front (past behind, present where the client stands, future ahead)

However a client could have **any** configuration at all, or a variation on one of the common ones. For instance, someone who doesn't really relate to time at all, might have a Time Line which is entirely behind them, running left to right, so that none of it is visible.

Some variations are cultural. For instance someone whose written language runs from right to left could have their future to the left and the past to the right. Someone whose written language reads vertically might have the past above them and the future below them - or vice versa.

The line may not even be straight. It could curve round the client or up to the right or left. It could spiral outwards or inwards, up or down. Or it may not even be a line, but a sequence of blobs suspended in space, or an infinitely long calendar with numbers - or anything else at all.

The main thing is not to assume anything and elicit the client's representation in as neutral a way as possible, without imposing or suggesting anything. You might even want to avoid mentioning "line" at all, but simply ask the client to tell you "what you see in your mind when you think about the past, the present and the future". For the purposes of the following I will assume it is a line of some sort.


### 8.1.17.2  Making the Future Visible

Having elicited the basic representation for the Time Line, the first thing to check is whether the part of the client's Time Line that represents the future is visible. If the purpose of coaching is to focus on creating the client's future, then no amount of goal setting, planning or visualisation is going to be successful if the client fundamentally has a problem seeing his future clearly.

To establish whether the future is visible or not, ask the client to see where the following points are on their Time Line: tomorrow, next week, next year and ten years time. Notice carefully whether the client can easily see these points clearly, or whether they have any trouble seeing them. Do they have to turn around to see it? Do they have to do something to the Time Line to bring these points into view? Are they clear or fuzzy?

Are these points even on the Time Line at all? Or are they floating, disconnected in some way?

Before doing any other work using Time Lines in coaching, the first job is to create a clear and visible Time Line for the client to work with.

If there are any visibility issues with the line, use EFT to correct these. For example:

> *"Even though I can't see anything more than 6 months away,..."*

> *"Even though my Time Line is behind me, ..."*

> *"Even though the whole line looks sort of fuzzy, ..."*

*"Even though the future doesn't really seem real,…"*

If the EFT does not correct the visibility problems (to the satisfaction of the client), it may be necessary to delve further and more directly into the client's beliefs about the parts of the Time Line that aren't clear.

Related sections:

8.1.18      Visualisations ⇩

## 8.1.17.3  Connecting to the Time Line

It is not uncommon to find someone with a clearly visible future but who nevertheless has problems with completion of goals because they are disconnected from their own Time Line. (I speak as someone this has applied to!).

In this case, the person's problem is not in creating amazingly ambitious plans, but in putting them into reality. In this case, creating a wonderful future can have literally nothing to do with them - they are standing at a distance watching it happen in an abstract way (e.g. as for Dream Goals).

It's important that the client connects with and feels themselves to be physically on their own Time Line. This can be achieved by asking the client to manipulate the location of the Time Line to ensure they are on it. If this is at all difficult or the image "flips" back to its previous state, then using EFT can be used to remove any resistance to staying connected. Some discussion about this may be needed to elicit the significance of "being disconnected" and whether the client feels this resonates with any other feelings they have about their life.

Some example setups might be:

*"Even though I feel disconnected from my own life,…"*

*"Even though I see myself as an observer of life,…"*

*"Even though I find it hard to be involved in life,…"*

*"Even though I like to keep my distance,…"*

*"Even though I want to connect but I don't know how,…"*

*"Even though I try to connect but then something makes me pull back again,…"*

Although this is extremely preliminary work, you are already discovering major insights into the client's beliefs about himself - his relationship to himself, to other people and his attitude to life in general. More importantly, the **client** is getting these insights and will be starting to evaluate whether these attitudes and beliefs are really serving him.

Related sections:

9.1.6.2      Dream Goals ⇩

## 8.1.17.4  Repairing the Time Line

Sometimes you or the client will discover "faults" on the Time Line, such as gaps or blocks which represent problems the client may be having with specific goals.

For instance:

- **A break** marking a specific life event, such as finishing a course of education, retirement, a wedding, a birthday or a divorce. A break implies that the event represents a kind of "ending" for the client.

- **A gap** beginning at a particular point, but the line resumes at a later point. This may represent a particular period of life that the client finds it hard to think about - either because of fears, or simply because it hasn't been thought about yet or because the client thinks of it as "dead time". Examples might be the period after an impending divorce or an expected bereavement (where the line resumes represents when the client believes it will be possible for him to start living again). Parents may have a Time Line which is empty but resumes magically when the youngest child becomes 5 or 16, or 18 or 21. It's even possible that the client is actually in the gap itself if they are now in the period of time that they defined to themselves as empty space - and it is often being in such a gap that draws people to seek coaching in the first place, since their very own internal representation of their direction and position in life is absent.

- **A wall** or screen at a particular point. This represents a different kind of belief to the break. It implies the existence of something beyond, but it just isn't visible. The wall represents some kind of block to thinking about anything past that point.

Whether a particular feature of the Time Line is a "fault" or not is defined by the client. If the client wants to create a new future of herself but sees a gap or a wall in the Time Line for the period in question, she is probably going to interpret the gap or the wall as a problem in achieving her goal. Before conducting any "repair" to the Time Line, the coach must check out whether the feature **needs** repair at all and if so, what the client would consider an appropriate repair. For instance does the client want the wall knocked down, or just made of glass so it becomes see-through? Does the client want to fill the gap with a seamless line, or does she want some other structure to fill it, such as a bridge?

By letting the client define the repairs you are allowing the client to exercise creativity and to literally create a new reality for themselves, but in a playful way. You also greatly increase the chances that the client's repair will be a workable solution back in the client's real life. Ultimately, all discussion about Time Lines, manipulations and repairs are about finding solutions to the client's problems around goal setting and achievement. But by working with the internal representation we are working with the energetic reality, therefore bypassing the client's rational "shoulds" and "musts" about their goals. It also bypasses client's judgements about themselves. Deciding to fix a gap in their Time Line with a golden cord or making a wall see-through doesn't have the same moral judgements around it that "writing a plan" or "making myself focus on the future" do.

EFT can be used to help make the repairs or to help decide what repairs to do. It can even result in having a repair happen spontaneously, using some methods the client didn't even think of - so they may finish doing some EFT, look back at the Time Line only to find that it has changed all by itself.

Since the Time Line is part of the client's energetic reality, applying EFT or any other energy technique to it can result in changes to the energetic reality and therefore to the representations, without the conscious mind having to even decide what needs doing. For clients who feel comfortable around these kinds of ideas and around the effects of EFT, you can work with them in this way explicitly. However most clients will prefer the idea of consciously choosing and deciding what to do and then using EFT to make that happen.

So here are some setups that you might use to effect repairs or other changes to a Time Line:

*"Even though the line is broken for that two year period, I deeply and completely,..."*

*"Even though I can't see past the wall,..."*

*"Even though I want to pull down that wall,..."*

*"Even though I want to find a way over the gap,..."*

*"Even though I don't know how to get over the wall,..."*

*"Even though I don't know how to fix the gap,..."*

*"Even though I can't imagine there not being a gap there,..."*

As always, these setups should be derived from what the client spontaneously says when you are discussing the Time Line and what they think needs to happen to it.

EFT can also be used to address any fears or doubts the client has about changing the representation:

*"Even though I'm afraid to see what's beyond the wall,..."*

*"Even though I'm afraid to be reconnected to the line,..."*

*"Even though I don't believe that fixing the line will have any effect,..."*

*"Even though I don't believe it's possible to repair the line,..."*

Although the focus of the work is the Time Line, don't be afraid to take the focus off it to discuss any insights or connections that the client gets relating to his real life. Ultimately, the Time Line is an elaborate metaphor (albeit generated by the client's own energetic reality) - so if it results in useful insights about the client's real life, then it's more than OK to go there if it relates to the client's goals.

Related sections:

| | |
|---|---|
| 5.4.3 | Principle of Goal Furtherance ⇧ |
| 8.1.9 | Metaphor ⇧ |
| 9.3.2 | Blocks as Avoidance ⇩ |

## 8.1.17.5  Placing Goals and Milestones on the Time Line

Assuming the client's future Time Line is clear, visible and free from any glaring gaps or blocks, it can now be used to assist in the achievement of the client's coaching goals.

In this use of Time Lines, we deliberately manipulate (under the client's guidance) the Time Line to include the achievement of the client's goals. By placing them on the Time Line in a way that feels good to the client, we effectively integrate their goals into their existing energetic reality.

As before, we are looking to bypass the conscious mind's "shoulds" and "musts" and instead create representations of the client's goals which seem to "feel right". (These will be checked against reality at a later stage and can be further manipulated if necessary).

This task can be combined with using The Compelling Way technique, to place a compelling image or representation of the goal at a particular point on the line.

As you work with the client to give the client's goal a presence on his Time Line, the aim is to make the goal good to look at (light, bright, colourful, welcoming) as well as being clearly accessible from the present. If the goal is very far away, it's a good idea to create milestones along the way and have them look appealing and achievable too.

Sometimes the client can do this work quite easily through discussion, but sometimes it feels difficult. EFT can help if this happens, again using setup phrases based on what the client says the problem is.  For instance:

*"Even though the goal won't stay put on the line,..."*

*"Even though I get a bad feeling when I see it there on the line,..."*

*"Even though it now just feels like a To Do list into the future,..."*

Reactions like these do not mean that the technique isn't "working". Reactions like these are precise descriptions (feedback to you as coach) about what problem(s) the client has with his goal(s). The Time

Line work has therefore been **successful** in getting the client to engage with the energetic reality of his relationship to his future and his stated goals, and his energy system is now responding and giving you information about how he really feels about the goals themselves. You are in exactly the territory that you want to be in as an EFT Coach - which is working at the level of the client's energy system and away from the client's intellectual beliefs and ideas about what he "ought" to be doing with his life.

Whatever problems or "bad feeling" the client experiences while doing the Time Line work can be explored and dealt with using EFT, just as you would explore any Aspect or Reversal.

Related sections:

| | |
|---|---|
| 6.2.3 | Psychological Reversal ⇧ |
| 6.2.12 | Aspects ⇧ |
| 8.1.4 | The Compelling Way ⇧ |

## 8.1.18 Visualisations

A classic coaching technique (taken from NLP) is to get a client to strongly visualise (or hear or feel) a desired future action or outcome. This gets the client used to the idea of how it will look/hear/feel to have achieved what they want.

But the success of the technique depends crucially on how firmly or vividly the client is able to create, maintain and then inhabit the scene.

If the image is fuzzy, blurred, distant or keeps disappearing or shifting to something else, then it's not going to provide the full sensory impact that is needed to make it effective. A coach with NLP skills can check for this by finding out the current image quality and asking the client to manipulate it (*"make it brighter, clearer, bigger, more colorful, steadier"*). While this is often at least partially successful, sometimes the client just can't make it as fully vivid as they would like or the coach would like. This either indicates that the client is resistant to the image itself and there is more work to do in overcoming blocks; or that they have a general problem in generating clear mental images in this way.

Whatever the reason, tapping while visualising is a great way to loosen any energetic blocks around seeing and feeling it clearly. And once the image is good and clear, the image is effectively the trigger for a Resourceful State and EFT is a great way to anchor the image. The setups you use are based exactly on whatever "trouble" the client is having with creating or maintaining a good, stable, positive image. For example:

> *"Even though it keeps going fuzzy, …"*
>
> *"Even though I can't really hear what's being said,…"*
>
> *"Even though it's very far away and I can't make it come nearer,…"*
>
> *"Even though it keeps flipping to a different image,…"*
>
> *"Even though I just keep thinking this isn't possible,…"*

Notice that along the way these statements are picking up not only different aspects, but specific reversals. This happens quite naturally as the client responds to the attempt to create the desired visualisation and then experiences whatever difficulties or objections along the way.

Once the visualised scene has been created in a way that the client feels happy with, you can use a Choices statement to explicitly and automatically bring the image to mind when it's needed - for example anytime the client feels self-doubt about the goal:

*"Even though I have this doubt, I choose to remember this image fully and vividly"*

As well as using visualisations to help with future events, visualisation can also be used to "remodel" past events (for instance, a job interview that didn't go well, or an argument with a member of the family).

In this exercise you are asking the client to try on a new "way of being" and a new viewpoint in order to try out one or more different possible responses to a past event. The ultimate purpose of this is to alter what's possible for the client when a similar event comes up again in the future. (As is the case throughout, the purpose of examining a past event in coaching is always in order to make a future goal more achievable).

Remodelling the past in this way can be achieved through conventional coaching dialogue, simply asking the client to visualise the scene and imagine what they would have done differently.

But, sometimes the client finds it hard to contact the new "way of being" necessary to construct a new response (i.e. they are stuck in the old "way of being" that produced the result they got). This kind of "stuckness" means that EFT is likely to be of use. Example setups might be:

*"Even though I think I was right to say that and I can't imagine saying anything else, ..."*

*"Even though anyone would have done that in the same situation, ..."*

*"Even though I can't imagine any other way to handle it, ..."*

*"Even though I don't think I would have dared to say something different, ..."*

*"Even though I was so angry and out of control by that stage,..."*

EFT can be used very effectively during the visualisation to remove any fears or other negative feelings that are triggered. In doing so, it eases the way for the client to create a positive, empowered and creative state where new possibilities for behaviour come more easily.

Having successfully "remodelled" the past event, EFT can then be used to anchor the new state of being for future access and use.

*"Even though a situation like this might happen again, I choose to remember exactly how this feels and how to be this way again"*

As well as using EFT, you can use any other kind of coaching structure that you and client like to reinforce the memory and the feeling.

Related sections:

6.1.12     Coaching the Past ⇧

6.2.8      The Choices Technique ⇧

8.1.1      Anchoring Resourceful States ⇧

9.3.7      Unsticking the Client ⇩

## 8.1.19 Key Points

- EFT can be used, like NLP, within a coaching context to access, anchor and consciously trigger resourceful states within the client. This involves getting the client to tune into how a resourceful state feels (either creating it from scratch or recalling in from memory) and then embedding and anchoring it for later use with EFT. This method can also be used to used to create and anchor new strategies for dealing with situations as a precursor to releasing negative emotions that are currently being used as resourceful states, such as anger or stress.

- EFT can be a good form of homework, especially for an issue which seems to need persistent application. The client needs to be given very specific instructions regarding exact setup statements, frequency and timing to ensure that they can achieve completion. EFT can be used to address specific issues, as support for other actions (to deal with anxiety), or to help structure Inquiry homework. Mirror tapping homework can also be particularly useful for building client self-acceptance and self-esteem in a persistent but gentle way.

- EFT can be used to assist in the creation, inhabiting and selection of new perspectives on a problem. Having chosen a perspective to be taken forward into action in the client's life, the Choices technique can be used to anchor the new perspective.

- EFT can be used to enhance the Compelling Way technique by increasing the vividness of the compelling scene created during the process, and by dealing with any "Tailenders" that might be attached to the goal in question.

- EFT can support the use of conventional coaching Structures and be itself used as a Structure. Conventional Structures (objects, images, sounds) can be used as a focus while tapping in order to remove Tailenders relating to the goal or commitment they represent. The Choices format can be used as a Structure to help remind or connect clients to feelings, ways of being, habits, commitments and goals.

- EFT can be used to help a client discover and clarify what Fulfilment means to them, by addressing any feelings, blocks or Reversals that exist around the concept. As for goals, EFT can help a client distinguish what they truly find fulfilling and what they think they should find fulfilling.

- Achieving Balance is about cultivating behavioural flexibility around the client's alternative activities and demands. Since client "stuckness" (lack of behavioural flexibility) is usually rooted either in a desire for control or a fear of some kind, EFT is a useful tool in this cultivation. Achieving Balance also entails saying No when necessary - and EFT can make it easier to cut through the fears, limiting beliefs or pseudo-values which make this hard to do.

- EFT can be a support during Process coaching in two ways. Firstly it helps build the client's confidence in exploring his inner state in a safe and supported way. Secondly it asserts the acceptability of the client in whatever emotional state they may be in. EFT can also support the coach in maintaining detachment and "being with" the client in their Process. Finally, it allows the client to return to a resourceful state at the end of a Process session, if they wish.

- Metaphors encapsulate for their user, not just the physics of the situation, but very much what is going on energetically. EFT offers an additional way of working with metaphor since the client's internal energetic landscape with respect to the problem can be acted on more or less directly, by asking about Reversals and fears implied by the metaphor.

- EFT can assist client and coach to generate ideas together and come up with new options. It can be combined with metaphor elicitation questions to take the client away from conscious processing and tap unconscious creativity.

- EFT can be a great support in ensuring that client learning is conscious and fully "locked in". Standard or SLOW EFT can be used to elicit consciously the learning from a situation; and the Choices technique can be used to anchor the situation with what was learned.

- Using EFT while focussing on a Peak Experience can be useful in eliciting more fully the memories around an event and in noticing any insights or connections that may be relevant to the current situation.

- The idea of Championing can be used to raise the power of Choices statements to whole new levels. The coach can help the client generate much bigger ideas about himself or about the Choice he is making. By using Championing to help clients create powerful Choices for themselves, they are effectively learning how to Champion themselves.

- In order for clients to Do something different, they also often need to Be something different. The Choices pattern allows clients to choose who they want to be - what qualities they want to express in particular circumstances and to loosen or eliminate any emotional blocks to achieving them.

- EFT can be used to assist in shifting what a client is "tolerating" in their lives, such as low grade irritations and habits which perhaps don't cause quite enough pain that they demand to be dealt with but which nevertheless together form significant blocks to progress with bigger goals.

- Using the client's Future Self as a source of reference or wisdom can be a powerful coaching tool. EFT can be useful at times when the client feels blocked from accessing that part of themselves, EFT can also be applied as though it were the Future Self doing the tapping, in order to come up with ideas or resources for the client.

- It is possible to work on the client's belief system indirectly by using EFT to redesign the client's Time Line. By "correcting" features of the Time Line in a way chosen by the client, it is possible to address indirectly the client's underlying beliefs which chose the original representation. In particular EFT can be used to ensure the Time Line is clearly visible, without obvious gaps, breaks or walls and that the client and his goals are firmly and clearly attached to it.

- The success of using visualisations in coaching depends crucially on how firmly or vividly the client is able to create, maintain and then inhabit the scene. Tapping while visualising is a great way to loosen any energetic blocks around seeing and feeling it clearly and then to anchor the image.

# 8.2  New Techniques

This section introduces ways of using EFT which are new to coaching, and some completely new variations of EFT developed specifically for a coaching context.

## 8.2.1  Enrollment

EFT can greatly enhance your ability to enrol clients, and is therefore a great thing to introduce at recruitment seminars or taster workshops.

It is relatively fast to get people using EFT and noticing results, so they will immediately "get" that you are able to help them achieve change in a painless way. This means it can be used directly to move clients to a state where they find it easier to say Yes to signing up with you (if that's appropriate for them) because you can start delivering right then, not just promising.

A great example to use in a taster workshop setting is the issue of change. Talking about change and people's fears about it is a perfect subject for a coaching taster workshop because it cuts to the heart of what coaching is about and starts participants thinking about what changes they would like to make - or fear making.

So, imagine getting your participants to rate their fear of change out of 10, and then doing EFT with them as follows:

> *"Even though I have this fear of change, I deeply and completely accept myself"*

How much would this reduce their fear around change and make it more likely that they want to sign up for a service which offers to help them make profound changes in their lives?

Is this manipulative? Of course it is, in the sense that you are deliberately having a positive impact on participants' emotional state in order to make them feel good about hiring you. If you're running a taster workshop you are doing so in the hope that some of the participants want to sign up with you. Your choice of coaching exercises and every word you say should be designed to demonstrate your ability as a coach and to make them feel more inclined to work with you. One could easily imagine conducting some other type of conventional coaching exercise around the issue of change without worrying whether that was "manipulative".

Is it unethical? Definitely not. EFT, by it's nature is totally explicit about what is happening and what's being worked on. You are not using secret embedded commands without them realising what you're doing. Neither are you hypnotising them or using mysterious non-verbal techniques to bring them into unconscious compliance. The participants are saying out loud and with full consciousness, what they are working on. They will know that doing EFT on "fear of change" is likely to reduce their fear of change. (And if you title your workshop appropriately that will in fact be what they are hoping and expecting to get.)

If they then experience feeling more open towards the idea of change as a result of your workshop they are then free to take whatever action they feel will move them in the direction they want - which might mean signing up with you - or it might mean actually taking some action in their lives straightaway. They have full and free choice about signing with you - you have simply demonstrated your skills in a powerful way.

If you do decide to use EFT as a demonstration tool in the hope of recruitment, do beware of the Apex effect. If you are already an EFT practitioner you will know about this well documented phenomenon whereby it is actually quite possible for EFT to work but for the client to find another "explanation" for the change (*"Well, you just distracted me"*, *"I think I was ready to change anyway"*) or to deny they even had a problem to start with (*"Fear of change? Me? Never had a fear of that."*).

So in fact it is very far from inevitable that workshop participants will find themselves "mysteriously compelled" to sign with you just because you did some EFT with them. But if you can give them other more "credible" or "conventional" coaching exercises on the same subject you may be providing them with material for their Apex effect to work with (*"I don't think it was the EFT I think it was that other exercise we did before the break"*).

You can help to counter the Apex effect somewhat by careful pre-framing of the exercise before it happens, and by getting participants to create some sort of evidence for their state prior to doing the EFT - such as writing down their ratings before they begin, or even writing everybody's ratings up on a flipchart or board. For some reason, people who are prone to the Apex effect in themselves seem to have no trouble perceiving the effects of EFT in others.

## 8.2.2   Co-active Tapping

So far I have presented many ways of using EFT for the coach and the client individually. And I have recommended that when the client is tapping for their own issues that the coach taps along in order to stay connected with the client.

However there is an even more powerful use for EFT within the coaching relationship, and that is Co-active tapping. This means that both client and coach tap together for the same thing, with it being made explicit that the coach is tapping too.

It has been observed by practitioners and coaches that when two people tap together for the same issue, somehow the effect is strengthened. But I am not talking here simply about adding in the coach's surrogate tapping to the client's self-tapping (I recommend not using surrogate or proxy tapping at any time during a coaching context - see Principle of Client Responsibility). I am talking about both client and coach taking an equal part in creating an EFT session that serves the client's needs. The client is equally responsible for the direction of the session, what setup and reminder statements are used and in specifying and achieving the outcome.

Co-active EFT carries with it the same benefits as co-active coaching: it makes the client responsible for his own progress, and it empowers him to continue making progress when the coach isn't there.

Co-active tapping may be useful when:

**Client and coach have a similar issue.** For instance, the client's issue is also the coach's issue and the coach has admitted that to the client. For instance, suppose a client comes to a call feeling somewhat down that day, and suppose that the client doesn't want today's current feeling to be the subject of today's coaching. Suppose also that the coach is also feeling a little deflated today (although ideally a coach should self-manage their state, sometimes circumstances prevent this from happening). The coach could suggest *"Well, I happen to be a bit like that too today, so let's work on this together and get ourselves in a more positive state of mind."* Note, there is no surrogate or proxy tapping going on here. The client is tapping for the client and the coach is tapping for the coach. However they are tapping for the same issue and for the same ultimate purpose - to prepare to resume coaching.

**The issue relates to the coaching relationship itself.** For instance, agreements, commitments, or even the general atmosphere of the relationship. Specific applications might include occasions when coach and client need to "make up" following a misunderstanding, miscommunication or any other event that threatens to hang over the relationship and would benefit from being "cleared". An example might be if a client misses a call. The coach might legitimately ask the client to account for himself and the client might feel somewhat guilty about it, but want to continue coaching. Assuming coach and client can sort out the issue in terms of logistics and any reparation involved and both are agreed they want to continue, then using EFT to clear any residual bad feeling around the incident can be a fast way to get the relationship back on track, restore trust, rapport and so on. Using the Both Of Us pattern would be appropriate here:

*"Even though this happened, I deeply and completely accept both of us."*

**During Idea Generation.** Idea Generation together is itself a co-active coaching exercise, with both client and coach trying to do the same thing at the same time i.e. looking for ideas and insights into a problem, generating perspectives and so on. It makes sense in this context to use EFT jointly to help the creativity process.

There are probably many more ways to use EFT co-actively and these will probably be revealed as more clients and coaches work together with EFT as a tool. The limit is only the creative imagination of clients and coaches.

Related sections:

| | |
|---|---|
| 5.4.6 | Principle of Client Responsibility ⇧ |
| 8.1.3 | Perspectives ⇧ |
| 8.1.10 | Idea Generation ⇧ |
| 8.2.13 | The Both Of Us Pattern ⇩ |

## 8.2.3   Starting a Session

Clients usually bring energy and thoughts from their everyday lives to the coaching session with them. This may or may not be relevant to the intended subject of the coaching. While it can be completely valid to coach based on whatever is "up" with the client right then, it's also possible that the client will want to make sure they are properly focussed on a specific coaching goal.

EFT can be effectively used to clear any lingering stresses, annoyances, or other emotional distractions, in order to help the client focus fully on the coaching session. This is a situation where the coach **must** check out with the client whether they want to use EFT to clear their state before beginning coaching, or whether they want to use their current state as coaching material.

For instance, if the agreed coaching goals involve work/life balance, and the client has come to the session in a stressed state because work has been particularly stressful that day, then this real life event may offer great coaching material since it relates directly to the client's goal.

But even if the client's state does directly relate to their coaching goals, it doesn't mean that you can't also use EFT as a way to calm the client before beginning work. There is no rule about this, and neither should there be. This is a case where you must truly "dance in the moment" with your client, with both of you using rapport and intuition to sense what seems right at this moment. The only rule I would advise is that the client should have the final say about whether to use EFT or not - because this rule applies to **any** use of EFT within coaching.  Remember, avidity (co-operative enthusiasm as part of a designed alliance) is the goal here, not "compliance".

Example opening statements for preparing for the start of a session might be:

*"Even though it's been a stressful day, I deeply and completely accept myself."*

*"Even  though I have all these distractions going on, ..."*

*"Even though focussing on coaching seems hard right now,..."*

Using a Choices statement might also be appropriate, assuming any extreme agitation or distraction has been calmed:

*"Even though I'm distracted, I choose to focus on coaching for the next hour."*

*"Even though it's been a really tough day, I choose to focus on my future now."*

After a while, when the client is familiar with these methods, you can ask them to do this clearing for themselves prior to the session. This is a nice gentle way to introduce clients to using EFT for themselves as self-support. It encourages their self-empowerment in a very real but unpressured way, and it reinforces the co-activity of the coaching relationship.

Related sections:

6.1.4        The Designed Alliance ⇧

## 8.2.4   Ending a Session

At the end of a session, EFT can be a good way to prepare the client to get back to their life. This is especially the case if the coaching has involved some emotional work by the client, with or without the use of EFT.

While calming and grounding at the end of a session is entirely optional and up to your judgement as coach, there is a good argument for making it a regular feature of your coaching - and that is some basic Stimulus-Response psychology: people are drawn to repeat experiences that feel good, and to avoid experiences that feel bad.

Coaching works best when it is a sustained relationship over many weeks or months. A longer relationship allows the relationship to mature so that even deeper work can be accomplished. A sustained relationship ensures that when the client experiences obstacles there is support and energy to see them through it. And thinking purely about good business practice for a moment, it pays to retain a client rather than have to recruit a new one.

So what makes a client want to stay with you for more than a few sessions? It's one simple thing - being coached by you feels good, and they look forward to doing it again. Notice that I did not mention achievement of goals as a reason for staying with a coach. A client may be making good progress towards their goals, but if they are not feeling good while they do it, they are unlikely to want to stay with you as a coach.

So helping your clients feel good (emotionally strong and calm, feeling empowered to take action towards their goals) is a pretty good habit to get into. And EFT is a great way to help that happen.

The use of EFT to end a session depends on the state the client is actually in - and choice of statement should always be determined by what's actually going on with the client rather than using a stock example. But there are two typical situations where EFT may be useful.

### 8.2.4.1   The Client is "Down"

Sometimes the coaching session ends at a point where the client is struggling with an issue or is experiencing realisations which they are finding unsettling. An example may be during Process coaching. I'm not talking about extreme levels distress or trauma - but more everyday examples that ordinary people experience every day with or without coaching going on, such as realising they really do have to start tackling their relationship issues because it's starting to affect their health or their career; or realising the cost that a particular habit has had on their lives.

Unless I believe that the client is in a resourceful state likely to lead to positive action and learning, this is not a state in which I choose to leave a client. However, the final judgement rests with the client - and there should be a co-active discussion about how the client is now feeling and how the session could most usefully be ended.

Assuming that the client does want to be brought out of the "down" state, then a round or two of "basic" EFT will relax and calm the client.

> *"Even though I feel <this way>, I deeply and completely accept myself."*

This can be a valid use of EFT if the client wants to feel better but also wants to have the process of working through the core issues themselves or in another way later on. Some clients - especially independent ones - appreciate the fact that the process isn't taken away from them.

It is also an option to do a more "thorough" EFT - addressing the root of the issue. But beware this can take a long time - perhaps as long as the entire coaching session - so it may not be practical as a session closer unless you are fairly sure you can nail the root issue in a few rounds (which may be possible if you have been talking around the issue for a while and picking up clues).

A hybrid option is to do some basic EFT to calm the client, and then set homework for the client to work on some of the deeper issues by themselves - if the client feels they want to and their proficiency with EFT is reasonable.

### 8.2.4.2  The Client is "Up" or "Scattered"

I remember one particularly enjoyable coaching session I had (I was the client) in which I discovered a state of being I called "The Blue Space" - which enabled me to view everything from a very detached and spiritual perspective and was a great place to visit for refreshment and general emotional re-grouping. At the end of the session I was really feeling rather lightheaded (in a very pleasant way) and wasn't really ready to leave The Blue Space yet, but immediately was required to come "down to earth" and resume a training course I was on.

You can bring your clients back down to earth in a very controlled way without in any way taking away the intensity or value of the experience they have just had, using EFT or selected meridian points.

Sometimes the client has just "been through a lot" during the session, and although there is no specific issue left unresolved, their energy system is feeling a bit "scattered" and could do with a bit of "pulling together" before getting back to normal life.

The following are useful for grounding an "up" or "scattered" client.

Assuming no extreme negative intensity is present, then you can go straight to using a Choices format. For instance:

> *"Even though I feel like this, I choose to be fully present with all my senses working fine"*

> *"Even though I feel like this I choose to feel grounded and present."*

> *"Even though I love being in the Blue Space, I choose to come back to earth now."*

But straightforward EFT can also be used:

> *"Even though I feel like this I deeply and completely accept myself"*

which will have a generally calming and balancing effect.

Alternatively, you can ask the client to tap or rub just the Under Nose and Chin points for a few seconds. These points relate to the Central and Governing Meridians which run up and down the font and back of the body. These two meridians together produce a general strengthening and energising feeling. And because they both run through the lower part of the torso, there is a general feeling of physical grounding and solidity produced.

Related sections:

## 8.2.5   What do you Want to Coach Today?

Sometimes in coaching there can arise a genuine conflict between "being with the client where they are" (also known as Process Coaching) and forwarding the client's agenda (Principle of Goal Furtherence). In my experience as a coaching client, it's one of the biggest pitfalls.

Having agreed on a set of coaching goals, it's all too easy to begin each coaching session by saying *"OK - so what's going on with you today?"* or even just *"How are you?"*. This leads straight to whatever is on the client's mind, what dramas have been going on in their life over the past week, and so on - and these things may or may not have anything to do with their goals.

A client you have rapport with is unlikely to say to you *"I'd rather not go into that, let's get on with the coaching"*. Having replied to your opening question, it is then all too easy to begin coaching based on that reply. Again, it can be very hard for a client to say *"Hang on a minute, this isn't what I want to be coached on."* And it's not just because they feel obliged to go along with the line of conversation - but because, by definition, this is the most important thing on their minds right now and so they are also eager to get into discussion about it.

Of course, the remedy for this problem does not necessarily require EFT. It only requires the coach to "hold the client's agenda" and seek agreement at the start of the coaching about what the client wants to have as the focus of coaching today.

But what happens if you ask the client and the client doesn't know? What do you do if the client is genuinely torn between "today's hot issue" and their wider coaching goals? If they are torn, there will probably be some "shoulds" and "oughts" operating - and of course there will be some emotional conflict. Also be aware that "choosing to coach today's issue" can provide clients with a wonderful way of indefinitely avoiding their main coaching goals.

EFT can be helpful in resolving such decisions. The first approach is simply to calm or clear today's issue, so that it is less insistent for the client (see Starting a Session) and then ask the question again.

But it is also possible to use EFT as a way to understand what's most important. Using a conflict pattern (see Conflicting Beliefs) is a good way of testing the question:

> *"Even though I want to focus on my goal **and** I want to talk about what happened today,..."*

I cannot tell you how much as a client and as a coach, getting genuine resolution on "what to coach" assists the development of the overall relationship. It builds huge confidence in the client that the time (and money) is being well spent on what's most important - and it builds confidence in the coach that they are truly gaining permission and serving the client's real needs.

## 8.2.6  Finding the Learning

Learning is the bedrock of the ongoing coaching relationship. It's the learning the client gets from his actions which result in the flexibility required to achieve the end goal as well as the growth and empowerment of the client as a person.

You can do a fair proportion of the important work in coaching simply by asking the question *"What did you learn?"*. But sometimes the learning isn't easy to find. Sometimes the client can come back with an answer that is glib:

> *"Well, I learned not to try that again!"*

or superficial:

> *"I learned I need to plan more carefully next time"*

or even just very defensive:

> *"I learned this is harder than I thought" (i.e. let's stop looking at the goal and start focussing on how inadequate I am.)*

Of course there are coaching techniques to get past these types of initial response (simply asking *"and what else?"* can achieve great things).  But what if the client seems genuinely stuck? Not just stuck in their bad feelings around the event, but stuck around seeing what learning there is to be noticed.

EFT can help - and it relates to understanding what learning is and what prevents it.

Learning **anything** involves a shift in viewpoint - whether it's how to solve a new kind of maths problem, learning how a different culture deals with a specific life event, or a new skill to use in coaching. Something that was outside your current universe of experience or knowledge suddenly becomes part of it. What was invisible or inaccessible has become visible and accessible to you. It's actually an expansion of consciousness.

But what about learning in the context of learning from a failure or event you were involved in? Again, it's about acquiring a new viewpoint on the situation. Specifically, learning in this context requires moving out of an "associated" viewpoint (e.g. reliving the memory of the experience, which triggers the bad feelings of "I failed") and into a "dissociated" viewpoint of seeing the experience from a different vantage point.

In conventional coaching there are techniques for achieving this. For instance, asking *"What would your Future Self say your learning was here?"* invites the client to consider the event from the point of view of 20 years in the future.  But sometimes (and I have experienced this myself as a client), the client is **so** strongly associated into the current experience that accessing the Future Self viewpoint or any other, is too difficult.

What keeps a client stuck in association with an event? Strong emotion. The very emotion that was triggered by the event has the client in its grip, and the intensity of it keeps the client's thoughts on a trammel line focussed on the negativity of the event. Cognition and emotion literally feed off each other and reinforce one another in a vicious cycle.

EFT is a great way to unstick the client and break this cycle, by reducing the intensity of the emotion around the event. Once the emotion is reduced, the client has a chance of getting out of the associated (attached) viewpoint and trying out other viewpoints. And this starts generating useful learning from the event which she can then use for future attempts.

Standard EFT can be used to target the association:

> *"Even though I keep seeing it the same way…"*

> *"Even though I don't think there is another angle on this …"*

…or the learning:

> *"Even though I can't see the learning in this yet…"*

…or any other fear or issue around finding the learning:

> *"Even though I'm afraid of what this might mean…"*

> *"Even though I don't want to learn anything from this…"*

> *"Even though I think it's X who should be learning from this, not me…"*

SLOW EFT can also be useful (perhaps as homework) to allow any learning to come through without having to delve around too much into what's stopping it. The client simply needs to focus on the relevant event while repeating "Learning" as the reminder phrase.

Sometimes the significance of the event is so great and the emotion so strong that it's clear the client will need time to mull it over. Rather than let the client off the hook, Choices statements are a good way of setting an intention to find the learning, but allowing it to not be right now. For example:

> *"Even though I can't see the learning right now, I choose to be open to seeing it soon."*

> *"Even though I'm afraid of what the learning might be, I choose to learn only what's safe and useful for me to learn right now."*

> *"Even though I don't think there can possibly be any learning in this, I choose to believe that some learning might be possible."*

It's important to remember that there is more at stake here than just the learning from this one event. You are educating your client about the importance of learning generally as a primary feature of what makes coaching work. Even if the client doesn't arrive at much learning this time, establishing an approach to looking for it, and making it a pleasant process, helps to prepare the client to be on the look out for learning in the future. The Choices examples above are likely to be helpful in this respect.

Related sections:

6.1.16     Action and Learning ⇧

6.2.8      The Choices Technique ⇧

6.2.9      SLOW EFT ⇧

8.1.2.3    Inquiries and Insights ⇧

8.1.16     Accessing the Future Self ⇧

9.3.7      Unsticking the Client ⇩

## 8.2.7   Minimising the Coaching Plateau

It is a common and well documented feature of the coaching relationship that after the initial excitement of the first couple of months has worn off, that clients enter what is termed a "coaching plateau". They may have made a great start towards their goals, but at some point they run out of steam. Real life starts to intrude, finding time for homework suddenly seems hard, they may become discouraged or the enormity of their goal starts to become real to them. In short, the honeymoon is over and the real work begins.

What was new, exciting and full of hope, has now become "business as usual" and therefore part of the scenery. On top of that though, some of the client's "writing on the walls" will be kicking in and starting to bo heard.

As a coach you may have successfully dealt with the client's Reversals and Gremlins around getting **started** with their project. But there are probably a whole lot of other Reversals around **continuing** with it over time, and more again around the idea of **completing** it. (This is probably why some people are great initiators but never seem to see things through, while other people are hopeless at innovation but are great at picking up someone else's project and finishing it).

Many coaches protect themselves from client disappointment by explaining the plateau to their client at the start of the coaching relationship. (What great "writing on the walls" is **that** for a new client? It's a bit like meeting a new romance and on the second date informing them that *"you will get very bored with me in about 6 months time and then we will have to do some serious work to make sure this works"*. It may be true, but what is the effect on the relationship **now** of saying it?).

And then when it happens, they simply point out to the client that "this is the plateau" and remind the client that this is where the real work begins. It's not an inspiring way to approach the problem. In fact it is likely to reinforce the client's existing negative beliefs about goal achievement (*"achieving goals is hard"*, *"this isn't going to be fun"* etc). Sometimes I even suspect coaches of **liking** the plateau as a kind of justification for the fun and enjoyment involved in the rest of their job - a kind of very insidious work ethic that says *"All worthwhile work must include some boring or difficult aspects to prove it's a serious thing."*

I believe EFT offers a way to minimise the effects of this problem and to help kick-start the client again. What is the "plateau" really a plateau of? It's probably fair to say that what has "plateaued" is the client's energy in relation to their goal. And since EFT is an energy technique, the EFT Coach is uniquely equipped to help the client regain their positive energy and get off the plateau and back into excitement and progress again.

Doing this effectively depends on the creativity of the coach. But the most important thing of all is **noticing** when it happens and addressing it in the coaching. Here are two specific ways to address the coaching plateau using EFT.

Related sections:

6.1.17      Gremlins ⇧

6.2.2      Working with the Client's Energy System ⇧

6.2.3      Psychological Reversal ⇧


## 8.2.7.1    Dealing with Niggles

Sometimes what looks like a "plateau" is actually a dip. Specific negative feelings are starting to creep in. Clients who have been having a good experience of the coaching so far can be reluctant to voice their negative feelings when they first arise, either to themselves or to the coach. But they "niggle" in the background and over time they show up as a general reduction in motivation and energy available for the coaching. By addressing these niggles head on, they don't get a chance to destroy the coaching.

Niggles can be about anything and may or may not be the real issue - but they all boil down to one thing - the client isn't enjoying the coaching process as much as they were - and the client will notice that feeling and will look around at possible explanations for that. Most often those explanations will be dissatisfactions with the coaching itself e.g.: the rate of progress being made, the money, the time etc. and can show up as questions to the coach *"So, how do you think I'm doing - how many more sessions do you think I'll need?"*, *"I'm getting a bit concerned about how much money I'm spending on all this."*

Doing EFT on such issues will either dissipate them, or bring forward the real issue behind it:

*"Even though I'm frustrated with our progress…"*

*"Even though the money bothers me,…"*

*"Even though finding the time every week is getting difficult,..."*

This needs to be done with sensitivity, however. Responding to a client's concerns about the coaching with an immediate suggestion to use EFT, can be taken to imply that they are somehow "wrong" for having the concern. Using EFT in this context should not be a substitute for open discussion with the coach.

Ultimately if a client is having negative feelings or concerns about the coaching then client and coach need to be re-designing the alliance to correct things. But clients can find it hard to tell their coach they're not happy - instead they end up just going through the motions for a while and then leaving. Using EFT to address the things the client **does** feel able to talk about can open the way for a lot more honesty from the client about what they really need from the coaching relationship.

## 8.2.7.2    Reconnecting with the Goal

It is the client's goal(s) that brought them to coaching and got them excited and into action initially. And it can be reconnecting with the goal(s) that can get the client off the plateau and enjoying the coaching process again.

What can happen is that once a goal has been defined and the necessary action planned out, the focus moves away from the end goal and onto the actions. Focussing on the actions can often take the coaching into less fun territory - like working through blocks.

While the client's initial vision of their goal may have been bright and shiny (after using The Compelling Way or some other visualisation method), the subsequent "less fun" work has taken the shine off a bit - and all this work and angst is becoming associated with the goal itself.

EFT can be used to "take a cloth" to the goal and make it shine again. This can be done by getting the client to list all the ways in which he now feels less than inspired by the goal. What you will be eliciting here is the client's "writing on the walls" that is relevant to making steady progress on a project and project completion. You will be looking for Tailenders and Aspects that have arisen in relation to the goal(s) that perhaps were not being triggered at the start of the coaching process.

Some issues that might come up include:

*"Even though I'm starting to realise what I've really let myself in for..."*

*"Even though it's normal for get the blues halfway through a project,..."*

*"Even though I'm not sure I've got what it takes to see it through,..."*

*"Even though I'm not sure it's all worth it anyway,..."*

*"Even though the end seems such a long way off,..."*

It's tempting as a coach to think *"But I thought we covered all the blocks and tailenders at the start"*. This is where it's helpful to understand Aspects and how they operate. You may well have covered these issues from the point of view (Aspect) of starting out on a **new** project. But thinking about these things from the viewpoint (Aspect) of being a few months in, can be entirely different. It really is a case of *"That was then, but this is now."* You need to stay with your client and deal with what comes up **now**. And that means looking at the goal again from this new viewpoint, seeing what fears, blocks or other problems present themselves and using EFT on those.

Related sections:

6.2.12    Aspects ⇑

6.2.15    Tailenders ⇑

8.1.4    The Compelling Way ⇑

## 8.2.8  Ecology Testing

*"An ecology check...is a close look at how your proposed action or change will affect the many interrelationships and interlocking systems in your life. ... It gives you a means of evaluating the outcome of your actions to ensure that they have the impact you want while checking for any undesirable consequences"* [4]

There's nothing more likely to put the dampers on a client's enthusiasm than doing an ecology check. I well remember a sample session with a coach (not a CTI coach!) in which he asked me what I would do if my plan to leave my job and start out on my own failed? It was an instant turn off. I did not want anyone putting me back in to the state of stagnation and fear that had prevented me making the move for years.

With hindsight I know that in his particular way, that coach was trying to understand what fallback plans I had in place. (I didn't have any! I barely had a plan for the success part!) His aim was probably to help me create a fallback plan, make my position less risky and probably help to secure my success in the long run. But right at that moment, my train was running on 99% enthusiasm and 1% realism - and his question was like pouring water on the coals it had taken me over ten years to finally get alight!

Unfortunately, if you want your client to achieve lasting change and to pick goals that will really enhance their lives (rather than simply shake them up), an ecology check somewhere along the line **is** essential and responsible. Your job as coach is not simply to see how brave, foolhardy, macho or ambitious your client can be before some aspect of his life (work, family, friends, health) starts pushing back and saying *"Hey - what's going on? Is this supposed to be helping?"*.

It is inherent to the idea of Balance coaching that ecology issues are addressed right from day one. A Balance coach isn't going to accept the client's single goal of setting up in business without also doing a wheel of life exercise to see what other issues are sitting out there. This discussion in itself can bring out many of the important areas of the client's life that could be impacted upon by the achievement of the goal.

However, sometimes the simple asking of a question like *"So how will it affect your marriage if you succeed at this goal?"*, can be enough to throw the client into a tailspin. Just the thought that it **might** have a negative impact could be enough for many clients to think *"Oh well, my coach thinks it might be bad for my marriage"* and perhaps drop their goal altogether. Many a business hasn't got started or a new job or promotion hasn't been applied for, for fear of the impact on family or personal life. But this isn't the aim of the coach's question. It really does mean *"Tell me what the possible impact might be, so we can work out how to manage that"*.

Now of course, a skilled coach will be able to think of many forms of language and pre-framing of the subject so that the client understands in advance what the questions are designed to do and why the coach is asking them. But even so, ecology checking can be a bit of an emotional minefield.

It is a minefield in the sense that this type of conversation usually occurs very early on in the coaching relationship, as part of the intake or goal-setting sessions. At this point, the client is unknown territory for the coach. If the aim is to anticipate the outcome of planned action, from the client's point of view, then the client's anticipated outcome is going to be based on a whole set of beliefs about himself, his abilities, his stamina, his worthiness, none of which have yet been properly explored by the coach.

These questions all have the potential to trigger these beliefs, any one of which might actually be a "killer block" to the whole enterprise. As a coach you may trigger a block like this and remain completely unaware of what that block might be - all you can see is a client who suddenly seems to have lost all interest in the goal or who takes themselves off to another coach who seems better able to share in their enthusiasm (as I did!).

EFT can be a great way of diminishing the emotional devastation (or even slight rocking) that ecology type questions can cause, while it is happening.

Perhaps the easiest way to use EFT in this situation is simply to tap along all the way through the conversation (or if tapping is too distracting, then holding the points in turn and moving point every now and again). Tapping while talking helps to minimise the emotional impact of anything difficult that is discussed - making it easier to consider the "sensible" questions but without putting a dent in the client's confidence.

But it also helps the process of answering the questions creatively. So perhaps the client starts thinking about how this business venture might affect his marriage - and while tapping suddenly sees not only what might be a challenge, but also how this could be minimised and even how it could be enhanced.

Here is one technique for getting the client to start becoming aware of his own ecology issues and without the coach having to ask questions which could be perceived as judgemental and which simultaneously reduces any "down" effect of considering them.

Give the client a set list of issues and ask them to do SLOW EFT on each item as Homework. The point of the set list is deliberate. It depersonalises the issues and removes any hint of personal judgement by the coach (i.e. *"I ask all my clients these questions"*). Secondly, by simply naming the areas, it totally avoids the need to use judgemental language in order to ask the question. This means the client may just as well come up with positive insights as negative ones. By doing them as Homework (the client writes down any thoughts or feelings that occur to them while they do SLOW EFT on each one) it is made extremely clear that these are client-generated ideas. Any negativity has not come from the coach - the coach is there to help work through the negativity but isn't the source of it.

The list of items can vary according to the field of coaching you are working in or the type of goal being worked on. For general coaching you could choose the areas on the classic Wheel of Life - or ask the client to tell you the 6-10 most important areas of their lives. Try to give the client as much physical space as you can to record their responses, but also try to limit the size of the worksheet to one side of paper so it's not overwhelming.

So the worksheet you give the client might look like the table below. I have deliberately avoided asking the client to focus on a question about their goal (e.g. *"What impact will this goal have on this area of my life"*), but on the fact of the goal itself. It's also useful to ask the client to write down the goal(s) they intend to focus on at the top of the sheet so that you know what it is and they don't switch aspects on themselves part way through the process. Whatever the client writes down is then material for the next coaching session.

This exercise assumes the client is familiar and comfortable with the use of EFT before they begin.


Instructions:

Focus on your chosen goal or set of goals while you do one complete round of SLOW EFT for each Life area. For each Life area, notice any thoughts, feelings, images or ideas that occur to you during the tapping and write them down on the right hand side.

| Life area | Results |
|---|---|
| Financial | |
| Partner | |
| Children | |
| Friends/Social | |
| Career | |
| Spiritual | |
| Health | |

Alternatively, you could use the Wheel of Life as a template, providing space for clients to write, and to record their starting satisfaction scores with each area, as shown:

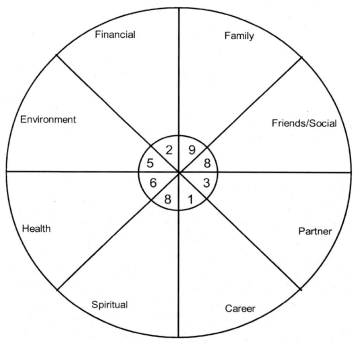

Related sections:

6.1.6 Balance Coaching ⇧


## 8.2.9  Dealing with Failure

*"When we are working with EFT, our paradigm always is Failure=Feedback and whatever the outcome of the test, it will clearly prescribe the next step that needs to be taken as a totally helpful and supportive part of the process…"* [4]

It's not that coaches want clients to fail - but when they do, failures can be one of the richest sources of learning and growth available (see Locking in the Learning). EFT can help reap the rewards of failure in several ways.

It's the coach's job to call the client to account when they fail or backslide on a commitment. But making this call can be hard for the coach to do if they happen to know how much it took the client to even make the commitment and how bad they now feel about failing. Some coaches don't explicitly call the client on their failure on the grounds that "the way they feel now is probably punishment enough". Coaches also tend to be caring people, good at seeing things from their clients' point of view and don't enjoy rubbing their clients' noses in it when they don't meet a commitment. Or worse, the coach may blame themselves for not doing sufficient work with the client beforehand to make failure impossible.

Having EFT up your sleeve is a way to call client's on their failed commitments while simultaneously offering a way to get the client off the ground and ready to have another go.

Related sections:

8.1.11     Locking in the Learning ⇧


### 8.2.9.1  Bouncing Back from Failure

During the coaching the client will be taking steps towards his goal through agreed actions. Sometimes, these actions aren't successful - or they aren't carried out at all - and the client has to report to the coach that they have "failed".

As an EFT practitioner, you will know that if a client makes a commitment and doesn't follow through with it, there is probably an energy problem somewhere (barring genuine emergency which physically prevented the commitment occurring). Energy problems are always present any time the client doesn't do something that will move them towards something they want (or say they want). And if it wasn't an energy problem that produced the failure (unlikely but theoretically possible), there surely will be an energy problem around the way the client now **feels** about his failure, the commitment he made to himself, about his goal and possibly even about the coaching process itself.

Addressing these feelings around the failure with EFT is a good place to start, before moving on to what actually happened and why the failure occurred. Asking the client to account for his failure while he is in a state of disappointment, self-blame, possibly fear at what you might say etc, is a way to reinforce how horrible, dangerous and generally not-OK it is to have failed. This is not what we as coaches want from the failure - we want learning and we want re-commitment to the goal. It's hard to get to that place from feeling angry, fearful and despondent.

EFT can help the client bounce back from failure faster by addressing any negative emotions around what happened.

*"Even though I failed, I deeply and completely accept myself"*

*"Even though I totally messed that up,…"*

*"Even though I knew I was going to fail all along,…"*

*"Even though I feel like a complete fool now,…"*

*"Even though I hate myself for messing it up,…"*

*"Even though I've always been a dud and this just proves it,…"*

The goal here is for the client to feel "zero" negative intensity when he thinks about the "failure". Usually this will be accompanied by a different attitude towards the failure e.g.

*"Well, I can always try again can't I?"*

*"Well, no-one died - it's not the end of the world."*

*"At least I learned something I can use next time."*

When you hear your client talking about the future instead of the event, you can be sure that the failure is effectively dealt with i.e. it's no longer holding them back emotionally. (This is a nice example where using EFT on a past event serves to quickly bring the coaching back onto focusing on the future).

However, failure is an area that seems to have the power to bring forth clients' deepest and most violent self-loathing and feelings of inadequacy. And so it is not uncommon for initial rounds of EFT to not clear the client's feelings completely. Whenever a rating falls and then sticks, it's a sign that the client has some emotional investment in maintaining this feeling - usually an underlying belief in their own inadequacy. Shrugging off a failure is incongruent with a belief system that expects to fail, think it deserves to fail etc, and so it may well be that the feeling of failure may stick at a 1 or a 2 if this is the case. Clearing this would require delving into the client's beliefs about failure in general (see section below)

Although the client's own words should always be used as the basis for setup statements, dealing with any kind of failure makes this especially important. However, clients usually edit what they say, so it is worthwhile as coach encouraging the client to express exactly what they are thinking and to use those words. If the client really cannot do this in your presence then set it as homework.

When the client learns that he can bounce back from failure quickly, he is more likely to take a risk in the future and attempt ventures that previously would have been impossible because of the fear of failure.

Related sections:

6.1.10    The Client Has the Answers ⇧


## 8.2.9.2    Clearing Past Failure

If a coaching client comes to the coaching with a particular goal in mind, the chances are that this is a goal that the client has attempted once or many times before, unsuccessfully. Even if there have been no actual attempts, probably the client has had the goal in mind for some time, and may be feeling like a failure simply for not taking action yet.

This can be a challenge, since the client comes to the coaching with a history of failure around the goal and possibly therefore some scepticism or negative feelings about the possibility of success this time.

But it is also a gift to the EFT Coach. Looking at what the client did before, perhaps many times, can be useful from two perspectives.

Firstly it gives both client and coach insights into the client's habitual behaviour patterns around this goal, signalling possible danger areas where the client might need more support this time. In other words it gives the coach advance warning about the types of block that need to be dealt with and EFT work can start immediately based on real information (rather than what the client thinks "might be" a problem).

Secondly, it offers a chance to deal with any feelings of failure set up on those previous attempts and which could be operating now. Dealing with failure before trying again can be effective in preventing another failure once the coaching gets under way. This is a most pro-active way of using EFT to assist in the coaching.

So some example setups might include:

*"Even though I've tried this before and failed, ..."*

*"Even though I know I should have done this years ago but didn't, ..."*

*"Even though the more I fail the more I think it's not worth trying, ..."*

*"Even though I think I must be a bit crazy to keep going with this idea, ..."*

*"Even though I've no idea what to do differently this time, ..."*

Related sections:

9.3        Blocks ⇩

9.4        Habits ⇩


## 8.2.9.3    Changing the Client's Relationship with Failure

As well as helping a client deal with specific failures along the way, or specific failure in the past, EFT can also be used to help change the client's relationship with Failure generally. This can happen incrementally to some degree simply by dealing with failures as they occur. But it's also possible to address the issue of Failure more abstractly.

At first sight this might seem like heading into "therapy" territory (examining why the client has their specific relationship to Failure, what past events may have set that up and so on) - but it is not. It is looking at the client's **current** belief system around an issue which is affecting the client's **current** ability to create the future he wants.

Using EFT in this way involves considering the client's energetic relationship to Failure quite apart from any specific failures that have occurred recently or in the past. In other words, for many people even hearing the word "Failure" is a trigger all by itself. Even discussing the possibility of failure becomes uncomfortable - which makes it hard to talk openly about risk, which in turn can cut off constructive planning towards a goal that the client feels is risky.

Indeed, there may be other words related to Failure which can be "triggers" in their own right and which may be part of the client's general relationship to Failure. Examples include: Loser, Risk, Poor, Weak etc. But each client will have a set of triggers unique to him.

EFT can be used to lessen the client's negative emotional reaction to all of these triggers.

*"Even though the word X makes me uncomfortable, I deeply and completely accept myself"*

The goal is for the client to be able to use the trigger word without feeling any negative intensity at all.

At first sight it might seem that reducing a client's fear of Failure might be doing him a disservice. If someone loses their fear of something, won't that make them more likely to seek it out and embrace it?

Actually it is this very type of thinking that creates millions of people who are afraid to fail - and therefore afraid to act at all. We've been trained to avoid failure as a self-protection mechanism - it's part of the "writing on our walls". It is this highly effective training that keeps people in jobs they don't like and which makes people hire coaches to help them take risks they feel unable to take on their own.

One of the strongest character traits of entrepreneurs is their unusual attitude to risk and failure. Entrepreneurial personalities consistently treat risk as a **necessary** precursor to success, and failure as an occupational hazard but not a reason to stop trying. Entrepreneurs in any field (whether business, social, academic or anything else) demonstrate that losing one's fear of failure does **not** mean seeking out failure or making it more likely to happen. And this is simply because there is a more dominant desire at work. Feeling comfortable with the idea of failure is balanced and far outweighed by the desire to succeed, and so the overall motivation is to succeed **despite** the possibility of failure.

Ironically, it is the people who retain a fear of failure who **invite** failure most strongly. When the fear of failure is strong, this fear can outweigh the desire to succeed, and so no action is taken and so success is not possible. Thus, fear of failure makes ultimate failure much more likely, since goals are never even attempted.

Related sections:

5.1         EFT isn't (Psycho)therapy ⇧

## 8.2.9.4    Failure = Feedback

Once the feelings around specific failures or "failure" in general have been cleared, the client will now be able to look at failure in a completely different way. First of all it will be a lot easier for him to be honest about what actually happened - he will be able to tell the story as though it were a movie that happened to someone else. This makes it a lot easier for client and coach to get to the truth about what happened. When the client can tell the unvarnished truth about what happened, learning is maximised (because alternative viewpoints are possible). And the truth about what happened makes a good basis for taking action to prevent the same problem happening again.

As a coach, you need to be learning too. You are looking for any Tailenders, blocks or Aspects that were involved in the failure and which weren't addressed before. It tells you exactly what work needs to happen before you ask the client to re-commit.

Perhaps the most difficult sort of failure to deal with in coaching is when the action concerned was preceded by a great deal of coaching work, preparation, or even EFT, to try and identify and clear possible blocks.

If the client "fails" under these circumstances, the coach knows how to get the client to bounce back - but what about the coach? Coaches frequently get so passionate about their client's goals that it's possible for them to experience any "failure" as much as the client, especially if the coach was involved in preparing the client for action.

But what does it mean if you use EFT to clear as many blocks as you and the client can think of, and the client still fails (assuming it wasn't for reasons outside the client's control)?

In all uses of EFT, this kind of "failure" means only one thing:- there are more Aspects to the issue which haven't been addressed yet. Gary Craig emphasises over and over again, that although someone may be reporting a "zero" for their issue in an EFT session, the **only** test of whether the issue is fully cleared is when the client goes back into real life and has to deal with the issue for real. Only real life - actually carrying out the action - will tell you whether there are any more Aspects that need clearing.

So when you send a client back into real life to carry out a step towards their goal, it is a test. It's an experiment to see whether the client can carry it out without blocks or fears occurring, or whether there are more blocks to be dealt with.

When a client comes back and reports a "failure", the ideal response of the EFT Coach is *"Really, how interesting, so what actually happened?"*. The client will know precisely how they felt, what triggered those feelings and so on, because they were just there. Having access to such a recent event in the client's life means the coach has great fresh material to work with. All that's needed is to work through the event, applying EFT for every identifiable trigger.

Viewed this way, all "failure" really **is** only feedback - that is, information to help the coach fine-tune their application of EFT.

And viewed this way, the client is to be congratulated on their willingness to try the action and **successfully** find Aspects that needed clearing.

Related sections:

| | |
|---|---|
| 6.2.12 | Aspects ⇧ |
| 6.2.15 | Tailenders ⇧ |
| 9.3.3 | Blocks as Reasons Why Not ⇧ |

## 8.2.10 Handling Success

Coaching should be about success. Planning for it, defining it, visualising it, taking action towards it. So when success happens in a client's life it deserves special attention. It should be providing the client with a taste of something so good that they will want more and be spurred on to achieve more of what they want. So here are a couple of EFT techniques for helping clients really taste and benefit from their own success.

### 8.2.10.1 Failure to Feel Successful

Believe it or not there are many clients - especially the high achieving or perfectionist ones - who are great at handling failure (they bounce right back, give themselves a good talking to and get right back on the horse all in one mighty leap), but are lousy at handling success. What I mean is, clients who having just completed a challenging homework assignment or significant milestone in their project, get congratulated by the coach and then just say:

> *"Yeah well, there's a hell of a way to go still"*, or

> *"Well, I think that just means it was easier than I thought, so it's no big deal"*, or even

> *"I really messed up that bit at the end, god what an idiot"*.

These clients are able to make their own successes feel like failures. In terms of their energy systems, they are confirming all their worst fears to themselves about their failings, their weaknesses and their ultimate worthlessness. It's a way to make their self-belief systems right, even in the face of the evidence.

If these clients have expressed any kind of interest in having more Fulfilment in their lives, the coach should be noticing and pointing out to this client that by dismissing their success in this way, they just missed an opportunity to experience Fulfilment. A coach should probably be curiously asking the client how they managed to do that to themselves after such a significant success. After all, what is the point of achieving these goals if it doesn't in some way add to the total amount of happiness, satisfaction or Fulfilment?

This can be a massive breakthrough for many clients who operate from this "way of being". Often it is moments exactly like this that turn the client's attention from Doing to Being as a goal to spend time on. They start to understand the personal cost of permanently being on their own case and never having time to smell the roses.

So assuming the client's response to this situation is that they are open to wanting to experience their successes more positively, what can you do and how can EFT help?

An NLP technique for enhancing the experience of positive events is to ensure that the client is in a state of association with respect to the event (they are experiencing it from within their own body, looking out of their own eyes at the thing they have completed or created). A state of association tends to put people more in touch with their feelings about a situation. Dissociated states on the other hand involve the person viewing themselves from the outside and the accompanying frame of mind is one of objectivity and intellectual distance - the very sort of viewpoint that invites self-judgement, self-criticism, seeing the action within the context of a longer project and so forth.

EFT can help people who find it hard to obtain and maintain associated states, simply by the physical act of tapping. Tapping really forces the person to feel the physicality of their body and inhabit it rather than drifting off mentally somewhere else. But EFT tapping will also help to loosen any resistances that the client has to allowing themselves to feel good about what they have done.

It is possible, (if the client is interested), to explore specific reasons (Reversals) for why the client doesn't allow themselves to celebrate their successes. The usual sort of elicitation questions would be used here, such as *"What would it mean if you were to just totally accept your success right now?"*. The answers you get back then form the basis for setup statements:

> *"Even though I'm afraid that I won't have any motivation to do anything if I stop and celebrate now..."*

> *"Even though I really don't **feel** like a success after doing that..."*

> *"Even though my parents always told me not to rest on my laurels..."*

> *"Even though I'm afraid I'll lose my momentum because celebrating equals stopping..."*

> *"Even though I don't think this really counts as a success because success is big things like winning an Olympic medal or getting a Nobel prize..."*

> *"Even though now I've actually done it, it doesn't seem like such a big deal after all,..."*

If this work results in any degree of movement by the client such that they begin to express and experience the feeling of success, following up with the Celebration pattern (below) can be used to further embed the feeling.

Related sections:

6.1.5     Fulfilment Coaching ⇧

6.2.3     Psychological Reversal ⇧

8.2.10.2  The Celebration Pattern ⇩

### 8.2.10.2  The Celebration Pattern

The above has shown how to deal with that situation where the client has succeeded but doesn't feel good about it.

It's equally important to know how to get the most from the time(s) that a client comes to a call flushed with success, feeling positive and on top of the world. If this is a rare event for the client (or even if it isn't), then it's important to fully acknowledge the success and the **feeling** of success. Right now, your client is fully "tuned in" to the feeling of success - so this makes it the best time to tap.

The "Celebration pattern" is a variation on the Non-Judgement pattern. It replaces the "problem" with a description of the good feeling, and the acceptance phrase is optionally altered to include either the client, the feeling itself, or both.

> *"I feel <good feeling>, and I deeply and completely accept myself and this feeling."*

So, for example:

> *"I feel really great about this, and I deeply and completely accept myself"*

> *"I really like this feeling, and I deeply and completely accept this feeling."*

> *"I'm feeling totally positive at the moment, and I deeply and completely accept myself and this feeling."*

But what are we tapping **for**? Isn't EFT about getting rid of problems?

When I first had the idea to tap as a response to feeling good, it was with the thought of carrying out a "pre-emptive strike" on any Tailenders that might possibly be lurking ready to bring me out of my good feeling, diminish it or otherwise make me feel differently about the good thing that just happened. For instance:

> *"Well, it was nice to feel good for a while, but that's not your normal state is it?"*

> *"You can't stay like that forever you know."*

> *"Well the thing that made you feel good has gone away now, so the feeling should too."*

This remains an excellent reason for tapping and is fully consistent with EFT practitioners' understanding of Tailenders and how they work. Which is nice in theory, but how does it actually feel?

But having actually experimented with it on myself and on other people, I have noticed a particular effect which I believe makes this particular use of EFT valuable to clients.

One person I did this with, reported absolutely no change of "intensity" of feeling good. But the "quality" changed subtly to *"...feeling more solid somehow - like I really believed it."* And this was after just **one** round of EFT.

It's as important here as anywhere else to use the client's own words to describe the feeling. However much you may be tempted to encourage the client to express their feeling more forcefully, by doing so you will invite bigger Tailenders. The purpose is not to change or increase anything here, only to consolidate and acknowledge.

Related sections:

6.2.3      Psychological Reversal ⇧

6.2.15    Tailenders ⇧

8.2.11    The Non-Judgement Pattern ⇩

## 8.2.11 The Non-Judgement Pattern

In coaching generally it's important to avoid judgement about what the client thinks, as far as possible. The standard EFT setup statement includes within it, an implied judgement, that the issue being worked on is "a problem". This judgement is expressed in the words "Even though". The linguistic assumption is that whatever follows these words is "bad" or "unwanted" in some way.

Within coaching, this is not always appropriate. Sometimes it clearly is - e.g. if a client identifies a block to progress or feels distress or fear when thinking about taking a particular action.

But sometimes the aim is simply to test an idea - such as a goal, or a value or a belief. In doing EFT focussed on these sorts of ideas, we are not trying to "get rid of them". But we do want to explore what insights are triggered in connection to them, or to find out if there are any negative emotions connected to them which could usefully be released.

In these cases, we can use the Non-Judgement pattern, which drops the use of "Even though" and changes the acceptance conjunction from "but" to "and", thus:

> *"I have this goal/value/belief, and I deeply and I completely accept myself"*

As soon as any insight or emotion comes up in response to this setup which does clearly seem like a problem, you can revert immediately to the standard setup statement e.g.

> *"Even though I'm not sure if I really want this goal any more, I deeply..."*

> *"Even though I think I got this value from my family, I deeply..."*

> *"Even though this belief is stopping me getting what I want, I deeply..."*

If no negative emotion or aspect is triggered, then this provides the client with extra confidence that the issue tested is not being motivated or influenced by any negative thinking.

On the second example above, you may think that even the fact of noticing that a value was inherited from one's family should also be a matter of non-judgement - in which case, continue with the Non-Judgement form thus:

> *"My family had this value and I deeply and completely accept myself"*

This shows how the need for stating the issue as a problem or maintaining non-judgement requires explicit thought at every stage and can vary according to what the client thinks about the matter.

This pattern is also a good way for clients to develop a "noticing" habit instead of a "problem" habit. Although EFT is good at releasing problematic emotions in the client, it does, nevertheless tend to focus the client on "what's wrong". Many coaches try to encourage clients to develop the habit of "simply noticing" what happens in their lives, how they feel and so on. Often this sort of detachment is what allows clients to take control of their situations, deliberately access resourceful states and find creative solutions. Using the Non-Judgement pattern of EFT regularly will develop this mind set quite effortlessly and may be of particular use in areas such as Spiritual coaching.

Indeed, for any coaches who have any lingering difficulty around the notion of EFT "fixing" a client, using the Non-Judgement pattern offers a complete solution. There is no reason why one could not use this pattern in all cases, even when both client and coach would agree that the client's current state is unwanted.

Related sections:

5.3.2      Fixing versus Changing ⇧

6.1.15    Accepting the Client Without Judgement ⇧

9.1.2      Validating Goals ⇩

9.5.9      Testing Values ⇩

10.15     Spiritual Coaching ⇩

## 8.2.12 The Doing and Being Pattern

Coaches shouldn't just be "professional nags". Successful coaching is not just about the results the client gets, it's also the degree to which the client learns in the process and how much more they take up the space of the Creative, Resourceful and Whole beings that they are.

So sometimes it's important not just to specify what a client is going to Do - but how he is going to Be while he does it.

Often in coaching, and in coaching books, Doing is **contrasted** to Being. The two concepts are usually taught by showing trainee coaches the **distinction** between the two. This unconsciously sets up an "either/or" view of these two aspects of experience, inviting the coach, and therefore the client, to focus usually on one or another at different times. Truly synthesising them is therefore made harder.

The Doing and Being pattern expressly targets both aspects at once, helping to synthesise them in the client's energy system. As well as serving to assert the client's intention on both counts, it also helps to elicit any Tailenders or conflicts between the two aspects which can then be addressed and dealt with.

Here are some examples of Doing and Being that a client might want to achieve simultaneously:

*"I'm going to clean out my office **and** have it be fun."*

*"I'm going to make that presentation **and** make it feel like a real buzz."*

*"I'm going to have that difficult talk with my ex **and** feel love while I do it."*

The Doing and Being pattern is a specific variation of the Choices pattern. The first part of the setup addresses the Doing, the Choice part of the setup addresses the Being aspect.

*"Even though I have to clean out my office, I choose to make it fun"*

*"Even though I have this presentation coming up, I choose to look forward to the buzz I'm going to get."*

*"Even though me and my ex have to talk about the kids, I choose to feel love while we do so."*

In cases where the thing to be done isn't seen as a problem by the client (i.e. it's something they are looking forward to), then you might want to drop the "even though" and combine it with the Non-Judgement pattern:

*"I'm going to go to the cinema and I choose to happily leave the ironing till tomorrow"*

*"I'm going to my gym class and I choose to enjoy letting my family cook for themselves."*

*"I'm going to accept this promotion and I choose to be my normal self with my old colleagues."*

Related sections:

6.1.1      The Client is Creative, Resourceful and Whole ⇑

6.2.8      The Choices Technique ⇑

6.2.15    Tailenders ⇑

8.2.11    The Non-Judgement Pattern ⇑

## 8.2.13 The Both Of Us Pattern

*"If you leave me, can I come too?"*

*Mental As Anything, 1981*

Almost all significant change in a client's life involves other people to some degree or another. And however much we might like the client to become a self-determining being, the fact is that "other people" are part of the ecology of the change that is being proposed. A lot of coaching can be around not just simply helping the client get from A to B, but with managing the process of negotiating with X, Y and Z about whether B is the right place to go, how fast to go and whether they can come too.

Fortunately EFT can help significantly in easing the transition of relationships, making communication with the other people involved smoother.

I use a pattern I call the Both Of Us pattern. It simply involves altering the acceptance part of the setup statement thus:

*"Even though <insert issue>, I deeply and completely accept both of us"*

Specific applications include:

When the problem is genuinely shared and both people are facing the same problem together:

*"Even though our finances are in a terrible state, I deeply and completely accept both of us"*

*"Even though we're so worried about our daughter, I deeply and completely accept both of us"*

When the other person is presenting an obstacle to progress:

*"Even though X is really making life difficult at the moment, I deeply and completely accept both of us"*

When you need permission or co-operation from another party in order to proceed:

*"Even though X won't co-operate, I deeply and completely accept both of us."*

*"Even though I really need X's support on this, I deeply and completely accept both of us."*

*"Even though I'm dependent on what X says, I deeply and completely accept both of us."*

When the problem is the client's needs and wishes versus the needs and wishes of another:

*"Even though I really want more time to myself, I deeply and completely accept both of us"*

*"Even though I need this and she needs that, I deeply and completely accept both our needs."*

This last application is a way to help clients who feel that focusing on their own needs is "selfish". It not only gives them a way forward which is explicitly not selfish, it also develops the client's confidence and comfort in expressing her own needs to herself. In this case, the Both Of Us pattern is a way of giving the client permission to focus on what she actually wants for herself while still including the other parties in a positive way.

What's important to understand here is that we are **not** doing EFT **on** or **for** the other party. The purpose is to loosen or release any negativity that the **client** may be holding towards the person in the situation. The purpose of including Both Of Us is not to "fix" the other person. It is to emphasise that no ill will is intended to the other party (the client is not going to achieve his goal "at the expense" of the other party). It also emphasises that the client continues to have power and responsibility for her own feelings and actions even though there is another party involved.

## 8.2.14 The Yes/No Commitment pattern

The CTI training includes a wonderful protocol for taking clients through the process of commitment. Part of the process involves not just saying Yes to what is being committed to, but also saying No, to whatever it is that is being left behind as a result of the commitment. For instance,

- Saying Yes to an exercise class means saying No to watching TV.
- Saying Yes to more time at home, may mean saying No to overtime at work.
- Saying Yes to developing self-esteem, may mean saying No to being around critical people.
- Saying Yes to this new project, may mean saying No to procrastination.

So successful commitment involves releasing something at the same time as it involves embracing something new.

I find this model of commitment particularly compatible with the use of EFT within coaching. In other words, it assumes and explicitly recognises that successful progress forwards often involves cutting the ties with what's holding us back. Until the action, activity or "way of being" which we need to say No to is fully released, no amount of saying Yes to the new activity will be successful.

This exactly the mirrors the use of EFT to release what's unwanted and the use of Choices to create and embed what is wanted.

So combining standard EFT and the Choices pattern will address both parts of the equation.

The first stage is to use standard EFT to reduce the attachment to what is being said No to (perhaps using several rounds and looking for aspects and reversals along the way).

> "Even though I find it hard to miss TV, I deeply and completely accept myself"

> "Even though I'm afraid to say No to Overtime, I deeply and completely..."

> "Even though it's scary to stand up to critical people, I deeply and completely..."

> "Even though I always procrastinate, I deeply and completely accept myself."

Once the fear or other negative attachment is reduced to a low level, the second stage uses Choices to assert what is being said Yes to.

> "Even though I find exercising difficult, I choose to go to my exercise class."

> "Even though I'm under pressure to do overtime, I choose to spend more time at home."

> "Even though <person> is critical, I choose to feel good about avoiding their company."

> "Even though I tend to procrastinate, I choose to get started on this project right away."

Although using EFT and Choices this way is effective, I have created a new pattern designed explicitly to assist the process of Saying Yes (committing) and Saying No (releasing). This pattern expressly links what is being said Yes to, with what is being said No to in the same sentence. The Yes/No commitment pattern is:

> "Even though I'm saying No to X, I ohoooo to say Yes to Y"

For instance:

> *"Even though I'm saying No to TV, I choose to say Yes to my exercise class."*

> *"Even though I'm saying No to overtime, I choose to say Yes to time at home."*

> *"Even though I'm saying No to spending time with <person>, I choose to say Yes to allowing my self-esteem to grow."*

> *"Even though I'm saying No to Procrastination, I choose to say Yes to seeing this project done."*

Apart from being somewhat faster and more direct than having to work through two statements, using this pattern has a distinct advantage over using EFT and Choices separately. By forcing the contrast between what the No option and the Yes option, any conflict between the two options, will be brought to the surface directly and can then be discussed in coaching or worked on using EFT.

Related sections:

6.2.8      The Choices Technique ⇧

## 8.2.15 Key Points

- EFT can greatly enhance your ability to enrol clients, and is therefore a great thing to introduce at recruitment seminars or taster workshops. Using the subject of change is a perfect subject for a coaching taster workshop and allows you to demonstrate that you are able to help participants achieve change in a painless way.

- Co-active tapping involves both client and coach tapping together for the same thing, with it being made explicit that the coach is tapping too. Co-active EFT carries with it the same benefits as co-active coaching: it makes the client responsible for his own progress, and it empowers him to continue making progress when the coach isn't there.

- EFT can be effectively used to clear any lingering stresses, annoyances, or other emotional distractions at the start of a session, in order to help the client focus fully on the coaching - subject to client agreement.

- At the end of a session, EFT can be a good way to prepare the client to get back to their life. It can be useful when the client is "down" after some deep emotional work (e.g. Process coaching); and it can be useful to "ground" a client who is feeling "up" or "scattered".

- EFT can be used to help decide whether to coach "what happened to me today", or to ignore that and focus on the client's goals. It can also help to find any connections or synthesis between the two. Maintaining focus where it's most useful is a good way to build the client's trust in the idea that they are being listened to and that they are spending their time efficiently.

- All learning involves a shift in viewpoint - an expansion in consciousness. Learning in the context of life experience, requires moving out of an "associated" viewpoint (e.g. reliving the memory of the experience, which triggers the bad feelings of "I failed") and into a "dissociated" viewpoint of seeing the experience from a different vantage point. But this can be hard when there is strong negative emotion around an event. By helping to clear the negative emotion, EFT can become an aid to learning.

- EFT can be used to help minimise the famous "coaching plateau". It can help to dissipate any "niggles" that come up during the coaching, and it can help to reconnect the client with their enthusiasm for their goal(s) by eliminating any Aspects or Tailenders that have arisen about the goal(s) since the start of the coaching process.

- Asking about possible impact of a goal on different areas of the client's life can be interpreted as negative judgement by the coach, or can trigger negative client beliefs concerning their ability, stamina or worthiness, any one of which might actually be a "killer block" to the whole enterprise. Use of co-active tapping while discussing ecology, or setting EFT as homework on a list of ecology issues can be a way to avoid any hint of negative judgement by the coach, as well as beginning the process of finding solutions, not just problems.

- EFT can be used to help clients bounce back from failures more quickly during coaching. It can also be used to deal with any previous failures in relation to the goal before the coaching started. And it can be used to alter the client's overall relationship with failure, so that it becomes treated at feedback, allowing his behaviour to be fine-tuned before trying again.

- Some clients have a hard time experiencing their own success, finding ways to make it feel like failure. EFT can help to loosen any resistances that the client has to allowing themselves to feel good about what they have done; and it can be used to undo any specific reversals they have about acknowledging their own success. Finally, the Celebration pattern can be used to embed the reality of success feelings.

- In coaching generally it's important to avoid judgement about what the client thinks, as far as possible. The Non-Judgement pattern, drops the use of "Even though", so that the focus of attention is not presented as or presumed to be a problem. This allows non-judgemental exploration of what insights are triggered in connection to the target issue, and to find out if there are any negative emotions connected to them which could be usefully released.

- Sometimes it's important not just to specify what a client is going to Do - but how he is going to Be while he does it. But often Doing is presented in contrast to Being, unconsciously setting up an "either/or" view of these two aspects of experience. The Doing and Being pattern expressly targets both aspects at once, helping to synthesise them in the client's energy system.

- Almost all significant change in a client's life involves other people to some degree or another. EFT can help significantly in easing the transition of relationships, making communication with the other people involved smoother. The Both Of Us pattern allows the client to expressly acknowledge and accept the presence and potential concerns of another party in relation to the client's goal(s).

- Successful commitment frequently involves releasing something at the same time as it involves embracing something new. The Yes/No Commitment pattern adapts the Choices protocol to expressly link what is being said Yes to, with what is being said No to in the same sentence, allowing any conflicts involved in the juxtaposition to be brought into consciousness and dealt with.

# 8.3  In the end, it's just one more tool

*"There are always a dozen different tunnels to go down with every client in every situation"* [2]

I remember "tool infatuation". Every coaching training class we would learn another great coaching tool. One day it was Perspectives (wild creativity married with reliable structure). Another day it was Future Self (a dream world of secret knowledge and infinite wisdom.) The day after that, perhaps Who Do You Need To Be? (oh, the heart-stopping moment of fear and anticipation, closely followed by streaming insight).

When you find a new coaching tool it's easy to think *"This is it - this is the **only** tool I'll ever need - my clients and I can run off into the sunset using this tool forever and ever..."*.

But of course it's not like that. Each tool has its place - its little painted outline on the garage wall of your mind - and its proper use. They have their "improper" uses too - when coaches add widgets, sharpen blades or even borrow one from the coach down the street, the possibilities multiply.

At the end of the day, you don't choose a plumber (or a programmer or a dentist) by inspecting his toolkit and asking which ones he uses most often. You assume he has all the tools needed for most jobs. You hire him for his ability to choose the right tool at the right time, and to wield it with skill in order to achieve the result the client wants.

Even if you feel somewhat infatuated by the possibilities of EFT (and I hope you are a little), you need to look at it and treat it as just one more tool. An extremely useful one that has the power to accelerate your clients' progress in ways neither you nor they can imagine at this point, but still just another tool.

We've seen a lot of what EFT can do, but in the end it is the skill of the coach wielding it - his understanding of its use and misuse in a coaching context, and his intuition in the moment - which will decide whether EFT is used as a precision tool or a cudgel.

Related sections:

8.1.3       Perspectives ⇧

8.1.14     Who Do You Need to Be? ⇧

8.1.16     Accessing the Future Self ⇧

# 9 EFT as a Key to Change

*"People come to coaching for many reasons, but the bottom line is change. ...to achieve the results they want, it's very likely [clients] will need to change attitudes, paradigms or underlying beliefs. The prospect of making this kind of interior change can be daunting. ... Part of the underlying purpose of coaching is to produce a stronger client who is capable of self-directed change"* [2]

The previous sections presented the tools for doing the job of coaching. Now we turn to the central tasks of coaching itself. (While there is inevitably an element of repetition, this is deliberate. Understanding something from two different angles helps to synthesise the information and embed it into your existing knowledge structure.)

Fundamentally, the job of coaching is to **facilitate change** - helping clients achieve positive transformation in their lives, which can be sustained after the coaching is over. Coaching without achieving change is like having a very expensive friend to talk to every week - very pleasant and perhaps even uplifting, but which leaves the client fundamentally the same person with the same life as when they started.

To me, one of the most significant measures of coaching quality is the extent to which the effects of coaching are sustained in the client's life after the coaching relationship ends.

It's my experience - both as a coach and as a coaching client - that both coach and client can believe that change has been made, only to discover months later that one's old ways have returned. Whereas the ongoing presence of the coach somehow allows the client to get past blocks to achieve desired changes in behaviour - when the coach goes away, the blocks remain and can rebuild themselves.

This is especially true when the coach appeals to client "willpower", incites their "courage", and provides structures for going through, round or over their blocks. These techniques may be effective for achieving a one-off action - such as applying to college, getting through an exam or going to the gym for the next six weeks. But for actions which need sustained repetition to be effective - such as those pertaining to exercise or diet goals, ongoing relationship issues, building a business or general work/life balance, these methods do not work in the long term.

Since change is the central purpose of coaching (and EFT), we devote a chapter to considering all the ways in which change can be blocked and hence all the ways that EFT can be used to tackle obstacles to change. Although the number of reasons a client can find to avoid or resist change is literally infinite (clients can be as Creative and Resourceful about ways **not** to do something as they can be about doing it), these reasons can be put under a few general headings: fears, blocks, habits and beliefs.

If you are an EFT practitioner - or have used EFT for self-help - you already know that EFT is one of the best change tools around. It shifts fears, blocks, habits and beliefs faster, more safely and non-traumatically than almost anything else currently known to the healing or coaching professions. If you are serious about wanting to help your client make changes - in their Doing or their Being - then EFT has to be seriously considered as a coaching tool.

Although I discuss fears, blocks, habits and beliefs separately here, they are actually strongly interconnected. (A block to progress may be tracked down to a belief which is preventing action or to a fear of the consequences. A habit may be a particular block to progress, which turns out to be driven by a need for security which is in turn a fear issue. And so on). But they are fairly distinct in terms of the client's experience of them and therefore how they present themselves during coaching.

The other main issue involved in successful facilitation of change is goals. Since getting goals clear is so fundamental to getting the sort of change the client actually wants, I discuss this first.

Related sections:

6.1.1     The Client is Creative, Resourceful and Whole ⇧

6.2.10    Where There is Willpower, There Are Blocks ⇧

# 9.1  Goals

Goals are at the heart of coaching. They are its destination and compass. So, it's an essential part of the coaching process to make sure that both coach and client are clear about the client's goals and therefore the aims of the coaching.

A goal can be thought of as the external manifestation of successful change. A goal cannot be started, progressed and then achieved unless the client has successfully negotiated the change necessary in himself to make it happen - even if the change was only temporary. At the very least, the client has literally "changed" from the person who had not achieved the goal into the person who achieved it.

But the change is usually even more profound than this. The change may be from the client who thought they couldn't achieve the goal into the client who now knows they can. Or from the client who didn't trust themselves to commit to a project to a client who now does.

Choosing the correct goal(s) to work on is therefore critically important, since it implicitly defines the type and degree of change that the client needs to undergo.

## 9.1.1  Clearing the Way

Some clients can be blocked around the very idea of goals. Even talking about goals can trigger things like fear of failure, fear of change, fear of rejection, worry about the effort involved and so on. This may even have been made worse by the constant emphasis on "goal setting" in many self development workshops, especially those aimed at the corporate market. After a few workshops and books which yet again failed to result in the client getting what they wanted, the very word "goal" can become a negative trigger.

Clearly, getting rid of these reactions to the subject of goals would be useful as a precursor to discussing the content of what those goals might be, since those reactions are going to prevent thinking clearly about what sort of goals the client actually wants.

You know you have a client who is blocked around the idea of goals and would benefit from some pre-work when:

- They tell you they find it hard to even know what they want.

- They tell you they have many goals but can never decide between them.

- They tell you they don't know where to start thinking about their goals.

- They tell you about things they have already started or achieved but even these don't seem to really count as valid goals.

Dealing with this kind of block with EFT is the same as with any other. And it is time very well spent. If either you or your client are eager to get on with the next stages of goal work, doing pre-work on these blocks is worth it in the long run.

As in all use of EFT, doing the EFT itself not only addresses the targeted issue (e.g. "how I feel about the idea of goals"), but often results in the client spontaneously coming up with solutions and ideas. It's as if the client's internal knowledge of what goals would be right for them has always been there and clearing away the blocks to seeing them allows them to be suddenly revealed.

The setups you might use in this context vary according to the client's current understanding of the block and how it feels to them. If the client is aware of specific triggers or fears that thinking about goals produces, these can be targeted directly:

*"Even though I have this fear of failure every time I start thinking about goals,..."*

*"Even though thinking about goals brings up this fear of change,..."*

*"Even though I'm afraid of being rejected if I start working towards my goals,..."*

*"Even though my heart sinks at the thought of goals,..."*

Having many goals can be an effective way to avoid really deciding and focussing on one. Alternatively, it could be that the goals are all valid for that person but the life purpose behind them hasn't been brought into consciousness yet. If the client has many goals and can't decide between them, target this specifically:

*"Even though I can never decide which goal to really focus on,..."*

*"Even though I have more ideas than action,..."*

*"Even though I find it hard to focus on one goal for very long,..."*

*"Even though it feels like focussing on one goal is neglecting all the others,..."*

If the client has trouble knowing where to start thinking about goals, this means they are generally blocked from even beginning to think about what they want. And having a part of the client blocking what the client wants, is a Reversal - or even a Massive Reversal. You will need to talk to the client to find out exactly what sorts of feelings they have around the possibility of discovering their goals - the client's own language will reveal what Reversals (objections, fears etc) are operating. Base the setups on what emerges from this discussion e.g.:

*"Even though I don't think it's possible for me to find a goal I really want..."*

*"Even though I think I'm setting myself up for disappointment if I start thinking about what I really want in life,..."*

*"Even though I think it's pointless to think about my goals because I'd never achieve them anyway,..."*

*"Even though I don't think I should be thinking about what I want when there is so much poverty and suffering in the world,..."*

*"Even though I just feel so wiped out most of the time even thinking about having more goals is exhausting,..."*

If the client tells you about goals they have already achieved or have made a significant start on, but still claim not to know what they want in terms of **future** goals, then this could be a sign that the client has issues around success and around the value of their own achievements. Such clients are never going to feel fulfilled no matter what goals they set themselves and achieve, until whatever it is that is blocking their ability to acknowledge their own success has been dealt with. Starting points for this work might be:

*"Even though I don't even value my own success,..."*

*"Even though I don't give myself credit for what I have done,..."*

*"Even though I think anything I've done doesn't count,..."*

*"Even though I think it's pointless thinking about new goals because I know that won't fulfil me either,..."*

*"Even though other people would probably think I'm a success, but I don't,..."*

Be aware that that doing EFT on these setups may not by themselves clear whatever is underlying the client's belief - but it is likely to generate ideas, memories etc which are at the root of the belief which can then be cleared with EFT.

Clients who have issues around acknowledging and experiencing their own success may also benefit from using the Celebration pattern.

Related sections:

6.2.3      Psychological Reversal ⇧

8.2.10.1   Failure to Feel Successful ⇧

8.2.10.2   The Celebration Pattern ⇧


## 9.1.2  Validating Goals

Where do client goals come from? Do they come from the client's "true self"? Or do they come from "shoulds" and "ought to's"? Or from their parents and teachers?

In my view, a coach should never just accept a client's goal without checking that it is congruent with the client's values and beliefs, or without exploring what's driving this goal and where it originated. (And this is why coaches so often go back to basics with a new client to establish values, life purpose and so on before starting work on goals.) But it's an extremely fine line between making a judgement about whether a client's goal is "true" for them; and objectively exploring a goal and what it means to a client.

EFT is a perfect way to test the validity (the internal congruency) of a client's goal while avoiding the coach making or implying any negative judgement.

Using the goal as a focus while doing EFT (especially SLOW EFT) will reveal any type of negative emotions or attachments to the goal. Sometimes these can be fears or insecurities about achieving the goal. But sometimes they can be negative feelings about the goal itself.

For instance, I can well remember the years of "wanting to do a PhD" but at the same time "wanting to write a novel". Both goals felt equally strong to me - but since they both involved serious commitment of time and energy, these goals competed with each other for my mental energy. If I had gone to a coach and said I wanted to do a PhD, my coach may well have been successful in getting me through the process of signing up and getting started with a PhD. It just so happened that one day - worn out with the inner conflict of these two massive goals - I asked myself the simple self-coaching question: *"If I had only 3 years to live, would I do a PhD or would I write a novel?"*. In that stark light, the novel won hands down and I realised that the "wanting to do a PhD" wasn't really my goal at all - but an expectation and implicit wish of my parents that I had taken on. Suddenly it was clear to me that writing a novel was my "true goal" - fulfilling my true desires and nature - and was in fact in conflict with what others wanted for me (or I thought they wanted for me).

It is important to coaches that they are coaching for a good purpose - that they are helping a client achieve what they **really** want. It's also important to clients that they expend their time and energy (and money) on achieving goals that **they** really want.

Now, it's hard to say to a client *"Are you sure that's really what you want?"* if you have picked up information about their values and personality which make their stated goal seem odd to you. EFT offers the perfect way to allow the real feelings around a goal to be explored.

You can quite legitimately suggest that a client does SLOW EFT while focussing on their goal as a way to elicit fears, blocks or other emotional obstacles to its achievement. It just so happens that one of the obstacles that might be revealed is the fact the client doesn't actually want the goal at all.

The relief that clients can experience when they finally let go of an ambition that wasn't really theirs, can be enormous and life-changing. In one of my introductory workshops I was demonstrating Psychological Reversal using muscle testing on one participant. She had a long-standing project ambition which wasn't going anywhere and was weighing heavily on her conscience. She tested "strong" to the statement *"I don't want to do this project"* and weak to the statement *"I want to do this project"*. We didn't even need to do any EFT. She turned to me and said *"I don't really have to do this project at all, do I? I can let it go."*

I don't usually use muscle testing when I'm doing EFT with people, mostly because I do most of my work over the phone. And it's not necessary to do so in order to help clients identify and release false goals. You can use EFT to test how much a client wants something:

First ask them to rate the degree to which they want their stated goal (the job, the PhD, the weight loss, the car, the boat etc).

Then apply EFT as follows:

> *"Even though I really want this goal, I deeply and completely accept myself"*

Then retake the rating. If the desire for the goal was based on any kind of negative emotion or belief (*"People will look down on me if I don't have this"*, *"I'll die poor if I don't do this"*) then the EFT will start to shift those negative emotions (the Tailenders to the statement of wanting the goal). And the effect will be that the client's rating of how much they want the thing will start to drop.

If on the other hand, the desire for the thing is being driven by genuine love of the thing itself, or is an expression of the client's true essence and life purpose, their desire rating will stay rock solid - or even increase, since negative emotions that were trying to limit their desire (fear, doubt etc) will have been shifted by it, making the goal easier to achieve.

This is such a wonderful and totally client-led way of getting true clarity on the client's goals.

---

**Warning:**

**Identifying false goals can seriously disrupt your client's life!**

Clients risk quitting their boring jobs, refusing to apply for promotions, giving up their academic studies, ending relationships and many other drastic and life changing actions. Use of EFT for this purpose should be done within the larger context of a safe and supportive coaching relationship, where the fallout of discovering false goals can be managed in an ecological way without simply ripping the carpet out from underneath the client and leaving them stranded. As a coach I believe you **must** have somewhere positive and constructive to go after this exercise (e.g. exploring the client's life purpose, finding new goals, working out a transition plan from his current life to a new life, and so forth).

---

Related sections:

### 9.1.3  Generating Desires

Where a client comes to the coaching with goals in mind, the best approach initially is to test their validity as described above.

But sometimes the client isn't at all clear about what his goals are. They may be drawn to coaching because of a general sense of dissatisfaction with their current life. Or they may know they want to change direction but don't know where they want to go. In this case, it's part of the coaching purpose to help the client understand what they really want.

Where the client really has no goals in mind - and assuming you have successfully Cleared the Way of any blocks around thinking about goals - the task is to help the client generate some.

This can be done in many different ways, including contacting the Future Self, getting in touch with Life Purpose, revisiting Peak Experiences to elicit values and so on. All of these conventional coaching techniques help the client to get a feel for their "goal requirements".

I personally believe that when a client starts out with vague or ill-defined goals, it is all too easy to channel the client down one particular route and get them working on some goal far too quickly. Getting into action too soon can appear productive to both client and coach - but unless it's on a goal that will really lead to client Fulfilment, it is a classic case of "much sound and fury, signifying nothing".

This doesn't mean that the client cannot start work straightaway on some essential feature of their life (such as organising their finances, joining a gym or preparing for a promotion) and then later think about their deeper goals. Achieving success on such goals can be important to build the client's confidence and their trust in the coaching process generally - so long as it is done with full consciousness and without making the mistake of thinking that organised finances or regular gym visits will by themselves result in lasting Fulfilment. (Of course, a client may hire a coach for just such a specific goal and that's fine - but the context we are working on right now is where the client has come to the coaching saying *"I don't really know what I want in my life and I'd like to find out."*)

A client's Life Purpose statement and values list will define a broad list of characteristics which any chosen goals need to be consistent with. But even knowing this does not necessarily mean that a goal or set of goals will automatically present itself to the client - sometimes more work needs to be done to generate options and to home in on the type of goal and eventually the specific goal(s) that the client will find fulfilling and want to take on as a focus for the coaching (and for their life!)

Here is one of my own examples.

My Life Purpose is around the theme of "expanding human consciousness".

This purpose can be fulfilled in many ways - and coaching, EFT, training and writing all pass my "validity" test.

So this gives me a flavour for the general area that my specific goals might lie. Writing this book on EFT and Coaching clearly fulfils the purpose. Designing a website for someone else's business clearly doesn't (even though I could).

But this doesn't tell me, what **kind** of coaching I would like to do (business or private? general or specialised?), or how much coaching compared to the other activities (what balance is correct?). It doesn't tell me what sort of training courses I'd like to run, or for which target group, or how many per year. It doesn't tell me whether I want to write books, short articles, newsletters, or whether the focus is on fiction, non-fiction or both.

In other words, knowing the broad parameters helps, (a lot!), but deciding on a **particular** project with particular content and in sufficient focus to allow planning and work to begin is a whole other task. And this is where goal generation assisted by EFT can be helpful.

Essentially the process uses EFT assisted Idea Generation combined with homework and very likely the use of SLOW EFT. Any other tools for expanding the client's imagination can be used and combined here also - such as visualising a future life. What's critical is that the client is under no pressure to decide or commit to any goals at this stage. The purpose is to expand the client's idea about **what's possible to want** (as opposed to what's possible to achieve).

Testing the validity and priorities of the options that are generated can come later. Right now the task is for the client to develop the art of "talking to themselves". This means talking to their "True Self", with consciousness about their Life Purpose, Future Self and values to find out what their true self wants for them.

As well as getting the client closer to understanding what they want, this process will tell you, the coach, what sort of belief systems are operating. For instance if a client says *"I'd so love working with children and I think it's worth it even if I'm poor as a result"* this tells you that the client has a belief that says *"I have to sacrifice financial wealth in order to do the work I want"*. These beliefs offer you a way in to help the client expand even further what they are really choosing for themselves.

Related sections:

| | |
|---|---|
| 6.1.5 | Fulfilment Coaching ⇑ |
| 6.2.9 | SLOW EFT ⇑ |
| 8.1.2 | Homework ⇑ |
| 8.1.10 | Idea Generation ⇑ |
| 8.1.16 | Accessing the Future Self ⇑ |
| 9.1.1 | Clearing the Way ⇑ |

## 9.1.4   Goal Clarification

Goal clarification is useful and necessary when the client has managed to generate a goal that passes the validity test (doesn't generate Tailenders), fits with his values, Life Purpose and so on, but which needs more definition.

For instance, using the techniques above I may have decided on a particular project of writing about Coaching and EFT. Although this already looks quite specific, there is more to do before it can be taken to the planning and action stages. Am I talking about a short pamphlet or article for my newsletter? A series of articles? Or a 250 page book? Is it for beginners or practitioners? When do I want to write it by? Will it be about the theory of two disciplines or a "how to" manual? Will I write it with someone else or by myself? Getting answers to some of these questions begins to make the final achievement more real, and starts to suggest steps that need to be taken.

There are two main ways of using EFT to help goal clarification: getting clearer focus on a goal, and choosing between or prioritising multiple goals.

Getting clearer focus is about getting more specific about what successful achievement of a goal would actually look like. This process of clarification is the bridge to making it happen. A lot of clarification can be done using conventional coaching dialogue and by the client simply writing down in detail how they want the goal to look when it's done. But this can be assisted with EFT in the following ways:

- Enhancing the visualisation (seeing it up close and in detail)
- Working with the Time Line (e.g. to travel to the future) to see when the goal fits best and what milestones are suggested along the way

- Undoing any fears or blocks that are triggered by thinking about it in detail (*"Oh my God, that looks much too ambitious!"*, *"How do I know anyone would even be interested in that?"*)

- Doing further validity testing if necessary

The second important clarification task is to choose between and/or prioritise multiple goals. For instance, to achieve the client's overall vision of a balanced life, she may identify that the following needs to happen: finding a new job closer to home, making more time for exercise and relaxation, starting a vocational course which will lead to her being able to set up her own business. Which one does she start first? Which is most important? Sometimes being clear about the goals sets up new conflicts about which one to start on first. And it can be this very conflict that sets up brand new blocks to actually taking action. It is possible to overload clients with too many new goals - all of which pass the validity test and which the client is fully motivated to start working on.

In my own example, I may also have the goals of building up my coaching and EFT practice, and running more training workshops. These both pass the validity test with no problem. But which should I do first? How can I maintain the focus I need to write a book if I have clients popping in and out all the time, or if I have to stop and write advertisements for workshops?

Of course some straightforward logistical planning should be employed too - and if that clarifies how to proceed then that's all that's needed.

What EFT can be used to help with is any emotional issues the client may be experiencing around having multiple goals to work on. For instance, if the client is in the gym but feeling guilty about not job-hunting, or if they are filling in a job application but feeling frustrated because they aren't working on a course assignment. This kind of stress reaction when in fact the client is making good progress on everything they need to, indicates underlying doubts, fears and anxieties, perhaps involving whether they are doing enough. Clearing anxieties about "what else needs to happen too" can be immensely helpful in allowing a client to pick the important thing(s) to start work on, and then be content to do that without worrying about the other things until it's time to do so. It also greatly enhances the client's sense of Fulfilment around the process of goal achievement - knowing they are doing the right thing and enjoying it.

So some example setups around clarification of goal priorities might include:

> *"Even though I have those other goals waiting for me too, I deeply and completely accept myself."*

> *"Even though I feel anxious thinking about the other goals, ..."*

> *"Even though I know I'm doing the right thing but I can't stop thinking about the other stuff, ..."*

> *"Even though it's hard to focus on just this one thing, ..."*

> *"Even though I know I'm doing as much as a I can but it never feels like enough, ..."*

Choices, as always, can also be employed usefully here:

> *"Even though there are other things to do, I choose to focus on this right now."*

> *"Even though there's always more to do, I choose to enjoy doing this part."*

Related sections:

8.1.17    Working with Time Lines ⇧

8.1.18    Visualisations ⇧

9.1.1    Clearing the Way ⇧

9.1.2    Validating Goals ⇧

## 9.1.5  Goal Reversals

Although I will cover Reversals again under blocks, dealing with Reversals about the client's goals directly is essential. I distinguish between Reversals the client has about the goal **itself** as an entity and Reversals the client may have along the way to achieving it.

For instance, a block or Reversal about a specific goal may be something like:

| Reversal type | How it may apply to a goal |
|---|---|
| Safety | "Having this goal threatens my financial security" |
| Identity | "I'm not the sort of person who goes after goals like this" |
| Possibility | "I love the goal - but it's just not realistic is it?" |
| Ability | "I don't have what it takes to do this" |
| Deservability | "I don't deserve to achieve this goal" |
| Social | "I don't know what my friends would think if I achieved this goal" |
| Ecology | "Achieving this goal would change my life completely" |

There is a significant amount of useful discussion that can be done on the client's goals which can help to bring them into sharper focus for both client and coach, and can begin to tell both client and coach where the likely blocks are going to be when the client starts working on them. Within EFT, this discussion would be termed "looking for Reversals". But in fact the questions that the EFT practitioner needs to ask to find Reversals are pretty much the same sorts of questions that a coach is interested in finding out before beginning work with a client on a goal - or later on in the coaching if blocks or resistance occurs. The EFT Coach can ensure this conversation takes place as **part** of the goal generation and clarification process rather than wait for the client to hit a wall in two months time and start asking then.

As well as looking out for client statements like those above, you may want to test for the presence of particular types of Reversal (either because you have an intuition, or because you have heard the client express a Reversal in a different context)

Here are the sorts of questions that are helpful:

| Reversal type | Opening question |
|---|---|
| Safety | What are you risking by going for this goal? |
| Identity | What would success reinforce about you? How would failing undermine you? |
| Possibility | How much do you believe you can achieve this goal? |
| Ability | Does this goal feel as though it's within your capability? |
| Deservability | Do you think you deserve to achieve this goal? |
| Social | How do you expect your friends and family will react when you achieve this goal? |
| Ecology | How will achieving this goal change your life? And what are the good points and bad points about what those changes might mean? |

Now, it is not compulsory to start diving in and doing EFT on the client's responses to these questions, at least initially. Their purpose are to help you as coach get a rounded feel about where the client is at with regard to this goal, and what general areas of resistance come up or recur. This information will be food for your intuition in later sessions when doing EFT on specific issues, and of course more generally in a coaching dialogue. The client's responses also help them to understand their own motivations and internal landscape around the issue for themselves. In a coaching context it can be the revelation of how the client really feels about a goal that can be the key to kick-starting progress.

Related sections:

6.2.3        Psychological Reversal ⇧

## 9.1.6   Dysfunctional Goals

Sometimes clients turn up to coaching with goals that are "dysfunctional" in the sense of being disconnected, ungrounded, or the client never seems able to achieve them or make progress. Or the achieving of them actually appears to be causing damage or distress! Although this is rare, I believe it's useful to be alert to them when they appear and to have some idea of how to progress.

### 9.1.6.1   Guiding Stars

I am indebted to Silvia Hartmann for articulating and explaining the terrible potential damage that can be self-inflicted in response to a Guiding Star[4]. A Guiding Star is a memory - but not a traumatic one. It's a memory that, in one instant, gave the client the exact feeling they were looking for - of feeling loved, of feeling fulfilled, of feeling happy, of feeling successful, of feeling important etc etc. So complete and perfect was the feeling that the memory becomes iconic in the client's mind. So much so that the client can literally spend the rest of his life trying to recreate that exact memory in order to once again feel loved, fulfilled, happy, successful or important. These wishes to recreate circumstances can of course show up as coaching goals.

Taking away someone's Guiding Star as an anchor and direction in their life, can be traumatic and severely disorienting to the person who has built their life around it. Silvia Hartmann counsels against even the most experienced therapists trying to "tap away" someone's Guiding Star without considerable thought and provision of aftercare and support. Trying to deal with them in a coaching context is therefore particularly inappropriate.

But nevertheless it is useful for an EFT Coach to know how to tell when someone's coaching goal seems to be driven by a Guiding Star.

The single strongest sign is if the client overtly seems to be trying to recreate a past feeling or past situation - as opposed to trying to create a new feeling or situation they haven't had before. Asking about your client's Peak Experiences - as you probably will do as part of the values clarification process, will most likely tell you what Guiding Star memory/ies are present. You can then be alert to when their description of their goals seem to more than closely resemble one of the memories they told you about just a couple of sessions ago.

If you know or suspect a Guiding Star to be at work you need to tread carefully. Silvia Hartmann warns against simply tapping away someone's attachment to a Guiding Star.  And in any case it is not your job as a coach to make a judgement about the validity of a client's goal and to suggest that it even needs "tapping away". If you suspect a Guiding Star at work, the best advice is to remain firmly focussed on the client's future. If it's becoming clear that the client's Guiding Star is becoming a problem within the coaching or causing distress to the client, then referral to an appropriate therapist is advised.

Related sections:

8.1.12      Peak Experiences ⇑

## 9.1.6.2    Dream Goals

Sometimes a client has had a goal for so long, perhaps since early childhood, that it has taken on "Dream Goal" status.

Dream Goals have some similarity to Guiding Stars - but with the important difference that the Dream Goal has never occurred in reality and has therefore not involved any actual people or events from the client's past and is less critically underpinning the client's sense of personal history, identity and body memory.

As a crude analogy, a Guiding Star may be likened to *"the one time I took heroin and it was bliss and now I need some more"*, while the Dream Goal may be likened to the desire for *"the glamour and all the things I've ever heard about how good heroin is"*. The person with the misguided ambition to take drugs is not in the same degree of danger as the person who actually has and who spends their life looking for more, destroying relationships and ruining their health in the process.

Dream Goals, while vivid in every detail, bright, colourful, close-up and positively glowing with compelling appeal, can often have one critical problem with them - they aren't connected to the client's future.

Instead of being anchored into the client's internal Time Line, the goal perhaps floats off to the side or above somewhere. Or the client may simply be unable to hold his Time Line and his Dream Goal in mind at the same time. The Dream Goal has become an unreachable paradise, for the client can travel along his Time Line for infinity and never get to a point where the goal is actually present.

Note that because a goal is also a Dream Goal does not define it as unrealistic or unachievable. It may be perfectly achievable - but its current location in the client's energetic landscape means that the client is not going to get to it from here - not without significantly adjusting their internal landscape, for example by manipulating their Time Line.

It is possible to get the client to put the goal on his Time Line and ensure that the events along the Time Line which lead to the fulfilment of the goal are clear and connected to the client's present, using conventional coaching dialogue or by using the methods described in Working with Time Lines.

But sometimes it's not so easy for the client to adjust the set of meanings around the goal that will allow this to happen. Sometimes the reason that a goal is disconnected is not merely an "administrative oversight" on behalf of the client's subconscious, or because the client has never got round to creating a plan for it. Instead the disconnection is maintained for specific emotional reasons.

Why would a client be resistant to moving his Dream Goal into reality? Isn't that what he hired a coach for? Well, if a client has had a dream for many years and has not managed to move it into reality by himself, then hiring a coach is a strong signal that there is some "reason why not" lurking in the client. Moreover, if the client has had this goal for many years, it has probably acquired emotional significance over that time.

In particular, the image of the Dream Goal may have been a sanctuary - a beautiful place to escape to or dwell at times of stress. It's the classic cry of *"This time next year, we'll be millionaires"* or *"When I win the lottery…"*. Bringing such a goal "down to earth" and making it just another event on the client's Time Line may seem like being robbed of the one beautiful place to be that the client could always go and reality could never intrude.

The Dream Goal image may have been allowed to be bright and clear on the underlying assumption that it is actually unobtainable for a variety of reasons. These reasons will be the classic Reversals we already know how to deal with e.g.

*"Well, it's not actually very realistic is it?"* (Possibility Reversal)

*"Well, it might have been possible 10 years ago when I didn't have people depending on me, but it would be too risky now"* (Safety Reversal)

A particular form of Reversal that can apply here is "Loss Reversal". In this case, the client may fear achieving the goal because it will mean they will **lose the dream** as a place to take sanctuary.

If this is the case then you, as their coach, actually become a threat, since you offer the prospect of **destroying** the Dream Goal by turning it into reality. This form of attachment to the Dream Goal can therefore turn up as resistance to the coaching process in general, failure to complete homework assignments or even personal friction between coach and client.

By hiring a coach, the client with the Dream Goal gets to externalise his internal conflict about the goal itself. It's partly down to your skill as a coach whether this is used as an opportunity to resolve these feelings about the goal or whether the coaching becomes another "reason why not" for the client to add to their armoury.

With all this in mind about the function of the Dream Goal and the emotional risks for the client associated with bringing it into reality, there are four things to be done in this case.

1. Take care to maintain the positive qualities of the goal as it is brought into the Time Line - it doesn't have to lose its glow, or its brightness. If the image does spontaneously become dimmer or less appealing, then this is a good sign that bringing it into reality may trigger feelings of "loss".

2. If the client's "reality" Time Line is a place of fuzziness and darkness, the risk is that the goal is made to take on the same qualities simply by bringing it into the same space. If this is the case, then work can be done on the client's existing reality Time Line to make it brighter, clearer, and so on, so there is less contrast between it and the goal. There will be less emotional need for a "sanctuary" if real life can be made brighter and more pleasant.

3. Work with the client on what happens **after** the goal is achieved. Seeing what is possible afterwards, allows the client to begin to contemplate life after the goal. It makes achieving the goal just one step along the journey, not the final destination.

4. Strongly connect the goal into the client's Time Line so that it can't detach itself again.

You might be wondering - wouldn't just doing some planning sort out this problem? Well, it might for goals that don't have such extreme iconic importance. But there's just no point putting plans on the client's real Time Line towards a goal that's not actually connected to the Time Line itself. You can't put milestones on a road that hasn't been built yet.

Related sections:

8.1.17    Working with Time Lines ⇧
9.3.3     Blocks as Reasons Why Not ⇩

## 9.1.7 Key Points

- Some clients can be blocked around the very idea of goals. Even talking about goals can trigger things like fear of failure, fear of change, fear of rejection, and so on - and those reactions are going to prevent thinking clearly about what sort of goals the client actually wants. EFT can be used to clear these blocks to thinking about goals generally, as a precursor to actually setting goals.

- EFT can be used to help clients validate their goal(s). Goals which are being driven by any sort of negative emotion will tend to seem less attractive after EFT because the negative roots will have started to be reduced. Goals which are expression of the client's true essence and life purpose will tend to seem even more attractive since any negative emotions limiting their desire (fear, doubt, etc) will have begun to shift too.

- Sometimes the client isn't at all clear about what his goals are - and it's part of the coaching purpose to help the client understand what they really want. EFT assisted Idea Generation combined with homework can be used to expand the client's idea about what's possible to want (as opposed to what's possible to achieve).

- Goal clarification is useful and necessary when the client has managed to generate a goal that passes the validity test, fits with his values, Life Purpose and so on, but which needs more definition. EFT can help with getting clearer focus on a goal, and choosing between or prioritising multiple goals.

- Clients may have Reversals about their goal(s) themselves as entities, and Reversals along the way to achieving them. Finding out what they are gives the coach advance notice of what needs to be dealt with during the coaching; and it helps the client understand their own motivations and internal landscape around the issue for themselves.

- Sometimes clients turn up to coaching with goals that are "dysfunctional" in the sense that they are disconnected, ungrounded or are even causing damage or distress. Guiding Stars are iconic memories of happiness and fulfilment that the client wants to recreate - but never can. Dream Goals are unrealised goals which the client's may have harboured since childhood, but which are not connected to the client's Time Line. Both require extremely delicate handling and are useful for coaches to be aware of when working with clients on their goals.

# 9.2  Fear

Fear is, of course, a block to action. But I have given fear a special section since ultimately, all the reasons a client will find to resist, avoid or slow down change are rooted in fear of some kind. (Which means all these things are addressable with EFT).

Once you understand how to eliminate fear using EFT, then you have simultaneously understood the necessary basics for clearing all other blocks and working with all other beliefs.

## 9.2.1  Clearing Fears

*"It's not enough 'not to be afraid anymore'. There is a realm beyond, in which you take delight in the activity/your body/your health/your work and your life. ...Accept nothing less."* [3]

All blocks are rooted in fear of some kind, but sometimes the client experiences the fear directly rather than as a block.

I tend to think of blocks as "masked fears". If the client is sufficiently in touch with his own processes that he is able to articulate what he is afraid of, you are one step further forward in clearing it.

Using EFT for clearing fears in a coaching context is exactly the same as clearing fears in any other context:

- Do any pre-work necessary (e.g. "the fear of the fear")
- Get an intensity rating for the fear, 0-10, tuning in to a particular image or memory if necessary
- Do standard EFT on *"Even though I'm afraid of X,..."*, or *"Even though I have this fear of X,..."*
- Take the rating again and repeat until zero, or...
- ...explore any Aspects of the fear that come up until all the Aspects are at zero and the overall fear is at zero.

(I am assuming that readers have basic familiarity with the Standard EFT protocol for addressing fear. If this procedure is not familiar to you then please consult one of the training manuals given in the resources section.)

It is likely but not necessarily the case, that the sort of fears you will come across in a coaching context will be significantly milder than the sorts of fears that appear in a therapeutic context. This has its advantages and disadvantages. Although milder in perceived intensity (perhaps producing a rating of 5 or less), they can be just as effective at blocking action.

For many people, even a slight feeling of unease (perhaps an intensity of 1 or 2) can be enough to stop action - or thinking about action - completely in its tracks.

As a coach therefore, you are interested in more than just the rating scale reported by the client. You are equally, if not more interested in the degree to which action is possible for the client. If the client's intensity rating for the fear in question is a 1 or even a half, but they are still uncomfortable about taking action, there is more work to be done.

Be aware also that it is possible for a client to achieve a true zero intensity for a particular fear and **still** not take action. This can occur when the fear is so long-standing that the client has a habit of avoiding a particular action which persists after the actual fear has gone. Or the fear has gone but the client's belief that "X is frightening" remains. If this occurs, you are in classic coaching territory and straightforward challenges to action may be effective at countering the habit or re-evaluating the belief. Alternatively use the techniques described under Habits or Beliefs below.

The one advantage of dealing with milder fears is that it is possible to give them to the client to work through as homework, confident that the client is unlikely to experience any strong feelings of distress. The list of fears should ideally be drawn up as part of the coaching session so that the coach can be made aware of them, and so that the coach can help the client create a comprehensive list of Aspects. You should then ask the client to give initial intensity ratings for each item. If there are any high ratings on the list (a 7 or above) then thoroughly check with the client whether they feel able to work with it alone. If not, it may be better to work with them on those fears. When working on fears especially, the client's feeling of safety is critical.

The list of fears and Aspects that the coach and client generates will look something like this:

| Fears about starting out on my own | Intensity | After EFT |
|---|---|---|
| Dealing with accountants | 5 | |
| Paperwork | 5 | |
| Financial stuff | 6 | |
| Having to cold call | 8 | |
| Fear of failure | 4 | |
| Not making the mortgage | 5 | |
| Embarrassment if I fail | 3 | |
| I won't get any customers | 5 | |
| I'm not good enough | 6 | |
| There's too much to learn | 2 | |

The list can pertain to a goal in general, or a specific action. So for instance if cold calling is necessary to the process of achieving the goal, coach and client might generate another list specifically for that:

| Fears about Cold Calling | Intensity | After EFT |
|---|---|---|
| People I don't know | 3 | |
| Not knowing how they'll react | 5 | |
| People getting angry or abusive | 7 | |
| People putting the phone down | 4 | |
| Not knowing what to say | 5 | |
| Feeling it's just wrong | 6 | |

It does not matter at all that some of these items might more properly be classified as Reversals, blocks or beliefs rather than fears - or even that they are Aspects of fears. In terms of the end goal (moving the client into action) all must be addressed. In fact it is likely if you start asking a client about their fears that it will prompt them to think generally of all sorts of "reasons why not". This is to be encouraged. Your understanding of the distinctions between fears, Reversals, blocks and beliefs is of no interest to your client.

Related sections:

6.2.5      Rating scales ⇧
6.2.12    Aspects ⇧
9.3.3      Blocks as Reasons Why Not ⇩
9.4        Habits ⇩
9.5        Beliefs ⇩

### 9.2.2 Phobias

Sometimes the fear around a block is so severe that it constitutes a phobia. As for all use of EFT within coaching, the decision whether to address a phobia (or anything else) depends on whether the phobia is preventing the client from achieving their stated coaching goals.

But sometimes clients will use the term "phobia" to describe something they dislike doing. For instance *"I've got a phobia about filling in forms"* or *"I've got gym-o-phobia"*.

It's helpful therefore to be able to distinguish between a true phobia and a lesser fear or a simple dislike of something. Don't be put off tackling a client fear or dislike simply because the client has used the term "phobia".

True phobias are characterised by the client entering a state of extreme fear at the thought of the feared object or activity, defined as mental terror and physiological symptoms such as shortness of breath, sweating, panic, inability to move and so on. For an extreme phobia that causes these types of reaction, it is wise to only tackle it yourself if you feel you have had adequate training in EFT to be able to avoid an extreme reaction.

For objects and activities that are really only a "strong dislike", these can be dealt with like any fear or block.

Related sections

5.4.3        Principle of Goal Furtherance ⇧


### 9.2.3  Fears About the Coaching

While most clients begin a new coaching relationship with high hopes and enthusiasm, sometimes a client will admit they have doubts or are otherwise afraid of what the coaching might bring up, or how challenging they are likely to find it. If these are expressed at the first session, then having EFT up your sleeve is the perfect way to address such fears and reassure the client that you care about their concerns and are not going to allow them to experience fear and distress needlessly. (This is one place where using full EFT at the first session would be entirely appropriate).


#### 9.2.3.1    Fear Based on Past Experience

A particular fear may exist if the client has previous experience of coaching or therapy (clients often don't distinguish between them even if therapists and coaches do) which either didn't work, or which produced reactions they found difficult. Clearing the feelings around these past experiences is an extremely useful relationship-building activity.

Incidentally, this is a prime example of a use of EFT which could be seen as "therapy" (even though this is a false distinction) in that it relates to the past, but has clear and obvious relevance to the clients **current** emotional state and readiness to be coached.

It is possible to provide the reassurance that clients need without at all having to go into or clear the past experiences themselves, by demonstrating how EFT works for a current and goal-relevant issue. It isn't your responsibility to undo the difficult or painful experiences associated with previous coaches or therapists - only to establish that you are different and it won't be more of the same.

Related sections:

5.1        EFT isn't (Psycho)therapy ⇧

5.3.1.1    "Therapy is About the Past, Coaching is About the Future" ⇧


### 9.2.3.2    Fear of Needing Help

Another more common fear (perhaps expressed as an objection) in relation to coaching is that of appearing or feeling "weak", "needy" or "dependent" by hiring a coach. A Gremlin that is common to many people in Western societies is the one that says *"You have to do it by yourself. If you get help, that's cheating."* This is unfortunately a by-product of our isolated, individualistic lives and an education system that favours competition over co-operation to achieve results. "Independence" is one of the most common pseudo-values you will come across as a coach.

But assuming that a client has overcome these concerns for just long enough to get into a session with you, if you sense any such fears or objections to the coaching then you will serve both your client and yourself by dealing with them very early on.

It's common to do a values elicitation fairly early on in the coaching relationship as they are generally a pleasant process for the client and are a way of the coach getting to know the client pretty fast. The coach will also be wanting to refer back to the client's values repeatedly in future sessions as a way of keep the client real and in touch with himself. You will therefore probably get a good early warning of any issues the client has around Independence, Strength and other values relating to the client's general attitude towards receiving "help". (Of course, it's also helpful with such clients to emphasise once again the co-active nature of the relationship and to remind the client that they will be doing **all** the work.)

Without even needing to go into any EFT, you can test these values and the possible effect they might have on the client's feelings about coaching by asking about them directly:

> *"So, if Independence is a key value for you, how does that affect how you feel about having a coach?"*

Apart from modelling for the client how you will be using values as part of the coaching (as a way of benchmarking the client's behaviours and choices), and demonstrating right from the start that you are not afraid to "get right down to it", it also gives you an opportunity to detect whether you have an Independence time bomb waiting to go off, perhaps at the point when the coaching is getting most critical. It can be the client's perfect excuse to leave the coaching relationship if the coaching is starting to actually get results - because the client can accuse the coach of taking away his need to feel he has done something by himself. This can turn up in many guises, but one is for the client to say *"Thanks very much coach, you've got me on track now so I've got what I wanted from the coaching and I can finish it by myself."*

By dealing with the client's objections to the coaching using EFT, you can avert this type of behaviour - so when the client does decide to leave the relationship, it's because the relationship has genuinely run its course.

As with all use of EFT (as indeed with all coaching), the client needs to believe that dealing with her objections are of value to **her**, rather than the coach.

The intake session should in any case address what success means for the client, what fears or obstacles are they experiencing right now in relation to the coaching. Useful questions for the intake session are:

> *"What needs to happen to make this coaching work for you?"*

*"What are your fears about the coaching process?"*

*"When you achieve something, what needs to be in place for you to really feel that you succeeded and to feel good about it?"*

If there is an Independence Gremlin anywhere in the client's makeup, it's likely to show up in some form to these questions. The dialogue might then go something like this:

*Client: "I need to feel like I really did something, that I did it and I can say That's Mine."*

*Coach: "What would get in the way of you feeling That's Mine about the goal we're going to be working on together?"*

This draws his attention to the fact that you will be involved in the process - which should trigger an Independence Gremlin if he has one.

*Client: "Oh, well, even though you're the coach, it's still going to be me who actually has to go and do it - it'll still be Mine when it's done"*

This response implies it may not be too much of a problem. But if the Gremlin has really had its cage rattled, the response might be:

*Client: "Mmm - yes - I do feel a bit weird about that to be honest. I wish I could just go and do this thing by myself but I've spent years and nothing's happened. So I figured getting it done with the help of a coach is better than not getting it done at all."*

If you get this type of response your alarm bells should be ringing! He has set up his feelings about coaching and achievement in such a way that not only is he determined not to feel good about his achievement when he gets it (he's already decided it's "second best" to doing it by himself), he is setting himself up to resent your role as coach for detracting from his success. With that kind of setup going on, it's going to be extremely hard to build true rapport and trust between you. He is going to resist really feeling a sense of co-active bond between you because you can't fully invest trust and easy-going rapport with someone who you secretly resent.

You need to sort out issues like this from the outset, with EFT or by any means at your disposal. But again, you need to get the client's genuine buy-in to addressing it - i.e. he sees it as a benefit to himself to deal with it. You can ask:

*Coach: "When you achieve this goal, I want you to feel fantastic about it. If you think having a coach will tarnish your success, we need to really look at that and deal with it so you get the positive experience you deserve. Is that something you'd like to work on?"*

There are many other fears and beliefs that a client could bring to the coaching and which have nothing to do with the particular goals they have in mind. Identifying and clearing them at the outset will pay dividends in the future of the coaching relationship.

Related sections:

6.1.17    Gremlins ⇧

6.1.18    Values and Pseudo-values ⇧


## 9.2.4   Fear of Change

Of all the infinite variety of fears that you will come across in coaching, fear of change is probably the one which probably every client has to some degree - and so it is given special attention here. In fact I will go so far as to say that if you can deal with a client's fear of change you have probably dealt with a major Reversal in the way of the coaching itself.

Starting by addressing a client's fear of change is, in EFT terms, doing "pre-work". It prepares the client for the real work of thinking about goals, taking action and so on, by reducing the fear that is a precursor to all those later fears.

You can help ease the overall coaching process by using EFT to work with the issue of change with your client right from the start and without referring directly to any particular issue. This can be done during the first session and connected to the discussion on designing the alliance - since the issue of who is responsible for what in the relationship cuts directly to the issue of change and whether the client is willing to make any. Alternatively it can be set as homework after the first session - perhaps with SLOW EFT, or perhaps with a Choice statement.

Doing this sets up the client's mind and energy system to expect change, and to feel more relaxed about change. It's hard to think of a more promising way to begin a coaching relationship. Discovering the client's attitude to change and having a technique which can improve it, could save a lot of time and heartache further into the relationship when the real changes start to happen.

Although EFT has the power to bring about amazing shifts in perspective and turn around long-standing emotional blocks in a very short time, this doesn't mean that the client always **wants** things to happen that quickly. Even if the client's general fear of change is reduced using EFT, the client may still have specific requirements for how fast he wants things to change in particular areas.

If the changes have potential to impact on areas that the client doesn't want changed (for instance his family relationships or his attitude at work), then you need to be able to offer EFT in a way that ensures the client maintains a sense of control over what happens when. It is their life and they have hired you to help them be **more** in charge of it, not less.

Now, all of these reasons that a client may have for limiting the pace or extent of change could all be seen as forms of Psychological Reversal. But even knowing that the Reversal **can** be dealt with, does not mean that it **should** be.

I believe that all use of EFT, whether by a self-help user or under the guidance of a practitioner, should be carried out **only** as a freewill choice by the recipient (Principle of Informed Permission). Using EFT with a client should never be like giving an injection to a patient "for their own good" or even "because that's the correct procedure for this situation".

In the context of coaching particularly, **all** uses of EFT should be carried out after full discussion with the client about the effects they want to achieve and what effects any changes are likely to have for them. Usually this will happen quite naturally between a client and coach who are in rapport, as part of the process of identifying goals, thinking about the person's whole life and agreeing how to spend the time on each session.

So, how can you manage the pace of change to match the client's wishes?

1.  Identify any fears or beliefs about the change under discussion and do EFT on these fears first, before even beginning EFT on the issue itself.

2.  Agree an acceptable degree of change for the client.

3.  Use creative EFT and/or Choice statements to limit the effect of the treatment to the degree requested.

The relief that clients have when you tell them they won't have their "problem" taken away all in one go can be immense. At one public demonstration I did for food cravings, one participant decided to work on his coffee craving. We were about to start tapping when he interrupted to ask me whether it was OK to **not** go to zero because he still wanted to have two cups of coffee a day. Accordingly I slightly adjusted the setup phrase to reflect what he had said. And his craving dutifully fell to a low but non-zero level.

Here are some examples of how clients might want to limit change, with possible EFT and Choice statements that would fulfil their requirements.

The client wants to decrease his anger at his boss, but not fully eliminate it - he wants some anger left over so he can tackle him about what happened, but still feel emotionally in control when he does so.

> *"Even though I have this anger at my boss, I deeply and completely accept myself, and I choose to keep 25% of it."*

The client wants to give up chocolate but doesn't feel ready to give it up completely. She decides that halving the amount of chocolate eaten will be OK for now.

> *"Even though I crave chocolate, I deeply and completely accept myself and I give myself permission to have half the amount I would normally have."*

The client wants to get over his social anxiety, but only gradually so his family can adjust with him. He thinks *"they wouldn't understand if I turned into an extrovert overnight."*

> *"Even though I have this social anxiety, I deeply and completely accept myself and I choose to release it gradually at the perfect rate for my family to deal with."*

The client has agreed to start work on his project but is worried about the impact of spending hours a day on it straightaway. He feels that would be too disruptive and he needs time to adjust the rest of his commitments. He also thinks *"I'm afraid it would just be another flash in the pan and I'd give up because it's too much and then I'd be a failure again"*. He decides that building up the amount of time slowly would work for him.

> *"Even though I'm afraid of disrupting my family with this project, I choose to start with 10 minutes a day and build up slowly in a way that makes me feel good and avoids disruption."*

However frustrated you may feel looking at these "client requirements", knowing how much more is possible for the client than they have asked for or clearly seeing the Reversals at play, these setups are only the first round of a longer process. Very often the result is that the client feels significantly differently afterwards and their requirements change to match. The point is not to "get to the right answer in the first round". The point is to be with the client where they are, fully accept them in that place and remember that the client is the best judge of what is desirable for them right now.

Related sections:

| | |
|---|---|
| 5.4.1 | Principle of Informed Permission ⇧ |
| 6.1.10 | The Client has the Answers ⇧ |
| 6.1.15 | Accepting the Client without Judgement ⇧ |
| 6.2.3 | Psychological Reversal ⇧ |
| 6.2.8 | The Choices Technique ⇧ |
| 6.2.9 | SLOW EFT ⇧ |
| 8.2.8 | Ecology Testing ⇧ |
| 9.5.5 | Beliefs about the Rate of Change ⇩ |

### 9.2.5   Key Points

- All blocks are rooted in fear of some kind - but sometimes the client experiences the fear directly rather than as a block. Using EFT to clear fears in a coaching context is exactly the same as clearing fears in any other context.

- The sort of fears that appear in a coaching context will be significantly milder than the sorts of fears that appear in a therapeutic context. Although milder in perceived intensity (perhaps producing a rating of 5 or less), they can be just as effective at blocking action.

- Sometimes the fear around a block is so severe that it constitutes a phobia (involving mental terror and physiological symptoms such as shortness of breath and sweating). But sometimes clients will use the term "phobia" to describe something they dislike doing. These can be dealt with like any fear or block.

- Sometimes a client will admit they have doubts or are otherwise afraid of what the coaching might bring up, or how challenging they are likely to find it. These can include the fear of appearing "weak" or "needy" by having a coach, or of the coaching not working due to previous experiences, If these are expressed at the first session, then having EFT up your sleeve is the perfect way to address such fears and reassure the client that you care about their concerns and are not going to allow them to experience fear and distress needlessly.

- If you can deal with a client's fear of change you have probably dealt with a major Reversal in the way of the coaching itself. You can help ease the overall coaching process by using EFT to work with the issue of change with your client right from the start and without referring directly to any particular issue. You can also use EFT to help manage the pace of change according to the client's wishes using Choices statements.

# 9.3   Blocks

Of all the applications of EFT within coaching, the clearing of blocks is by far the most obvious - and also the easiest. However, the term "block" actually covers a wide range of psychological processes and client experiences, so here we cover the most common, to enable you to recognise more easily the type of block you may be looking at and help you home in on a suitable way of using EFT to clear it.

In one very important sense however, you do not need to classify blocks in this way or know which type of block it is before you can deal with it. If you are an EFT practitioner you will already know that you can deal with any emotional issue purely by following the thread of language given to you by the client. If a client says *"I have this block around giraffes"*, you don't have to look up "the giraffe reversal procedure" before you can start work.

I define a block as any resistance the client has to taking the action needed to achieve his goal.

Any procrastination in taking an action or doing homework, any avoidance of talking about an issue relating to a goal, any expressed fear of achieving the goals, any doubts about their ability to carry out a goal, any worries about what other people will think of them if they do or do not achieve their goal - all these are blocks.

They are all negative emotional responses to the thought of achieving their goals. It may be experienced by the client as fear, anxiety, doubt, worry, inertia, lethargy, forgetfulness or self-sabotage (such as being late, making crucial mistakes etc). Whatever label the client puts on it and whatever behaviours accompany it, it's all the same thing: **some part of the client doesn't want to achieve the goal**. And this is acting as a brake on the process of action or even thinking about action.

I have said above that at the root of **all** blocks, is fear of some kind - of what will be lost, of what it might change, of failure, of rejection, of looking stupid, of being the centre of attention etc etc etc. And if it's a fear of any kind, EFT can help.

You may notice some overlap or fuzziness between this section on blocks and the next section on beliefs. Very roughly I define blocks which can be felt in terms of "intensity levels" when working with EFT (e.g. as one can notice the intensity of issues such as fear, anxiety, frustration and so on). I then define beliefs as more mental phenomenon which are usually not experienced as physical intensity, but as "degree of truth" or "level of conviction".


## 9.3.1   An Energy View of Blocks

I remember one coaching session I had (I was the client) in which I was repeatedly expressing some self-doubt with respect to a particular task. My coach very cleverly gave me a pen to represent my self-doubt and asked me to throw it over my right shoulder to get rid of it. Every time I expressed self-doubt again, she would hand me another pen and it too would be thrown over the shoulder. This happened about half a dozen times until eventually I stopped expressing self-doubt.

Within the context of the coaching dialogue, this was an effective strategy for moving the coaching along and stopping me getting bogged down in the self-doubt. It was certainly successful in terms of stopping me expressing my recurring self-doubt to this coach. But was it effective in **reducing** my self-doubt? Did I learn not to have self-doubt? No. I was still thinking it and feeling it. All I had learned was that I was wasting my time expressing it to the coach.

At the time this seemed to be an effective way of dealing with my block. But looking back at this interaction from an energy and EFT perspective, I understand it in a completely different way. You can "push past", "throw away", "go round" or otherwise avoid a persistent emotional block - but unless you release it directly, it will still be there and will still have the power to be a block at any time in the future.

From an energy viewpoint, blocks exist for real reasons, relating to past fears and experiences and ongoing belief systems. Often, blocks exist to protect the client from some feared threat to the self (either physical, or perhaps to the identity or belief system of the person). Ignoring or circumventing a block merely threatens an already threatened system. And this simply reinforces the system's belief that the block is necessary to create safety.

Since blocks are fear-based, EFT has the power to address a block directly and shift the energy and beliefs that relate to it.

Using EFT to shift blocks to action is not only more sustainable in terms of future action, it also **feels easier** and more **pleasant** to the client than exerting willpower or screwing up courage. This creates a sense of pleasure at making change - so more change seems like something to look forward to, not something to avoid. If a coach can help to create a client who is more and more open to change, rather than more and more resistant to it, both client and coach are going to see more action, and ultimately more success.

Related sections:

6.2.10     Where There is Willpower, There are Blocks ⇧

9.2.1       Clearing Fears ⇧

## 9.3.2   Blocks as Avoidance

Although blocks have their roots in fear, not all blocks are expressed directly as fears. More often the fears are "masked" and appear as the variety of ways someone may find to avoid doing or thinking about a specific goal.

Possible avoidance tactics include:

- Feeling "blank" about the issue

- Procrastination

- Lots of thought but no action

- Distraction activities (TV, games, socialising)

But these tactics aren't the blocks themselves. They are only the symptoms of the block. But even knowing this, EFT can help. EFT allows work to begin at the level of whatever symptom is presenting itself. Often, the process of beginning the tapping begins the process of revealing related Aspects and uncovering what lies beneath. In other words, you do **not** have to do any analysis of "what's really behind this behaviour" before you can begin useful work - and you don't have to ask the client to either.

So even if the client can't give you any "Reasons why Not" (see below), you can still start work based on the surface symptoms e.g.:

> *"Even though I just feel blank when I try to think about it,..."*

> *"Even though I just keep putting things off,..."*

> *"Even though I've got all these plans in my head and never do anything,..."*

> *"Even though I always seem to have something else to do,..."*

Related sections:

6.2.12     Aspects ⇧


## 9.3.3   Blocks as Reasons Why Not

If we define a block as "a reason why not" with respect to the client's goal, then we can deal with any block as a Psychological Reversal.

We looked at some common types of Reversal in the section on Clearing Fears, but there are many more - an infinite number in fact limited only by human ingenuity to find reasons for not doing something. Here is a more comprehensive list of Reversals, not all of them common, but all of them possible.

| Reversal type | Example client statement |
|---|---|
| Safety | "Losing this fear would be dangerous" |
| Identity | "I don't know who I'd be if I achieved this"<br>"I don't want to be the kind of person I'd need to be to do this" |
| Possibility | "It's not possible for this to happen" |
| Ability | "I don't have what it takes to do this" |
| Deservability | "I don't deserve to get over this problem" |
| Social | "I'm scared what my family will think if I start doing this" |
| Ecology | "This would turn my whole life upside down" |
| Poverty | "I could end up with nothing if I try this" |
| Imagination | "I don't have the kind of imagination needed for this." |
| Physical/Health | "What's the good of being wealthy if I drop dead from stress?" |
| Permission | "I don't think my husband would allow me to neglect the house" |
| Children | "The kids have to come first until they've all left school" |
| Security | "I can't do anything that risks my pension" |
| Mortgage | "I'm totally stuck while I have this mortgage hanging over me" |
| Age | "I'm too old / too young to do this" |
| Race | "No one will ever accept someone White/Black/Asian succeeding at this" |
| Religion | "I don't think that kind of success is consistent with my religious values" |
| The Unknown | "I can't start if I don't know where it's all going to lead" |
| Control | "At least I'm in control of my life as it is right now - that will disappear if I take this on" |
| Loss | "I've got too much to lose by trying this" |
| Commitment | "I know it's possible but the commitment just scares me" |
| Phobic | "If I do this it will mean more air travel" |
| Pioneer | "If I knew other people had done this it would be OK, but being the first one really scares me" |
| Attention | "I don't want to be in the spotlight if this succeeds" |
| Fame | "I want to write the book but I don't want the fame that goes along with it" |
| Privacy | "I don't want to lose the privacy my family currently has" |
| Parents | "I don't want to end up like my parents" |
| Failure | "I don't think I could handle it if I failed" |
| Disappointment | "I don't want to set myself up for more disappointment in my life" |
| Doing OK | "Life is actually OK - why rock the boat?" |
| Starting | "If I could just get started I'd be OK after that" |
| Progress | "I'm great at getting started but I just fizzle out after a while" |
| Completing | "I can get things 99% done but that last 1% is the killer" |

Since the EFT protocol includes treatment for any Reversal at the setup stage, it's not necessary to "work out" what type of reversal it is - you simply need to listen to what the client is saying, notice whenever they are giving you a "reason why not" and use their own words to formulate a setup statement. (Do **not** the above labels as the basis for setup statements e.g. *"Even though I have this Pioneer block,…"*)

Related sections:

6.1.10    The Client has the Answers ⇧

6.2.3     Psychological Reversal ⇧

9.2.1     Clearing Fears ⇧


## 9.3.4    Shortcut Reversal Correction

There is a shortcut for correction of Reversals which avoids having to do the full EFT procedure. The shortcut reduces the time needed from a minute or so to about 15 seconds.

The setup statement of the EFT procedure is the part that corrects possible Reversals in preparation for the tapping that follows. Performing the correction then allows the subsequent tapping to have an effect on the client's energy system and release other aspects of the issue from their body/mind/energy system.

This means it is possible to perform **just** the setup statement with the client (*"Even though….I deeply and completely accept myself"*) one to three times while rubbing the sore spot (or tapping the side of the hand if that's what the client is used to).

The aim here is to simply get the client's energy system in a proper alignment such that the coaching dialogue can be productive once again. Often, doing a Reversal correction is enough to allow the client to approach his goal from a more positive angle.

We know that doing the setup statement by itself can produce profound results, simply by putting the client back into a correct energy alignment.

One of Gary Craig's favourite demonstrations is to muscle test a workshop participant with relation to a particular long-standing issue (e.g. depression, weight loss, addictive craving). He tests them on the statement *"I want to get over this depression/weight problem/craving"* and then again on the opposite statement *"I don't want to get over this depression/weight problem/craving"*.

If they are reversed then the person will test weak to the first statement and strong to the second one. He then performs the correction (doing the setup statement while rubbing/tapping) and then repeats the muscle test. Usually the person is astonished to find they now test strong to the statement *"I want to get over this problem"*. I've had this experience myself when demonstrating Reversal during workshops.

Gary is also to be observed on some of his later videos apparently doing nothing but a string of setups, each setup addressing a different Aspect of the issue.

I believe (but cannot definitely prove) that using the shortcut correction  works best on clients who are already very familiar with the full EFT procedure since they have a body memory of the full procedure which is "anchored" to the setup statement.

So how and where might you use the Shortcut Reversal correction within coaching? And how do you know if it's worked, especially if you are not familiar with muscle testing?

If a client has just given you a string of reasons why they "can't", "won't" or "musn't", then you can do an extended Reversal correction, consisting of a series of setups covering all the reasons the client has just stated. Or you can perform a catch-all correction such as:

*"Even though I have all these problems to deal with,..."*

*"Even though there are so many reasons why this is difficult..."*

*"Even though I just seem to be on a downer about it all right now,..."*

You do not need to muscle test to know whether it worked or not. You will be able to tell simply by how the client is being. If they are still expressing negative language relating to the **specific** thing you corrected for, then it didn't work and you need to do it more thoroughly and perhaps do one or more full rounds of EFT.

If the client is still expressing negative language but about something different, then the correction may well have worked but they have switched to a different Aspect that they are Reversed on.

If the client stops expressing negative language and starts being able to view things differently and start seeing solutions, then you can be confident that the correction worked pretty well.

By the way - when the client starts giving you one "problem" after another, this **isn't** the client being awkward. This is the client's subconscious mind realising that it can get all these Reversals dealt with and giving them to you one by one to deal with. It may not feel much like it, but in a way this is the client's subconscious co-operating with you!

Related sections:

6.2.3      Psychological Reversal ⇧

6.2.12    Aspects ⇧


## 9.3.5   Unknown Blocks

Sometimes a client just knows they "feel blocked" but have no idea about what might be causing it. There are two possibilities here: either the cause is genuinely not available to them at a conscious level, or it might be but they are afraid of delving into it for fear of what they might find. In either case, persisting with questions like *"If there was a fear behind this block, what might it be?"* might work - but equally could just produce resistance or answers that the client hopes (consciously or unconsciously) will be enough to stop you asking any more questions.

(If clients do have ideas about what is behind a block they are usually only too eager to tell you their theory.)

There are three approaches you can take in this situation:

The first method involves applying EFT to the block directly:

*"Even though I have this block, I deeply and completely accept myself".*

Since success in EFT is enhanced by being specific about the issue, this may or may not produce any results. I would expect it to perhaps take the edge off the block, but perhaps not much more (although that is a generalisation and people have had successes with EFT this way). If it doesn't get anywhere, move onto the next method.

The second method involves applying EFT to the problem of not knowing what's causing the block:

*"Even though I have no idea what this block is about..."*

This approach can generate insights and give clues about where to go next. But if the client is really fearful of exploring what's behind the block, then EFT can be used to address this fear:

> *"Even though I'm afraid to know what this block is about,..."*

And of course it's also possible that this approach produces no ideas right now at all - sometimes clients come back the next week with a realisation about something, which is of course useful, but somewhat delayed.

The third method involves doing EFT on how the block **feels**. In this approach you ask the client to notice any bodily sensation that accompanies the block. This can include what might be thought of an "non-sensations" such as feeling "empty", "blank" or "numb". The answers are then used in EFT setup statements:

> *"Even though it feels like I'm trying to walk forwards but something else is pulling me backwards..."*

> *"Even though it feels as though I have lead weights in my shoes..."*

> *"Even though it feels like someone is in my head screaming No! every time I start to make progress..."*

> *"Even though I get this empty feeling inside when I think about it..."*

For people who don't connect with their bodily feelings very easily, you might try asking them how the block **looks**, or even how it **sounds**. (Depending on their preferred sensory modalities, clients will generally come up with an answer that already fits their preferences - asking a neutral question such as *"What is it like?"* doesn't assume any particular modality). EFT can be as easily applied to these images or sounds as to the feelings.

> *"Even though it looks like a huge black wall that goes on forever,..."*

> *"Even though it's like a sheet of glass, so I can see my goal but can never get to it,..."*

> *"Even though it's like horrible white noise over everything so I can't think clearly or hear what anyone's saying,..."*

All these feelings, images or sounds are of course, metaphors, and we have seen earlier how to use metaphor to explore a problem, generate a solution in the language of the metaphor and then translate it back into the client's real world.

These metaphors not only give us energetic material to work on with EFT, they also invite further lines of enquiry such as:

> *"Who is it that's pulling you backwards? Can you see them? What do they look like?"*

> *"What would need to happen to get the lead out of your shoes? What shoes could you wear instead?"*

> *"Whose voice is it that's screaming No? If you could ask the voice what would be OK for you to do, what would it say?".*

> *"Where is the emptiness? What does it want? What would fill it?"*

> *"What is the black wall made of? Can it be moved or altered in any way?"*

> *"How thick is the glass? What happens if you try to break it?"*

> *"Where's the white noise coming from? Could you turn the volume down somehow?"*

All these answers suggest different coaching or EFT-assisted methods to deal with them. The "person pulling me backwards" might turn out to be the client's Gremlin - and so we are into some Gremlin work.

The "lead in the shoes" example might lead on to the client's beliefs about his own abilities so we might do some more EFT on that:

> *"Even though I don't think I can take the lead out by myself…".*

The "screaming voice" example might lead to some conflict resolution work (*"Even though I want this and I don't want this…"*) or you might bring in a more powerful voice such as the client's Future Self.

As with all metaphor work, we are working almost directly with the client's energetic state, and bypassing the conscious mind's beliefs and strategies aimed at preventing the client getting past the block.

At the end of whatever EFT or coaching tools you use to work on the block, you need to refer back to the original block and find out what difference the work has made:

> *"How does the block feel now? Has it altered in any way?"*

Sometimes the process of working with the block in this sort of creative and safe way will have made it easier for the client to continue in that mode for a while longer - perhaps making connections or finding insights to the origin of the block. Sometimes the client is really none the wiser about what caused it originally - but if it has gone away or even just loosened its grip a little, the client can now begin to make progress.

Related sections:

6.1.17     Gremlins ⇧

8.1.9      Metaphor ⇧

8.1.16     Accessing the Future Self ⇧


## 9.3.6  Multiple Blocks

Sometimes the client will give a litany of reasons, doubts and fears why they are having trouble achieving their goal.

> *"it's hard to find time between work and family commitments"* **and**

> *"I've never done this before"* **and**

> *"It's probably just an unrealistic pipe-dream from when I was a child anyway"* **and**

> *"My husband is very sceptical about me doing this"* **and**

> *"My sister's going to be SO jealous if I do this my life won't be worth living"* **and**

> *"I'm going to be up against everyone else at work trying to get the same thing"*

**and, and, and**…

This type of litany can be as overwhelming for coaches as it is for clients. Conventional coaching techniques such as "Bottomlining" (*"So what's the real block here?"* or *"So, what do you want?"*) can be ways to get the client away from listing their Reasons Why Not and onto focussing on what they are going to do about it. It's also a way for a coach to stop feeling overwhelmed by the magnitude of the problem and to get started on an area they feel more comfortable with - getting clients into action.

But when a client gives an EFT Coach a list like this, they are handing over, on a platter, all the blocks that need to be addressed so that they can make progress. It's as though the client wants help opening a complicated box with many locks, and hands you the bunch of keys at the same time. Using "Bottomlining" in this situation can be likened to refusing the take the keys and then asking the client *"So - do you want to get this box open or not?".*

Fortunately, EFT allows you to deal with a litany of blocks in an orderly fashion, never feeling overwhelmed and gaining all the learning and self-empowerment the client could ever wish to have along the way.

In EFT, all these different blocks would be regarded as Simultaneous Aspects of the problem. All these fears, beliefs and doubts are operating on the client at the same time. If she's not thinking about one of them, she's thinking about another.

If you study Gary Craig's training videos and/or if you take a practitioner training, you will learn in detail how to deal with Aspects thoroughly and elegantly. But briefly, we deal with Simultaneous Aspects as follows:

1. List all the items in the litany explicitly on paper.

2. Ask the client to give a rating out of 10 for each one to indicate which ones have the most influence on preventing her make progress with the goal. Zero indicates that this isn't in the way at all, 5 indicates that it's somewhat in the way, and a 10 indicates it has the power to stop progress altogether.

3. Pick the item with the highest rating to start work on first.

4. Work on each block in turn from highest to lowest.

5. You can either do a full EFT round on each item, or use the Shortcut Reversal correction and then check the intensities again.

For example, the list might look like this:

| Block | Severity |
|---|---|
| Finding time between work and family commitments | 8 |
| I've never done this before | 5 |
| It's probably just an unrealistic pipe-dream | 5 |
| My husband is very sceptical | 3 |
| My sister will be jealous and my life won't be worth living | 4 |
| Everyone else at work is trying to get the same thing | 9 |

And the first round of EFT will be:

> *"Even though everyone else at work is trying to get the same thing,..."*

In a way, this is also achieves what Bottomlining might achieve - it tells coach and client what the biggest problem is. When the client, perhaps for the first time, can clearly see what the "biggie" is and sees that logically this is the best place to start work, then the client can start to see the goal as a tractable problem - which invites, optimism, hope and generally a different energetic state in regard to dealing with it.

Working through the list may take several sessions. It may be put aside for a while and then brought out again if the client begins to struggle in a particular area. But the list provides a structure and something to refer back to and help track progress, even if no actual action is yet being taken towards the goal.

As with Aspects in EFT, sometimes what the client thought were Aspects seem to collapse or reduce as a result of work done on the biggest ones. Therefore new ratings need to be taken for each block before beginning work on it. Don't assume that because three weeks ago the client rated a block as a 7 that today it will still be at a 7. You need to stay current if you are to "dance in the moment" with your client.

By the way, taking the time to write down and rate each of the client's perceived blocks to progress, is a deeply accepting act on the part of the coach. It signals *"I'm interested in understanding your problem and how it feels to you."* It also signals *"What you think and feel is important and useful and worth my time".* This helps build the relationship of trust with your client and actively models Acceptance for them from the start. It also tells them that they are free to tell you about any new blocks they discover and that this will be treated as **useful information**, rather than resistance to the process and potentially a sign of "uncoachability".

Related sections:

| | |
|---|---|
| 6.1.9 | Coachability ⇧ |
| 6.1.15 | Accepting the Client Without Judgement ⇧ |
| 6.1.21 | Bottomlining ⇧ |
| 6.2.12 | Aspects ⇧ |
| 9.3.4 | Shortcut Reversal Correction ⇧ |

## 9.3.7   Unsticking the Client

Sometimes the client is so completely stuck in one particular viewpoint, that it is useful simply to unstick them from where they are without particular regard (yet) to where they will end up. Indeed, sometimes the client is so stuck, you can't even begin to have a proper coaching discussion with them concerning goals, visions, life purpose or anything else.

When the client is "stuck" they can rarely see past the present. The present (what's happening around them and how they feel about it) consumes them.

They may seek out coaching with no particular goals in mind, except getting rid of the stuckness. Or if they do have some goals they can tell you about, they seem vague, disordered and even the client doesn't seem to really connect with them strongly. Alternatively the client's "goals" can be just more evidence of their "stuckness" and typified by *"Things that will get me away from all this"* such as moving house, leaving a job, leaving a relationship, emigrating and so forth, or perhaps Dream Goals with no real connection to their future.

Getting a client unstuck can be a challenge when neither coach nor client yet have a handle on what the client **does** want instead. And in the absence of any lead from the client, it's a particular challenge to prevent the coach's judgement or opinion appearing in the form of suggestions.

EFT offers a way to begin the process of unsticking that steadfastly follows (and discovers) what the client wants.

Either standard or SLOW EFT can be applied to the stuckness either directly to the issue the client feels stuck about (if known) or to the feeling of stuckness itself:

*"Even though I feel totally stuck around my career right now…"*

*"Even though I can only see one possibility for this relationship…"*

*"Even though I can't see any way out of this business problem…"*

*"Even though I don't really know what I want…"*

*"Even though I have this stuck feeling…"*

Get the client to tune into either the specific issue or area of life where they feel stuck, or on the physical feeling of stuckness if there is no specific area.

If the client is really stuck, it's possible that they get no particular flashing insights or ideas on the first round or two of EFT. But watch carefully for physical signs of release (yawning, sighing, burping, relaxation of posture and so forth). Severe stuckness may have many different blocks and fears operating at the same time. The client's energy system may be so closed down and blocked that a significant amount of tapping will be needed to get the energy flowing again so that the emotional and cognitive effects can start to come through. If you observe physical release, you can be sure that **something** is starting to shift, even if much more shifting is necessary before unsticking at the cognitive level actually becomes apparent.

If you have reason to suspect global or massive Reversal operating (see Psychological Reversal) then do not be surprised if one session doesn't magically unstick them in all ways. Persistence may well be required, and EFT should be given as homework. However, even though you may be convinced that global or massive Reversal are at work, there is almost always **some** issue that you can apply EFT to for which there is no Reversal in place. Pick an issue that is unrelated to their stuckness. A physical issue or breathing are good examples. If you are able to demonstrate to the client that EFT can work in one area - however trivial or unrelated to their problem, then it is easier for them to believe that EFT could work on their "big" issue and they are more likely to do EFT homework. And simply being given hope is a great aid to the process of "unsticking" generally.

But assuming the client is not massively or globally reversed (i.e. is only reversed on this specific issue), then tapping for the stuckness is very likely to bring about thoughts or feelings in relation to the stuckness. New thoughts or ideas relating to the stuckness is what you are looking for as a coach. As soon as a client generates a new idea about something they are stuck with - however far it may be from a solution - the closer they are to getting unstuck.

For instance, suppose a client taps on "feeling stuck in my career". During the EFT, perhaps he laughs and says *"I can't believe I've been stuck for so long!"*. There is no solution, or even the beginning of a solution in this response. But this idea is a massive shift. Suddenly the client is able to look at his overall situation from the **outside** - a good sign that the client has shifted perspective from *"I'm just stuck and that's the way it is"* to *"Look how long I've been stuck"*.

Finding it funny is also highly significant. The presence of humour is always a sign that the client is looking at the problem in a different way to before. It's useful to understand the full significance of these apparently trivial remarks and reactions in order to track the progress that is being made in the unsticking process. (Being able to feed these "small but significant" shifts back to the client also helps them to trust the process and motivates them to continue). Being able to help the client find alternative perspectives is the key to unsticking clients. Once you have signs that the client is able to view his situation from **any** different perspective (even if it's just to laugh at the situation), you are in a position to do some more structured Perspectives work with him to start generating one that might contain a solution.

Related sections:

6.2.3       Psychological Reversal ⇧
6.2.9       SLOW EFT ⇧
6.2.11      Persistence ⇧
8.1.2       Homework ⇧
8.1.3       Perspectives ⇧
9.1.6.2     Dream Goals ⇧

## 9.3.8  Parts

Clients seek out coaches because part of them wants change and part of them doesn't - and they want someone to sort out the part that doesn't. (If all of them didn't want change they would not seek out a coach. If all of them did want change then they wouldn't need one).

The idea of "Parts analysis" and "Parts integration" comes from the realms of counselling and psychotherapy - and it has also made its way into other disciplines such as NLP. Even if you have never had any training in these areas, it's a fair bet that before too long you will find a client saying to you *"There's a part of me that's really scared about doing this"*, or *"Well, part of me wants to and part of me doesn't"*. Simply by following the language, being curious about who and what these different parts are and using standard coaching techniques it is possible to achieve very successful outcomes.

If you fear that doing this takes you into realms for which you are unqualified, let's consider use of the Future Self concept. The Future Self can also be thought of as a "Part" of the client - because it is. So if you are comfortable with getting the client and his Future Self talking to each other and finding solutions to problems, then getting other Parts to talk to each other or to the client is not such a big leap.

But another way to deal with "Parts" is simply as a different sort of Reversal (or block). Thus we can address "Parts" using absolutely standard EFT setups:

> *"Even though there's a part of me that's scared of doing this…"*

> *"Even though part of me wants to just run away and not bother…."*

It's possible that both "Parts" have viewpoints that seem equally valid and neither one can be judged by client or coach as being "the Part I want to get rid of". Where this happens, it's not possible to say where the Reversal is. It may not lie in either of the identified Parts, but in the resulting conflict. Using the Conflict pattern[3] simply places both viewpoints together in the same setup and allows the energy system to sort out the relative truth of each.

> *"Even though part of me wants to do a PhD and part of me wants to write a novel,…"*

> *"Even though part of me wants a career and part of me wants to be with the kids,…"*

Or the Non-Judgement pattern may be used:

> *"Part of me wants to do a PhD and part of me wants to write a novel, and I deeply and completely accept myself."*

> *"Part of me wants a career and part of me wants to be with the kids, and I deeply and completely accept myself."*

In fact this is another sort of goal validation and is likely to help clarify the motivation behind the goals wanted by the different parts.

If the "Parts" involved appear to have identities and/or the client seems able to speak from either Part alternately, then using the Both Of Us pattern might be appropriate. For instance:

> *"Even though Part of me wants to finish my degree and part of me just wants to take a job and start earning money, I deeply and completely accept both of us."*

> *"Even though part of me hates my job and part of me loves it, I deeply and completely accept both of us."*

You can also direct the acceptance onto one of the Parts directly, as opposed to "myself" as a whole. The Part can be referred to as "it", "him", "her", "that part of me" or even a name if the client already has a label for it.

*"Even though there's this part of me that just wants to give this whole thing up, I deeply and completely accept it."*

*"Even though the Casanova in me wants to ignore the warning signs and just run off with this woman, I deeply and completely accept Casanova."*

So you can freely adapt the standard pattern, the Non-Judgement pattern, the Both Of Us pattern - or make up your own pattern to deal with Parts. The important thing is to follow the client's language and use a setup which accurately reflects how the client sees the situation and which talks to the Part in a way that is natural for them.

Having shown how to deal quite easily with Parts, I'll come back for a moment to the subject of Gremlins. It should now be clear that a Gremlin can be treated just like any other Part of the client that doesn't want what the rest of the client wants. And if a client finds the concept of a Gremlin useful and talks in those terms, then this is a perfectly acceptable term to use in their EFT setup statements also.

Unfortunately, the notion of the "Gremlin" has taken on moral overtones amongst many coaches. The second a client starts to express his fears or doubts about an action the response of some coaches is to say *"Am I coaching your Gremlin now or am I coaching You?"*. The intention is to have the client "drop" the Gremlin and be coached from their "true client self". In energy terms this is really just sweeping trouble under the carpet. In my view it fails to "coach the whole person". I hope this section shows that the Gremlin need not be ignored or "noticed into submission", but can be accepted and dealt with quite straightforwardly like any Part of the client. To demonstrate, here are the last two setups recast to focus on a client's Gremlin:

*"Even though my Gremlin wants me to give this whole thing up, I deeply and completely accept it."*

*"Even though my Gremlin wants to ignore the warning signs and just run off with this woman, I deeply and completely accept the Gremlin."*

Related sections:

6.1.2      Coaching Addresses the Client's Whole Life ⇧

6.1.10     The Client Has the Answers ⇧

6.1.17     Gremlins ⇧

8.1.16     Accessing the Future Self ⇧

8.2.11     The Non-Judgement Pattern ⇧

8.2.13     The Both Of Us Pattern ⇧

9.1.2      Validating Goals ⇧

## 9.3.9   Blocks to Commitment

When a client is giving a commitment to a particular action, the coach needs to make some assessment of how strong the client's commitment is. This is important for all clients - but especially for clients who have a history of failing to meet commitments. For them to experience failing in a commitment that occurred as part of the coaching process not only reinforces their belief that they find commitment hard, it also reduces their trust in the process of coaching to make the difference (even though dealing with the client's failure can be effectively dealt with using EFT).

The keys to the whole issue can often lie in the client's attitudes and beliefs about his commitment. The degree to which a client really feels committed to a course of action is dependent on all the remaining blocks and resistances he has towards the goal itself. So testing the level of commitment is another way of looking for blocks that need to be addressed.

As discussed elsewhere, EFT can be used first to test the client's belief in his own commitment:

- Overall feeling: *"On a scale of 0 to 10, how committed do you really feel to this?"*

- Anticipated success: *"On a scale of 0 to 10, how likely is it that you will fulfil this commitment?"*

- Fear of failure: *"On a scale of 0 to 10, how afraid are you that you won't fulfil this commitment?"*

Asking the question in different ways like this allows different aspects of the client's attitude towards the commitment to be triggered. For instance, if a client answers with a good high score to the first two, but with a low score for the "fear of failure" aspect, it is likely that although right now the client is experiencing a high level of commitment, it is probably based on courage and willpower, rather than actual desire and expectation of success.

I described earlier how willpower and courage are really only necessary if you fundamentally doubt your ability to take the action easily and without particular effort. And where action is based on willpower (i.e. fighting one's own energy system in order to achieve something), at some point the effort is likely to fail - especially if the required action needs to be sustained across a long period of time in order to achieve the goal (for instance, improving health and fitness, study towards a qualification, writing a book, etc).

By eliciting all the client's feelings about a commitment and clearing them with EFT, you not only enhance the chances of the client fulfilling their commitment this time, but also of building their confidence in their ability to fulfil commitments in general.

Related sections:

6.2.10    Where there is Willpower, There are Blocks ⇧

8.2.9     Dealing with Failure ⇧


## 9.3.10 Key Points

- Blocks are negative emotional responses to the thought of achieving goals. Whatever label the client puts on it and whatever behaviours accompany it, it's all the same thing: some part of the client doesn't want to achieve the goal. And this is acting as a brake on the process of action or even thinking about action.

- From an energy viewpoint, blocks exist to protect the client from some feared threat to the self. Ignoring or circumventing a block merely threatens an already threatened system and reinforces the system's belief that the block is necessary to create safety. Using EFT to shift blocks to action is not only more sustainable in terms of future action, it also feels easier and more pleasant to the client than exerting willpower or summoning up courage.

- Blocks can be expressed as types of avoidance rather than as fear directly. Possible avoidance tactics include: feeling "blank" about the issue, procrastination, lots of thought but no action, and distraction activities such as watching TV. EFT allows work to begin at the level of whatever symptom is presenting itself, even if it does appear to be a mask or avoidance tactic for something deeper.

- I define a block as "a reason why not" with respect to the client's goal - so any block can be dealt with as a Psychological Reversal. There are many types of Reversal - limited only by human ingenuity to find reasons for not doing something. The EFT protocol includes treatment for any Reversal at the setup stage, so it's not necessary to "work out" what type of Reversal is present.

- There is a shortcut for correction of Reversals which reduces the time needed to about 15 seconds. It involves performing just the setup statement with the client (*"Even though....I deeply and completely accept myself"*) one to three times while rubbing the sore spot. The aim here is to simply get the client's energy system in a proper alignment such that the coaching dialogue can be productive once again.

- Sometimes a client just knows they "feel blocked" but have no idea about what might be causing it. EFT can be used to work on the block directly, or on generating insights about what the block might be, or on how the block feels physiologically. Sometimes progress can be made without ever knowing what the block was really about.

- Sometimes the client will give a litany of reasons, doubts and fears why they are having trouble achieving their goal. A list of blocks can be dealt with straightforwardly as Simultaneous Aspects of an issue. The logicality of this approach allows the client to start seeing the goal as a tractable problem - which invites optimism, hope and generally a different energetic state in regard to dealing with it.

- Sometimes a client is so stuck, you can't even begin to have a proper coaching discussion with them concerning goals, visions, life purpose or anything else. EFT offers a way to begin the process of unsticking which steadfastly follows (and discovers) what the client wants. EFT can be applied to the stuckness either directly to the issue the client feels stuck about (if known) or to the feeling of stuckness itself.

- Clients seek out coaches because part of them wants change and part of them doesn't - and they want someone to sort out the part that doesn't. Parts can be dealt with quite straightforwardly as blocks or reversals.

- When a client is giving a commitment to a particular action, it's useful to know how strong the client's commitment actually is. Testing the level of commitment is another way of looking for blocks that need to be addressed By eliciting all the client's feelings about a commitment and clearing them with EFT, you not only enhance the chances of the client fulfilling their commitment this time, but also of building their confidence in their ability to fulfil commitments in general.

# 9.4 Habits

If clients are going to make long term life changes and achieve new goals, they are almost certainly going to have to alter their habits. The reason is straightforward: their current lifestyle and habits have not produced the results they want - so keeping those habits intact is unlikely to produce those results in the future. As someone said *"Do what you always did - Get what you always got"*.

But people's habits are very hard to change. Most people use routine and habit to give them a sense of control over their lives and a sense of security. The most threatening thing is change - and in a world where change seems to be thrust upon us almost daily, the creation and maintenance of personal routines and habits are an inoculation against this modern plague.

It is rare in my experience simply to be able to point out to a client that if she is to achieve a particular goal then one of her habits needs to be changed, and for the client to say *"Of course! I never thought of that before - I'll change from tomorrow"* - and then they do.

It **can** happen of course - but it's rare. Even if clients can see the logic of altering a habit (for instance when they get up in the morning, whether they have breakfast, what they do when they first get to work, what they have for lunch, when they come home etc), it is often very hard work to change it and keep it changed.

Of course habits can be thought of as simply a type of block. But they are also more than that. The blocks we have looked at previously may be thought of as a reason for **inaction** (a Reason Why Not). However habits are harder to overcome because not only is there a "Reason Why Not" at play (i.e. preventing the client from taking positive action towards a desired goal), but there is also an existing momentum in the opposite direction.

To address a habit successfully, requires not only dealing with the underlying blocks (in all the ways already given above), but also requires dealing with the structure, momentum and associated emotional attachment of the habit itself. And these can vary in particular ways.

Related sections:

6.2.8      The Choices Technique ⇧

6.2.11     Persistence ⇧

8.2.14     The Yes/No Commitment Pattern ⇧

9.3.3      Blocks as Reasons Why Not ⇧


## 9.4.1   Types of Habit

Habits can be placed on a spectrum according to the degree of negative intensity experienced as a result of trying to change them. (By the way - I am sure there are other ways of conceptualising and characterising habits, and I do not mean to contradict them - but here is one way which provides a way in to deciding the best way of using EFT to deal with a particular situation.)

- Zero-intensity habits are those which are carried out without thinking and for no other stronger reason than that's what the person has always done. The prospect of altering them or stopping them feels totally neutral and indifferent.

- Low-intensity habits are those which are carried out without thinking but the prospect of changing them does cause low levels of unease or feeling unsettled. The unease is usually produced not by the content of the habit itself, but the process of change.

- Medium-intensity habits are those which are pursued primarily for the content of the habit itself (e.g. watching TV, dressing or bathing rituals, regular social arrangements) so that altering or stopping them results in significant feelings of deprivation as well as unease about changes to the structure of one's life.

- High-intensity habits are also pursued for the content of the habit (chocolate, alcohol, drugs, compulsions). But additionally they are pursued for the tranquilising effect it has on an underlying anxiety. Extreme levels of anxiety or even panic can be triggered at the thought of having to alter or stop them. In fact, these are addictions.

Assessing what sort of habit you may be dealing with is therefore fairly simple. You ask the client about the prospect of altering or stopping the habit in question and observe the reaction. If you get agreement straightaway the chances are it is a zero-intensity habit. If there is any resistance or reluctance then take a rating out of 10. The words you use for this can vary. A couple of examples are:

> "On a 0 to 10 scale, what level of anxiety do you feel when you think about changing this habit? (10 is extreme anxiety)"

> "On a 0 to 10 scale, how difficult would you find it to change this habit? (10 is extremely difficult)"

Having decided roughly what intensity of habit you are dealing with, use one of the clearing strategies given here.

## 9.4.2  Zero-intensity Habits

*Most people would rather die than think;*

*In fact most do.*

*Bertrand Russell*

The key features of zero-intensity (rating true zero) habits are:

- They are carried out without thinking.
- The person feels no resistance (anxiety, unease, panic etc) to the suggestion of swapping it for a different habit or simply stopping it.

An appropriate response from a client who is considering the idea of altering a zero-intensity habit might be:

> *"Well, sure I could - not sure if I'll remember though, because it's not something I pay attention to very much."*

> *"Wow that's easy - is that all I have to do?"*

Examples might be:

- Putting on the left shoe before the right shoe
- Having dinner at 7.00 instead of 8.30
- Doing the laundry on a Saturday instead of Sunday
- Taking a bath instead of the usual shower
- Checking the answer machine before checking the email
- Walking up to the shops instead of driving

(Whether these examples are really zero-intensity for a particular client will need to be checked out - but let's assume they are for the moment.)

The method for clearing them with EFT involves targeting and making use of the two key structural features of the habit.

The antidote to "unthinking" habits is thinking. Or to put it another way, increased attention and awareness. Attention will have been increased simply by discussing it of course, but to make sure the habit is cleared requires maintaining attention until a new, preferred habit takes its place. Really the only "problem" for the client is remembering to notice.

Since there is no intensity around the habit it is appropriate to use a Choices format which will serve to anchor the new, preferred habit into any occurrence of the new one. And since "remembering" is a problem, we also need persistence over time - such as repeating it morning and evening for a week, or even longer. Any additional Structures that will help the client remember (such as setting alarms, writing notes to himself, rearranging something) can be added in too.

Example Choices statements might be:

> *"Even though I usually have dinner at 8.30 I choose to eat at 7.00 so I can get to sleep more easily."*

> *"Even though I usually do the laundry on a Saturday, I choose to work on my project instead."*

> *"Even though I usually take a shower, I choose to relax and take a bath on Fridays."*

*"Even though I usually check my email first, I choose to check my phone messages first."*

*"Even though I usually drive to the shops, I choose to walk instead."*

The Choices statement doesn't have to be a stark contrast between the old habit and the new one. It can be embellished with whatever other features the client likes as a way to emphasise the appeal or benefits of the new chosen habit. For instance:

*"Even though I usually do the laundry on a Saturday, I choose to give myself the time and peace to enjoy working on my project instead."*

Related sections:

| | |
|---|---|
| 6.2.5 | Rating Scales ⇧ |
| 6.2.9 | The Choices Technique ⇧ |
| 6.2.11 | Persistence ⇧ |
| 8.1.5 | Structures ⇧ |

## 9.4.3   Low-intensity Habits

The key features of low-intensity habits (rating 1-4) are:

- They are carried out without thinking.
- The person feels mild resistance (such as unease or uncertainty) to the suggestion of swapping it for a different habit or stopping it, or experiences mild unease in the process of changing it.
- The attachment to the habit may be as much about the idea of change as about the content of the habit

An appropriate response from a client who is considering the idea of altering a low-intensity habit might be:

*"That might feel a bit strange for a while but I'll give it a go."*

*"Well, it feels like giving up a kind a tradition, but I guess it won't hurt that much."*

Examples might be:

- Wearing a wristwatch on the right hand instead of the left.
- Not buying the Sunday paper.
- Socialising with colleagues after work instead of getting home in time for the soaps.
- Being five minutes early for every appointment instead of five minutes late.
- Switching the TV off instead of having it on by default.
- Switching from listening to news radio first thing in the morning to listening to a music CD.

(Again, you'd need to check the actual intensity for your client)

The method for clearing low-intensity habits with EFT is similar to that for zero-intensity - except that the intensity needs to be addressed before proceeding to the Choices statements. Straightforward EFT is needed, based on the way that the client expresses the intensity to you e.g.

*"Even though this is going to feel weird for a while,..."*

*"Even though I'm losing a tradition,..."*

*"Even though I'll feel a little bit deprived,..."*

Once there is no intensity around the habit (ideally zero, but no more than a 1) it is appropriate to move on to using a Choices format as described above. Persistence is recommended as before and additional Structures may also be useful.

For example:

> "Even though I usually like to watch the soaps, I choose to build better relationships with my work colleagues."

> "Even though it's so quiet and weird without the TV on, I choose to have more peace and quiet in my life."

Related sections

6.2.9      The Choices Technique ⇧

6.2.11     Persistence ⇧

8.1.5      Structures ⇧

9.2.4      Fear of Change ⇧

## 9.4.4   Medium-intensity Habits

Medium-intensity habits (rating 5-7) may not be full blown physical addictions, but they certainly have an addictive quality to them. And they need to be dealt with in a similar way to addictions in order for the client to make progress.

The key features of medium-intensity habits are:

- The object of desire tends to force itself into the client's mind frequently - remembering to notice is not a problem.
- The person feels medium levels of resistance (such as anxiety, anger or frustration) to the suggestion of changing it.
- The intensity is focussed more on the content of the habit than the idea of change.
- The client experiences craving and/or anxiety prior to the habit and temporary relief or calm afterwards. (i.e. the habit serves as tranquiliser)

It is the presence of craving and anxiety which means that we are talking about addiction, not simple habit.

A typical response from a client who is considering the idea of altering a medium-intensity habit (or who is asked to commit to an action which they know will necessarily disrupt their habit) might be:

> "This is going to be a real challenge."

> "What am I going to do when I get stressed out if I can't do this?"

> "It's one of my few pleasures in life."

> "It will be a big sacrifice but I guess it's worth it"

Examples might be:

- Giving up chocolate (ice-cream, TV soaps…)
- Not going clothes/gadget shopping at the weekends until the debt is cleared.
- Only drinking alcohol at weekends.

- Going to bed by 11.30 even if there is something good on TV.

- Not answering the phone if there's an assignment to be completed.

Habits like these have the power to override our other plans - or even prevent us from even **making** other plans to achieve what we want. And it is also at this level of intensity that clients may be rather reticent to confess to such habits at all, making them hard to know about and therefore deal with.

When a coaching client fails to do their Homework and make progress on their project, it's instructive to ask what they did instead. What activity seemed to be more urgent to them than doing the thing that was so important that they hired you to help make it happen and are spending 30-60 minutes a week talking to you about? The answer(s) to the question may reveal some addictive habits. And if the client can recognise them as such, they can be dealt with using EFT.

The method for clearing medium-intensity habits with EFT is considerably different to that for no-intensity and low-intensity. The principle difference is the need to address the feelings of craving and/or anxiety that accompanies or precedes the habit.

Addressing the craving or anxiety associated with the habit is covered thoroughly in Gary Craig's trainings and in most EFT source books, including [3].

If the object is to simply stop a particular habit, then dealing properly with the craving and anxiety may be all that's needed. Only if the client wants or needs to replace the habitual element of the activity with a new activity would you then proceed to do some Choices work as described above.

So, for instance, in the case of the "going to bed by 11.30 example", you may successfully break the compulsion to watch late night TV using standard craving procedures. But once that has been done, there is still some further work to do (Choices statements or other Structures) to ensure the client adopts the new habit of going to bed by 11.30, as opposed to finding some other late night activity instead such as internet shopping, reading, home improvement projects etc.

Related sections

6.2.9      The Choices Technique ⇧

8.1.5      Structures ⇧

## 9.4.5  High-intensity Habits

High-intensity habits (rating 8-10) are what we would call true addictions and can be for substances, activities and even people.

"Addictions" is one word almost guaranteed to make most coaches hold up their hands and say *"No - that's therapy - find a therapist and come back when you've dealt with it"*.

And yet how many coaches do we see specialising in Weight Loss as a specific and highly legitimate area for coaching? We know that beliefs and behaviours around food fit all the classic definitions of addiction. And sometimes addictions apply to extremely specific foods and beverages.

There are coaches specialising in quitting smoking - using only coaching techniques with no additional "therapeutic" tools and no medical supervision. (If you don't need medical supervision to be allowed to smoke, why would you need it to give it up?). I've also seen "Sobriety Coaching" and "Recovery Coaching" offered to alcoholics who have given up drinking but want additional support to help them stay that way.

And then what about non-substance addictions and compulsions such as playing computer games, shopping, cleaning, nail-biting, hair-pulling, repeatedly checking that the gas is off? Although these are perhaps not health-threatening, they can cause disruption, distress and, of most relevance to us here, can prevent other goals being achieved.

For serious addictions that have the potential for serious harm to the client (such as alcohol, drugs, self-harming, anorexia or bulimia and so on) the client **must** have the appropriate level of medical or psychological treatment and support in place in **addition** to any work they may want to do with you as a coach. (The only exception is if you have a background that clearly qualifies you to work with such clients).

The key features of high-intensity habits (rating 8-10) are:

- The object of desire tends to be almost constantly on the client's mind - remembering to notice is not a problem.
- The person feels high levels of resistance (such as outright panic) to the idea of "losing" the content of the habit.
- The intensity is focussed primarily on the content of the habit (i.e. strong fear of **not** having it, combined with strong desire to have it).
- The client experiences intense craving and/or anxiety prior to the habit and temporary relief or calm afterwards (i.e. the habit serves as a tranquiliser).
- The client anticipates future cravings and/or anxiety before they even occur and makes provision in advance for access to the habit content (i.e. there is fear of the fear).

The intensity of craving and anxiety means that we are talking about full blown addictions here. A typical response from a client who is considering the idea of altering a high-intensity habit might be:

> "There's no way I can do that - let's move on."

> "That's just not reasonable to try and do at the moment."

> "I have far too much stress going on already without that."

> "I really don't see what harm I'm doing just having some chocolate - I'm only flesh and blood after all."

> "I thought coaching was about making your life better?"

Examples might be:

- Giving up chocolate / smoking / alcohol / gambling
- Not calling my ex who I'm still desperately in love with
- Stopping shopping and hoarding and doing a complete de-clutter of the house

The method for clearing high-intensity habits with EFT is the same as for medium-intensity habits, except for making sure to deal with the "fear of the fear" first.

Again, this is covered thoroughly in Gary's trainings and in [3] and [4] as well as practitioner level training. The important principle is not to attempt to work on the addiction directly until the client is completely comfortable doing so. This can mean a considerable amount of pre-work on the fear of the fear.

I have said above that as a coach you probably should not be dealing with severe addictions (and certainly not with life-threatening or medical addictions) without appropriate support. It is appropriate for you to refer your client to specialist help in this situation. But there is one very critical way you can positively assist while remaining in a coaching capacity - and that is to help the client take the necessary action to consult the necessary specialists. When the anxiety is so high, even seeking help feels like a threat.

If coach and client agree that there is an addiction / addictive habit / compulsion (you don't have to argue about terms - just look at the intensity rating!) which needs specialist help but the client is experiencing a block around seeking that help, then it is entirely appropriate to coach the client on the issue of taking that action, including using EFT.

You can treat the problem as a block to action:

>*"Even though I don't really want to deal with this problem right now,..."*

>*"Even though part of me wants to get help and part of me wants to ignore it,..."*

Or you can deal with it as a fear (or rather, the fear of the fear):

>*"Even though I'm afraid to even start looking at this problem,..."*

>*"Even though I'm afraid of the process I'll have to go through,..."*

And of course you can address any specific Aspects related to either:

>*"Even though my career is at stake if I don't deal with this now,..."*

>*"Even though this is damaging my relationship,..."*

>*"Even though my partner has the same problem,..."*

>*"Even though I went for help before and it was a horrible experience,..."*

The other way you can assist while staying in a purely coaching capacity is to set relaxation homework for the client and to ensure they know EFT well enough to be able to deal with stress effectively. If anxiety levels are contributing to the craving (and they do), then helping to keep general anxiety levels down will all ultimately make it easier for the client to get the specialist help they need and/or give up by themselves. I would recommend finding a way to build in persistent tapping (i.e. daily over several weeks) into the homework of such clients, even if the subject of the tapping is nothing to do with the addiction directly. This will produce cumulative relaxation effects which will be generally helpful to whatever the client is trying to achieve in other areas.

Related sections

6.2.11     Persistence ⇧

6.2.12     Aspects ⇧


## 9.4.6   Turning Habits into Options

Sometimes what the client wants or needs is not to overturn a habit completely and never do it again, but to be able to do it **sometimes**, at times when it serves them and with full consciousness and choice.

This applies when the habitual action isn't actually an activity which is harmful in itself. For instance, the habit of getting the Sunday papers and reading them in bed could be a wonderful way to balance the frenzy of a hard week at work. But if the client is looking for ways to find time to study, or spend more time with his family, then this activity could be a time-waster.

Similarly, the client may want to watch TV sometimes, eat chocolate sometimes, eat late sometimes, have a drink after work sometimes, and so on.

One solution to this is to use time-specific Choices which allow the client the flexibility of choosing when to undertake his "habit" and when not to do so. This is the ultimate in Balance and behavioural flexibility. The activity that was previously a habit remains available to the client as something he may **choose** to do to relax or as a reward for achieving some other goal, or simply to provide variety.

The format of a time-specific Choices statement is:

*"Even though I usually <old habit>, I choose to do <new habit> <specify time>"*

Some more specific examples might be:

*"Even though I usually just have salad for lunch, today I choose to have desert too."*

*"Even though I normally check my phone messages first, right now I choose to check my email instead."*

*"Although I normally walk to the shops, I choose to drive there on Saturdays when I have a lot to carry."*

The statement starts out by affirming the positive new Choice that the client now has as his default behaviour.

The "time" element of the statement states when the client intends to do the old activity and is a way of limiting the time spent doing it. It makes it explicit that this is a one-off, fully conscious choice, not the beginning of a slippery slope back into the old habit. Making the Choice consciously like this also serves as permission, thus avoiding guilt or other anxiety.

It goes without saying that this type of behavioural flexibility will not be appropriate for high-intensity habits (addictions) which have not yet been fully cleared or where the activity involves immediate harm such as smoking or taking drugs.

Related sections:

6.1.6      Balance Coaching ⇧

6.2.8      The Choices Technique ⇧

8.1.7      Achieving Balance ⇧

## 9.4.7   Key points

- Habits can be thought of as simply a type of block. However habits are harder to overcome because not only is the client blocked from taking action towards a desired goal, but there is also an existing momentum away from it.

- Habits can be placed on a spectrum according to the degree of negative intensity experienced as a result of trying to change them. The intensity determines the strategy for breaking the habit.

- Zero-intensity habits are those which are carried out without thinking or "by default" and which produce no anxiety or unease at the thought of stopping them. Persistent use of Choices statements are used to cause the client to both notice and remember to do something different.

- Low-intensity habits are also carried out without thinking, but there is mild resistance (such as unease or uncertainty) to the suggestion of changing it. The method for clearing low-intensity habits with EFT is similar to that for zero-intensity habits, except that the intensity needs to be addressed before proceeding to the Choices statements.

- Medium-intensity habits may not be full blown addictions, but they certainly have an addictive quality to them and need to be dealt with in a similar way to addictions. The object of desire tends to force itself into the client's mind frequently and the person feels medium levels of resistance (such as anxiety, anger or frustration) to the suggestion of changing it. There is a need to address the feelings of craving and/or anxiety that accompany or precede the habit, before proceeding to the use of Choices to install a new behaviour.

- High-intensity habits are what we would call true addictions and can be for substances, activities and even people. The person feels high levels of resistance (such as outright panic) to the idea of "losing" the content of the addiction. They may also feel extreme intensity at the prospect of even working on the issue. The method for clearing high-intensity habits with EFT is the same as for medium-intensity, except for making sure to deal with the "fear of the fear" first.

- For serious addictions that have the potential for serious harm to the client such as alcohol, drugs, self-harming, anorexia or bulimia and so on, the client **must** have the appropriate level of medical or psychological treatment and support in place in **addition** to any work they may want to do with you.

- Sometimes what the client wants or needs is not to overturn a habit completely and never do it again, but to be able to do it sometimes, at times when it serves them and with full consciousness and choice. One solution to this is to use time-specific Choices which allow the client the flexibility of choosing when to undertake his "habit" and when not to do so. This is the ultimate in Balance and behavioural flexibility.

# 9.5  Beliefs

> *"A man convinced against his will, is of the same opinion still."*
> Samuel Butler (1610-1686)

People generally aim to keep their behaviour and choices consistent with their conscious or unconscious beliefs. A departure from internal consistency generally produces a feeling of unease or "something feeling wrong", which immediately prompts a desire to return to consistent action.

Therefore, attempting to effect client change simply by altering their behaviour is doomed to failure - either now, or later. The only exception is if the behaviour **itself** produces a change in belief (such as *"I can't do it"*). Lasting behaviour change can only occur when any underlying belief structures have also been changed, so that internal consistency can be maintained.

Being able to identify and alter beliefs is therefore a crucial tool in the overall process of achieving change.

Fear or other emotional distress tend to "feel bad" in a fairly tangible way to clients (which is what allows us to measure the intensity using rating scales). Similarly, clients also tend to be very aware of blocks or habits stopping them from achieving what they want, even if they don't know why they have them. And this awareness is what prompts clients to seek out "therapy" or coaching to deal with them.

But beliefs don't have the tangible intensity of fear or distress. Neither do they have the obvious symptoms of blocks and habits. This is because, by definition, nobody chooses to adopt a belief unless they already believe it. The belief itself doesn't produce feelings of unease - only the prospect of behaviour that is inconsistent with the belief.

In other words, there isn't (usually) a part of the client looking at his beliefs and saying *"Oh I don't like the way that belief feels - let's find a coach or therapist to deal with that"*.

It is therefore, perhaps uniquely, the privilege of the coach, to be in a position to help clients question and shift beliefs - and EFT is a great tool for helping with that. Throughout we still use a 0-10 rating to measure the client's strength of belief as described earlier.

Most people would rather not alter their beliefs if they can help it. And it's certainly true that belief change isn't the primary function of coaching. If a goal can be achieved within the framework of the client's existing belief system, then life is going to be a lot easier for both client and coach. But if a client wants a goal but finds one of their beliefs is an obstacle to that, then suddenly the belief becomes noticeable, and can be targeted for change. Ultimately it's the client's call whether they want to work on a belief or leave well alone.

Related sections:

6.2.5    Rating Scales ⇧


## 9.5.1   The Structure of Beliefs

Beliefs usually come with a "reason" attached, either explicitly or implicitly. And it is usually the "reason" which is the key to altering the belief.

Examples of beliefs with **explicit** reasons include:

*"I'm over 50 now, I'm not going to find a really good relationship at this age."*

*"My husband will leave me if I start asserting myself, because men don't like bossy women."*

*"I can't go it alone now because I've got the mortgage to pay."*

*"This business idea is risky because one in three businesses fail."*

Examples of beliefs with **implicit** reasoning might be:

*"Thinking I can write a novel is just unrealistic isn't it?" (Because writing novels is hard)*

*"Being open-hearted in a new relationship leads to heartbreak" (Because last time I was open-hearted I got my heart broken)*

*"Saying what you really feel is dangerous" (Because when Mum said what she really felt, Dad left)*

*"Wanting to be financially comfortable is OK, but wanting to be rich is not" (Because rich people aren't nice people)*

*"I should be running my own business by now" (Because everyone else in my family did so by my age)*

Sometimes clients are consciously aware of their implicit reasoning and sometimes they are not. And it can often be EFT which brings the reason to the surface and allows it to be cleared.

Sometimes the reasons are themselves beliefs, embedded down to many levels:

*"It's wrong for me to get a massage"*

because

*"I should be spending any spare money I have on the children"*

because

*"The children should always come first"*

because

*"The children are more important than me"*

because

*"Everyone is more important than me"*

because

*"I am useless"*

because

*"Dad told me I was useless".*

Eventually the "becauses" lead down to a statement that isn't a belief, but the actual evidence (the memory, the event, the statistic, what someone said) on which the belief was concluded.

(In a therapeutic context the practitioner would try to get right back to the evidence and clear that as a way of fully clearing all the beliefs that spring from it. In a coaching context, this is not necessarily the aim, although it can happen quite spontaneously as the work progresses. For instance, if the client's goal is to achieve better life balance and it has been agreed that getting a regular massage would be a useful contribution towards that, then it's only important to do **enough** EFT to allow the client to feel fully comfortable about arranging a massage.)

I present this structure simply so that when you are doing EFT with a client on a belief and the client seems to come up with more beliefs as a response, you will recognise what is happening and be on the lookout for the evidence statement if it appears.

I am **not** suggesting that an appropriate strategy in coaching is to keep asking "Because?" in response to a belief until the evidence statement is found. In fact I think it is actually **inappropriate**. Asking "Because?" is the same as asking "Why?" - which takes us into analytical therapy territory.

It's also inappropriate for another reason - which is that the answers the client comes back with in response to repeatedly being asked "Why?" may not be entirely reliable if the client isn't really consciously aware of where a belief comes from. Asking a client directly "Why?" asks the client's conscious mind to "come up with a plausible answer". In contrast, EFT tends to bring up new and relevant information quite spontaneously without the conscious mind having to be involved and without the coach/practitioner having to ask explicitly.

As well as the internal structure of beliefs, most beliefs don't exist in isolation - they interconnect with other beliefs.

Some beliefs are outcomes of higher level beliefs:

*"I believe that people with poor educations have a disadvantage when it comes to being successful. I had a poor education so it will be hard for me to be successful."*

Other beliefs are the bedrock for lower level beliefs.

*"If I stop believing that I don't deserve success, then maybe I also have to believe that I deserve to have love in my life, and I ain't ready for **that** one yet."*

This understanding about the structure of beliefs will now form the basis for working with them in the following sections.


## 9.5.2   Clearing Limiting Beliefs

*"It's become clear to me that defining beliefs are the root of all evil in terms of not getting positive results in your life."* [8]

Having understood the structure of limiting beliefs, we can now define a strategy for dealing with them.

Before you start work, it's vitally important to get ratings for the initial strength of belief. (It's vital all the time, but especially so for beliefs where there may be no actual "intensity" as such).

If you don't have a rating to start with, you might have the client begin the EFT with a certainty level of 9, and finish with a certainty level of 6 - a significant change and an indication that the EFT is having an effect.

If you simply ask *"Is the belief still there?"* then most people are likely to say Yes to a belief as strong as a 6. This could mislead you and the client into thinking that the EFT hasn't had an effect and to abandon that line of work or accept the belief as "valid" after all.

Once you have a rating, start work on either the belief itself, or the "reason" supporting it.

You can start with either depending on your intuition, but if the "reason" is consciously known then this is as good a place to start as any:

> *"Even though I'm over 50 now, I deeply and completely accept myself."*

> *"Even though one in three businesses fail, I deeply and completely accept myself."*

> *"Even though I've got the mortgage to pay, I deeply and completely accept myself."*

> *"Even though men don't like bossy women, I deeply and completely accept myself."*

The setup can be varied to emphasise the belief status of the "reason":

> *"Even though I **believe** men don't like bossy women, …"*

This can act as a particular prompt to the subconscious to question the acceptability of this reason.

If the reason propping up the belief can be weakened then it's likely that the conclusion (belief) that was resting on it may be weakened too.

If the "reason" isn't consciously known, or having addressed the "reason" already, then do EFT on the belief itself.

> *"Even though I thinking writing a novel is unrealistic, …"*

> *"Even though being open-hearted leads to heartbreak, …"*

> *"Even though saying what you really feel is dangerous, …"*

Likely responses to doing EFT directly on the belief include one or more of the following:

- The client's strength of belief rating falls
- The client starts to notice exceptions or other logical flaws to the belief
- The client gets an insight into the "reason" for the belief
- The client remembers the underlying "evidence" for the belief

Another strategy for clearing beliefs is to address the feelings the client has about having the belief or their reasons for not wanting to release it (i.e. Reversals):

> *"Even though I hate having this belief round my neck, I deeply and completely accept myself."*

> *"Even though this belief keeps getting in the way, …"*

> *"Even though I can't seem to shake this belief even though I know it's rubbish,…"*

> *"Even though I'm scared of not believing this because I don't know what I'll end up believing instead,…"*

These types of feelings can be produced as a result of directly addressing the beliefs or the reasons as described above. When the client expresses feelings behind the belief in this way you know you are on to something, because the client has moved from the level of cognition to the level of emotion i.e. nearer to the root source of the issue.

The process of looking for Reversals and noticing Aspects works exactly the same way for beliefs as it does for emotional intensity issues. After tapping for any Aspects or Reversals, always return to the original belief statement and get a new "strength of belief" rating.

If you were working on the belief as a route to making progress on a goal, then also check back and look at the goal and look for any changes about how that now feels. Does taking action feel any easier? Does the goal overall feel more achievable? By checking back to the ultimate purpose of the work (achieving the client's goals) you not only Hold the Client's Agenda very explicitly, you also see what other work remains to be done, either on this belief, or some other Aspect.

Related sections:

| 6.1.14 | Holding the Client's Agenda ⇧ |
| 6.2.3 | Psychological Reversal ⇧ |
| 6.2.5 | Rating Scales ⇧ |
| 6.2.12 | Aspects ⇧ |
| 9.5.7 | Improving Goal Believability ⇩ |

## 9.5.3   Changing Beliefs Safely

*"Most people will find it easier to change a behaviour if they can be reassured that it doesn't involve them changing at a belief or identity level".* [4]

Most people's sense of self is based on a complex structure of beliefs about who they are, where they fit into society, what they are capable of, what's possible and so on. Even if you and your client have identified a belief that would be better replaced or modified, there is a danger of pulling down a client's internal support structure too quickly.

Belief change **can** occur quickly in clients who are already comfortable with the idea of beliefs as essentially transient structures which don't relate to their underlying essence as a human being. However, few clients have this degree of emotional or spiritual maturity. And even for those who do, there is rarely a benefit in simply removing a belief, since it creates a vacuum just waiting to be replaced by something else.

Nature abhors a vacuum, and so do clients. Taking something away from their identity - even if it was negative - can still produce a sense of loss, especially if it relates to the structure of their daily life (such as a habitual activity).

Understanding the ecology of beliefs and dealing with them safely is critical not just to the happiness of your client but to the long term effectiveness of the coaching.

Fortunately there is an inbuilt safety mechanism when using EFT. EFT tends not to release any belief structure until its emotional roots (the client's emotional reasons for having the belief) have also been released along the way. This means that by definition, once the belief is cleared there are no attached emotional factors - such as "sense of loss" - likely to pop up and be a problem.

But even with that inherent safety mechanism it's a good idea to check that the following conditions are met before starting any tapping:

- That the client has already understood the negative impact that the belief is having on their lives (what it is stopping them doing, having or being).

- That the client has begun to see the logical flaw in the belief itself (perhaps its inconsistency with other beliefs they have, or examples where the belief clearly isn't true).
- For the client to be looking forward to the benefit possible once the belief is released (a specific thing they can now have, be or do which they couldn't before, such as a coaching goal).

Clearly these conditions will always be met if the coach is following fundamental coaching principles: involving letting the client find their own solutions (The Client Has the Answers), not judging the client (Accepting the Client without Judgement) and keeping the client focussed on the future (Holding the Client's Agenda).

So for instance, if a client identifies a particular belief which is directly preventing him from achieving a particular goal, it is always the client's choice whether they want to retain the belief and adjust their goal, or whether they want to release the belief and achieve the goal. The coach should make no assumption about which decision is correct.

In fact this is goal validation from a different viewpoint. The client may legitimately and correctly decide to drop a goal because it is inconsistent with a strongly held belief or value. And the client may legitimately refuse to "test" the belief directly using EFT if he does not wish to. But in cases where the client would actually like to know how to resolve an inconsistent belief and goal, EFT can be used.

The setup can address the belief directly:

*"Even though I have this belief, I deeply and completely accept myself."*

Or it can address any additional feelings or worries surrounding the belief:

*"Even though I'm not sure if this belief is valid, I deeply and completely accept myself."*

*"Even though I'm not sure what will happen if I lose this belief, I deeply and completely accept myself."*

*"Even though this belief has cost me so much in my life, I deeply and completely accept myself."*

And of course the Non-Judgement pattern is perfect to use here where the client is undecided about whether the belief needs to be changed or not:

*"I believe that being successful means losing my privacy, and I deeply and completely accept myself."*

Related sections:
6.1.10    The Client has the Answers ⇧
6.1.14    Holding the Client's Agenda ⇧
6.1.15    Accepting the Client without Judgement ⇧
8.2.11    The Non-Judgement Pattern ⇧
9.1.2    Validating Goals ⇧
9.4    Habits ⇧

## 9.5.4  Beliefs about Beliefs

*"Those are my principles. And if you don't like them, I can change them!"*    Groucho Marx

In both coaching and EFT it is helpful for the client to develop a change in perspective on beliefs themselves - where they come from and how they work. This is because it is hard to achieve behavioural flexibility and resourcefulness unless there is a belief flexibility underlying that.

Behavioural inflexibility tends to be associated with people who see their beliefs as "fixed" and which "must be obeyed". In this view of beliefs, the beliefs end up dictating behaviour regardless of whether the outcome is what the person actually wants. Often the only consolation that the person gets is knowing they "did the right thing". It's the classic case of "I'd rather be right than happy".

To achieve true behavioural flexibility (where the person can choose different responses at different times in order to achieve what they really want) beliefs need to be viewed differently - as "chosen" and "modifiable" if it's not working to help achieve a goal, allow a value to be fulfilled etc. In this view of beliefs, the person is in charge and the beliefs serve the person. The person drops any vested interest in "being right" or "being consistent with my beliefs" as the most important consideration.

Now, there is a danger that the prospect of seeing beliefs as mutable and choosable according to what someone wants, looks as if it could lead to a moral meltdown with people just going after whatever they want without worrying about the consequences (as expressed in the Groucho quote above). This isn't so - and in fact the **opposite** becomes possible with this viewpoint - such that the happiness and welfare of human beings can be placed above the handed down judgements and restrictive codes of previous generations.

Taking it at a more spiritual level: all beliefs are judgments of one kind or another about what is right or wrong. They embody assumptions about what is better than what, and what should be done. We also know that such judgements lead to all manner of human misery: prejudice, discrimination, violence and war.

So how can EFT help? If you have a client who keeps on running into her own beliefs as reasons why she can't achieve her goals, and those individual goals are proving somewhat resistant to being modified, then another tack you can take is to back up a step and work on the belief about the beliefs.

In particular you can look for what the client believes will happen if beliefs aren't obeyed. Answers to the question: *"What would happen if I did just change my beliefs"* can be used in setup statements e.g:

> *"Even though I think society would break down if people didn't follow beliefs…"*

> *"Even though I would feel all at sea with myself if my beliefs started changing all over the place…"*

> *"Even though going against my beliefs makes me feel awful, even though it didn't come from me…"*

> *"Even though I think I'd be betraying my parents/religion/nation, by going against this belief…"*

> *"Even though I think without beliefs we'd be no better than animals…"*

Now, working at this level should only be done after a considerable amount of time when there is very good rapport and trust and the client isn't going to start thinking you are the devil in disguise. It needs to happen in the context (as all EFT and all coaching) of making headway towards a goal.

The client must already have come to a realisation that they have several beliefs which have been preventing him from making progress and he has already begun the process of attempting to modify individual beliefs. Without an existing relationship, good rapport and clear evidence of the cost to the client of maintaining his beliefs, then diving in and working on someone's beliefs about their beliefs will cause only unease or outright panic. Undermining client's beliefs with no clear direction and alternative structure being put in place just messes with their sense of identity and possibly even their grip on reality.

This is advanced self-development work and only to be undertaken with clients who know that examining and questioning their own beliefs can be done safely because they have developed an strong sense of their underlying self independent of their beliefs. Repeatedly asserting one's self-acceptance regardless of one's beliefs would probably be a good foundation for developing this sort of sense.

Related sections:

9.5.6.2    Hand-me-down Beliefs ⇩

10.15      Spiritual Coaching ⇩

## 9.5.5   Beliefs about the Rate of Change

Many people, including coaches, have Beliefs about how long change takes - or rather how long they think it **should** take.

But it is important to take account of clients' different levels of comfort with regard to change and to allow change to unfold at a rate that feels OK for them. I have had experience of doing EFT sessions with people for a very specific issue which I believed would only take one session, with perhaps a follow-up just to check for loose ends - and found that it extended to several sessions.

Initially, there was a part of me that felt that perhaps if I'd been a better practitioner I could have helped the issue resolve faster; but there was also the part of me that accepted that things take as long as they take. When I found clients saying to me after a few sessions things like *"Well I guess after 3 sessions it's reasonable for this to be clearing up now, isn't it?"* that I began to suspect something else going on: that some people start out with ideas about how long the change should take - and that this has an influence on how long it actually **does** take.

And there is of course a strong ecological reason for **not** making drastic alterations to a client's energy system (and therefore their behaviour patterns and the structure of their life) - because even if the energy system can be adjusted quickly (and it can), other features of the client's life may not - especially when there are other unchanged energy systems to be taken into account, such as bosses, colleagues, family, friends and so on.

It should always be the case - but especially in coaching - that the client gets to decide what rate of change he actually wants. This relates to potential areas of Reversal such as safety, possibility, fear of change itself, control and so on.

As with any coaching goal, the client gets to say not only what the goal is, but the timeframe over which he wants to make progress. Client beliefs about the "correct" rate of change is therefore one area of beliefs that you probably shouldn't start attacking with EFT, at least not while progress is going along at a reasonable rate.

Having said that, sometimes it is the coach's job to "raise the bar" on the client's expectations of themselves - either because the coach believes the client is capable of more than he is committing to, or because his intuition tells him that the client is deliberately making things more drawn out than necessary in order to avoid dealing with certain aspects of the project.

So assuming the coaching relationship is well enough established in terms of rapport and trust so that the coach can "raise the bar" in a way that the client will understand as supportive and Championing rather than criticism, you can use EFT to address the client's belief about possible and desirable rate of change. Working on a client's beliefs about the rate of change will clearly complement any work you may do on the client's fear of change generally - and both might be addressed together. For instance:

> *"Even though I think true change needs to happen slowly over time, I deeply and completely accept myself."*

*"Even though I need to change slowly for the sake of the people around me,..."*

*"Even though change that happens quickly must be superficial,..."*

*"Even though I think fast change is counter-productive because it's too scary to change all at once,..."*

Related sections:

5.3.5      "Anything that works that fast must be superficial" ⇧

6.2.3      Psychological Reversal ⇧

8.1.13     Championing ⇧

9.2.4      Fear of Change ⇧

9.3.3      Blocks as Reasons Why Not ⇧

## 9.5.6   Common Types of Problem Belief

As with fears and blocks, the variety of beliefs that a client may have or want to deal with is infinite. The following serve as illustrations and examples of some recurring categories of belief that commonly come up during coaching at some time or another. The method for dealing with each type is the same as that given above.

As we discuss each type of belief you may well find yourself thinking: *"Well, this is a block rather than a belief"* or *"Isn't the root of this belief really a fear?"* or even *"Isn't this belief really a type of habit in disguise?".*

As I said right at the start of this chapter, the distinctions between fears, blocks, habits and beliefs can be somewhat fuzzy and they all interconnect and give rise to each other in strong ways. This is because in EFT terms, emotion is the common denominator for each one.

I have separated them out in terms of how a client may initially present them to you. Once you start working with the fear, block or belief you will (and should) find yourself flowing with ease between the different sorts of entity in order to get to the bottom of the issue.

### 9.5.6.1   Self-limiting Beliefs

Self-limiting beliefs are any beliefs that tell the client what they can't do, what's impossible for them, what's not available to them and so on. Almost by definition, any belief that you or the client identify as being a problem or obstacle in achieving the client's goal(s) will be a self-limiting belief.

Examples:

*"That's not possible at my age."*

*"I don't have what it takes."*

*"That area is pretty much sewn up - there's no room for newcomers"*

*"Only one in a million succeed at that"*

*"Success will mean working even harder."*

*"I don't know if I could really handle it if I were really successful."*

## 9.5.6.2   Hand-me-down Beliefs

Most people have beliefs that don't even belong to them. They have no personal evidence or data that generated them. They have never directly thought about them. They may not even be aware that they are present.

They simply have the effects that all beliefs have - and that is to act as a filter on incoming data and to dictate that later beliefs and current behaviour must be as consistent as possible with them.

Hand-me-down beliefs can be inherited from many sources:

- Family traditions
- Individual family members
- Cultural traditions
- Linguistic traditions (expressions, sayings)
- Educational systems
- Religions
- The Media

Just because a belief is "inherited" does not mean that there is no personal emotional attachment to it. In fact it can be quite the opposite. Simply noticing the attachment that people have to family heirlooms or cultural traditions is sufficient evidence for that.

In these cases, bringing the attachment into conscious awareness can **increase** the resistance to releasing it. For instance, knowing that a limiting belief is one that is also strongly held by a beloved other person, or a respected religious institution, can create a sense of guilt or disloyalty at the thought of questioning or changing the belief, which may be expressed as:

> *"I'm not just defending this belief for myself you know - it's for my whole family/tradition/race/humanity/life as we know it."*

It can be the questioning or rejection of inherited beliefs that can be at the root of long-running family feuds, institutional schism and the bitterest of internecine strife. It's at the root of the idea *"My country, right or wrong"*.

For the individual, the issue very often boils down to a choice between "individual conviction based on personal experience" and "social belonging".

It's important to understand that evolutionarily speaking, the human need for group acceptance long precedes and instinctually outweighs the much later development of conscious thought and articulated belief. So normally, the odds are stacked against the winning of individual belief over social pressures (hence the effectiveness of peer pressure in securing individual compliance). But there is one glimmer of hope.

The evolutionary benefit of social belonging is survival. With the group you have a much better chance of survival than as an outsider. And any survival issue has fear as it's root.

This offers us a specific suggestion for how to handle "hand-me-down" beliefs using EFT and that is to address directly the fears associated with losing group acceptance:

> *"Even though I'm afraid of being rejected by my family if I stop believing this,..."*
>
> *"Even though I think I will become an outsider,..."*
>
> *"Even though I don't want to risk the support and help of my family,..."*
>
> *"Even though I'm scared what my <religious cleric> would think of this,..."*

Of course you do need to have some evidence from your client that belonging issues are relevant before you start. But understanding the direct Reversal that the fear of losing social acceptance can have on the releasing of an inherited belief, may be helpful in helping you target that specific Aspect if it arises.

Related sections:

6.2.3        Psychological Reversal ⇧

6.2.12      Aspects ⇧


### 9.5.6.3   Identity Beliefs

Identity beliefs are beliefs which define the client to themselves. They tell the client Who They Are, or rather Who They Think They Are and are characterised by the use of "I am".

Examples:

>  *"I'm a slow learner"*
>
>  *"I'm important"*
>
>  *"I'm unimportant"*
>
>  *"I'm not good enough"*
>
>  *"I'm the sort of person who…"*
>
>  *"I'm an addictive personality."*

Identity beliefs can be hard to eliminate or modify since the client's sense of self is so directly at stake.

It's especially important in these cases to fulfil the guidelines described in Changing Beliefs Safely particularly on the point of the client having understood the cost of having this belief so far.

A particular sub-category of identity beliefs involves the labels the client uses about themselves. These labels can be based on many aspects of identity that follow the phrase "I am":

>  *Occupation:*     *"I'm a graduate / manager / doctor / cleaner / writer…"*
>
>  *Gender:*          *"I'm a man / woman / transsexual…"*
>
>  *Religion:*        *"I'm catholic / protestant / jewish / atheist…"*
>
>  *Origin:*          *"I'm Scottish / African / British / Texan…"*

These identity labels, once stated, then require the client to restrict what they say and do afterwards to be consistent with that, in their terms.

Of course if your client **is** a female doctor from Scotland, then approaching the identity beliefs in the way shown so far is going to be inappropriate (*"Even though I'm a woman…"*, *"Even though I'm a doctor…"*, *"Even though I'm Scottish…"* all sound ridiculous).

Usually, if there is a problem with such beliefs, the problem is not that (for example)

>  *"I am **Scottish**"*

which is just a factual statement about where someone comes from, but that

>  *"I **am** Scottish"*

so the person has to be consistent with what they think "being Scottish" means.

In a case like this where no judgement can or should be made about the content of the belief/fact in question, use the Universal Belief Antidote described below.

Related sections:

9.5.3        Changing Beliefs Safely ⇑

9.5.10      The Universal Belief Antidote pattern ⇓

### 9.5.6.4   Conflicting Beliefs

Often the problem lies not in one particular belief but in the fact that two conflicting or contradictory beliefs are held at the same time.

Example:

> "I need to work and bring in a good income for the family, and I should be with my growing child in it's early years."

Conflicts can be addressed using the Conflict pattern described in [3]. The basic format of the Conflict pattern is:

> "Even though <1$^{st}$ belief> and <2$^{nd}$ belief>, I deeply and completely accept myself."

For example:

> "Even though I'm a scientist and I believe in God,…"

> "Even though I'm a woman and I believe men are better at X,…"

> "Even though I believe we are made in god's image and I believe that being gay is a sin,…"

> "Even though I believe in being loyal to my employer and I believe in being responsible for my own career,…"

> "Even though I believe you have to be very disciplined to be successful and I believe you need to have lots of freedom to be happy,…"

As with all uses of the Conflict pattern[3], juxtaposing the conflicting issues (feelings, problems, beliefs) invites resolution or even synthesis.

A particularly intense form of conflict occurs when either belief looked at individually looks valid and strong; but then so does the other one as soon as that one is looked at. I call these "Necker-cube Beliefs". A Necker-cube is a well known visual illusion in which the edges of a transparent 3D cube are shown as lines (see below). In the diagram, the brain can see either the bottom left corner as the "front" of the solid object, or the upper right as the "front" - but not both at once. Each view, when it is seen, looks completely convincing - until the viewer "flips", either deliberately or spontaneously, to the alternative viewpoint.

Some beliefs operate like this. Sometimes conventional coaching methods can be successful in getting a client to see an alternative viewpoint or belief about an issue. But the old belief hangs around because it still has emotional reasons and evidence connected to it which have not been addressed by the intellectual exercise of finding an alternative viewpoint.

When a client's belief system has this pattern, the client has to work very hard to keep viewing the issue from the viewpoint they have chosen.

Sometimes consistently choosing the same viewpoint can, over time, result in the older belief being overwritten by the new belief. This can happen when the old belief has not especially strong emotional charge attached to it, but was really the result of habit, inherited or unconscious beliefs which had arisen by "default".

But when the old belief has strong emotional charge attached to it, overwriting it can be extremely difficult, because the emotional events or evidence which created the old belief are still present.

Examples:

> *"I should be slim"* **and** *"I should accept myself as I am"*

> *"I need to provide for my financial future"* **and** *"Relationships are far more important than money"*

> *"I need to bring in income for the family"* **and** *"I should be with my child in it's early years."*

These are classic Balance issues - where both beliefs may have significant or even total validity taken individually, but somehow they seem to create conflict and the client finds it hard to know which to give precedence.

The first level of resolution is to apply EFT to each belief individually (see Clearing Limiting Beliefs).

Assuming both beliefs test as valid (i.e. the client's conviction stays solid after application of EFT), the next stage is to generate a "Balance solution". It could be some form of synthesis that incorporates the essence of both beliefs into an over-arching belief. Or it could be insights into the specific situations where the different beliefs are valid. Or it may generate creative ideas for managing how to divide attention of resources between the two in order to honour both.

The format is as for Contradictory Beliefs, using the Conflict pattern[3].

> *"Even though I should be slim **and** I should accept myself as I am, ..."*

> *"Even though I need to provide for my financial future **and** Relationships are far more important than money, ..."*

The Non-Judgement pattern may also be used in cases where the client feels confident that both beliefs have strong validity.

> *"I believe in science and I believe in God, and I deeply and completely accept myself."*

Related sections:

| | |
|---|---|
| 6.1.6 | Balance Coaching ⇧ |
| 8.2.11 | The Non-Judgement Patterns ⇧ |
| 9.5.2 | Clearing Limiting Beliefs ⇧ |
| 10.15 | Spiritual Coaching ⇩ |

## 9.5.7 Improving Goal Believability

Goals which are perceived as being believable have a better chance of actually being achieved than goals which do not. The subjective believability (or achievability) of a goal (from a client's point of view) is a product of the client's current belief system and therefore amenable to change using EFT.

It's vital that working on believability occurs only **after** both you and client are absolutely sure that the goal is valid and wanted. A lot of reasons why a client might say a goal isn't believable are really ways of saying they don't **want** the goal at all - which is a totally different problem.

It's also vital that you, as coach, don't get dragged into the client's (or society's) beliefs about what is "realistic", "achievable" or "difficult" and in so doing inadvertently confirm the client's subjective believability to be lower than it needs to be.

For instance, I might firmly believe as a coach, that "*Setting up in business is hard*", or "*One in three new businesses fail in the first year*", or "*Entrepreneurs have a different sort of personality to most people*".

Now, these reasons appear to be perfectly justified, based on the facts, and very "realistic". But logically, **none** of them prevent the goal of successfully running my own business as being **fully** achievable, **even if they are all completely true**!

In fact it's more likely that with these "reasons why it might not be achievable" operating in my belief system, the final achievability of the goal is actually reduced.

To illustrate, take the example of tossing a coin. I cannot guarantee that I will get a head if I throw the coin. But this does not prevent it from being fully achievable. In fact, if I am prepared to throw the coin many times, I increase my chances of eventually getting a head. Or if I sneakily place a piece of gum on the tails side of the coin I can make it more likely to land heads up. So we can start to generate a list of conditions which, if fulfilled, increase the chances of achieving the goal.

To improve goal believability, first ask the client about either achievability or believability to see what negative beliefs are lurking around the goal itself:

> "*On a scale of 0 to 10, how believable does this goal feel to you right now (where 0 is impossible and 10 is easily believable)*"

> "*On a scale of 0 to 10, how achievable does this goal feel to you right now (where 0 is impossible and 10 is easily achievable)*"

Next, if it is anything less than a 10, apply EFT:

> "*Even though this doesn't seem believable, I deeply and completely accept myself*"

> "*Even though this doesn't seem achievable, I deeply and completely accept myself*"

The aim is to get the rating up to a 10 or as close as possible to it.

If it "sticks", then you need to ask the client why it's sticking (i.e. "*What's stopping it from being achievable?*"). This will elicit the client's beliefs about why it's not achievable e.g.:

> "*I haven't done it before, so I won't really know till I've done it.*"

> "*No-one's ever done it before so I won't know till I've done it.*"

> "*I'm not convinced I'll really follow through with it.*"

> "*Well, X is a big unknown at the moment and that's not under my control*".

> "*I don't know if I trust myself to do it.*"

Clients will almost always interpret the question "*Is it achievable?*" as "*Will **you** achieve it?*". And their rating out of 10 will almost certainly include their estimation of how likely the goal is to be achieved. (This response is also about wanting to be internally consistent. They don't want to say that something is fully achievable and then fail to achieve it - because then that looks as if it is a problem with them, rather than a problem with the goal.)

Apply EFT to whatever answers come up for this:

*"Even though I haven't done it before, ..."*

*"Even though I'm not convinced I'll really follow through with it,..."*

*"Even though, X is a big unknown and that's not under my control, ..."*

Also notice that these answers can take you back into the familiar territory of fears, blocks and beliefs. This is absolutely fine. As long as ultimately you bring it all back to the targeted belief it doesn't matter what other Aspects are covered along the way.

And of course, if there are beliefs about the achievability of the goal which really do look like a brick wall, there is always the Universal Belief Antidote which can be applied to ensure that if there are any other possibilities that haven't been thought of yet, that these can be invited to make themselves known.

Related sections:

6.2.12     Aspects ⇧

9.5.10     Universal Belief Antidote Pattern ⇩

## 9.5.8   Strengthening Positive Beliefs

A positive belief can be an important resource for a client. And clients will typically have less resistance around the idea of strengthening an existing belief than of undoing a negative one. It will feel like an incremental change to the existing state of affairs rather than a radical re-ordering of their identity and assumptions about the universe.

Most clients will have **some** positive beliefs about **some** aspects of themselves but which they rate as less than a 10 on the strength of belief scale. This occurs when clients have Tailenders connected to the belief (negative beliefs which are triggered by thinking about the positive one).

For instance, the client may believe that *"I'm capable of succeeding"* but nevertheless have trouble actually exhibiting the kind of success they want in their life.

In fact, the Tailenders that are stopping the client report a 10 on their chosen belief and stopping them fulfilling it, may themselves be rooted in other negative beliefs. So by strengthening a positive belief the client is almost certainly chipping away at some negative ones.

The process for strengthening an existing belief is:

- Get a rating for the strength of belief now.
- Find the Tailenders to the belief and apply EFT to them.
- Check back to the rating for the belief until it is at least a 9.
- Reinforce with a Choices round, if appropriate.

For instance, for the example positive belief mentioned above, some Tailenders might include:

*"But I never get the time to make it happen."*

*"But other people are even more capable than me."*

*"...if I could just get myself started."*

*"...if I could just decide what I really want."*

*"But I don't have the knowledge I need."*

*"But succeeding means a lot of work and stress."  etc*

Having addressed these Tailenders, a suitable Choices round might be applied either to a specific Tailender :

> *"Even though I'm afraid of the stress involved, I choose to find a way to succeed."*

or to the overall belief involved:

> *"Even though I haven't succeeded yet, I choose to begin my success now."*

Related sections:

| 6.2.15 | Tailenders ⇧ |
| 6.2.8 | The Choices Technique ⇧ |
| 8.1.1 | Resourceful States ⇧ |

## 9.5.9   Testing Values

Values can be forceful motivations to positive change, acting as internal benchmarks and success criteria. Indeed this is the way that values are principally viewed and used within coaching.

But they can also be as much hindrances to change as they can be a help. This is perhaps strange news to coaches who swear by using client values as a primary reference point for coaching.

It's true that eliciting and referring back to client values is an immensely powerful coaching technique.

But there is a basic problem with values - and that is that they are intricately bound to beliefs - and we already know how problematic beliefs can be. That is why I deal with values here, in the overall section on beliefs, rather than giving it a section of its own.

Just as people like to behave consistently with their beliefs as far as possible, so they also like to behave consistently with their values as much as they can. People also filter their experience and make judgements about what's around them based on these values. Functionally therefore they have the same effect as beliefs and so I deal with them here as a particular form of belief.

The following sections present the ways in which values and beliefs can interact, and then present techniques for testing the validity of a client's values.

### 9.5.9.1   True Values, Limiting Beliefs

A client who holds a value, also holds a belief. A value is a belief about Who You Are, or perhaps Who You Would Like to Be. But the belief is not only *"I believe in <value>"* or *"I am <value>"*. In practice there are also likely to be many beliefs **around** that value.

For example, if your value is Compassion you do not merely hold "Compassion" in your belief system as an abstract entity disconnected to anything else. Holding "Compassion" as a value influences your beliefs about a whole lot of other things. For instance:

> *"Compassion is always better than Violence."*

> *"Compassion is the correct response to someone in pain".*

> *"Compassion means giving money to charities."*

> *"Compassion means turning the other cheek and forgiving my neighbour."*

Similarly, if you hold a value of Independence, you might have some of the following beliefs:

*"Independence means doing everything myself."*

*"Losing my Independence means losing my identity."*

*"Independence is Freedom."* (tying it to another value)

*"Independence can only be achieved by living alone."*

I hope you can instantly see the sort of limiting beliefs that it is possible to have operating, even if the value involved is itself entirely desirable and "correct" in terms of the client's true essence.

In her wonderful book "Return to Love", Marianne Williamson says *"I shudder to remember now how Angry I used to get when people wouldn't sign my Peace petition"*. Clearly Peace was a core value for her then and still is. But in between that event and writing the book, she had clearly dropped a belief that used to produce Anger in her when other people did not share her value or would not comply with her request.

Thus a particular value may not be "false" just because there is a faulty belief attached to it. So now we can start to think of values as perhaps some kind of affirmation, with all the attached beliefs behaving like Tailenders. As with beliefs, challenging client values is not the primary function of coaching. But we do need somewhere useful to go in situations where a client finds one or more of her values in conflict with her goal(s), or with another value. EFT offers a way to find out the negative emotional roots behind this sorts of conflict so that the client can get clarity about their true values.

Related sections:

6.2.15     Tailenders ⇧


## 9.5.9.2    Testing a Value in Isolation

In this application you are looking out for any Tailenders or objections that arise in response to the value itself. It is only appropriate to do this test if the client himself isn't sure whether the value is correct and wants to clarify.

The format is the Non-Judgement pattern, but can be expressed in whatever variation the client prefers or finds most natural. For instance:

*"I have this value, and I deeply and completely accept myself."*

*"I value Independence, and I deeply and completely accept myself."*

*"Independence is important to me, and I deeply and completely accept myself.""*

Using SLOW EFT instead of Standard EFT, perhaps as Homework, can help the client get deeper insights into what the value really means to them, what else it is connected to, where it originated and so on.

By applying EFT in this way, we are not aiming for a specific outcome in terms of how it may be transformed. And we are certainly not assuming that it will be "cleared" or disappear as a value. We are only "loosening" it in terms of how it fits within the client's energy system. Where it "falls" or "comes to rest" is up to "gravity" and the terrain of the rest of the client's overall belief and energy system. It's like pushing a rock off the top of a mountain. You know it will move, but can't predict the path it will take or how far down the mountain it will go.

Any of the following outcomes are possible, and maybe still others:

* The client may remember when they first acquired the value (helping to identify whether it belongs to them or is "hand-me-down")

* The client may come up with objections to the value or situations in which they realise it wouldn't apply

- The client may find clarity about why the value is important to them or what's at stake for them if they don't fulfil it (i.e. reinforcing the value)

- The client may stop identifying with the value so closely - it may seem more distant or remote - just another quality among many qualities that are useful at different times.

Related sections:

| 6.2.9 | SLOW EFT ⇧ |
| 8.2.11 | The Non-Judgement Pattern ⇧ |
| 9.5.6.2 | Hand-me-down Beliefs ⇧ |

### 9.5.9.3   Testing a Value against a Goal

It's easy to think that by not questioning a client's values, that this is part of "Holding the Client's Agenda".

But the ultimate agenda in coaching is never what the client happens to be thinking or feeling right now - but the client's stated goals. Values (or any other sort of belief) are not right or wrong - but they can be judged to be moving the client further towards or away from their stated goal.

When a value is discovered which is preventing movement towards a desired goal, then either the goal must be changed, or the value must be changed. The alternative is stagnation and stalemate - and no action. Most clients come to coaching to help move them on with things they've been stuck with for a while - and so it's a fair bet that there is a belief or value conflict going on at some level.

There are two format options for testing a value against a goal. The first is Standard EFT and is appropriate when the client acknowledges the conflict between the value and the goal as a problem:

> "Even though this value seems to conflict with my goal,...."

But if the client (and coach) do not want to make a judgement about this even being a problem, perhaps having a synthesis in mind, a second format is the Conflict pattern[3] combined with the Non-Judgement pattern. For instance:

> "I value Freedom and my goal is to find a new relationship,
>
> "I value Security and my goal is to leave my job and start my own business"
>
> "I value Love and I need to challenge my partner about her behaviour."

As above, the outcome is unknown and not to be "aimed for" in any sense. The task is to observe carefully the emotional and cognitive reaction of the client (and preferably for the client to observe their own reaction) and see how they now feel about the value, the goal or both.

As well as the outcomes possible when testing a value in isolation, this particular test also holds the possibility of finding a solution whereby both value and goal can be fulfilled.

Related sections:

| 9.5.6.4 | Conflicting Beliefs ⇧ |
| 8.2.11 | The Non-Judgement Pattern ⇧ |
| 6.1.14 | Holding the Client's Agenda ⇧ |

## 9.5.9.4 Testing a Value against another Value

Sometimes a client finds himself with two apparently conflicting values in respect to a particular goal.

So for example, suppose a client has stated that he believes *"I am someone who values family loyalty"* and on the basis of this identity (his belief about "Who He Really Is") decides not to proceed with his dream to sail round the world because it would cause problems for his family.

This dilemma could be addressed by using Conflict resolution and tapping on the desire to sail versus the desire to be with his family (there is often more than one variation of EFT that can be used) but let's suppose that the issue of values is of interest to the client.

The following fictional dialogue illustrates how a dialogue to clarify competing values might unfold.

> Coach: *"So when it comes to family loyalty, is that a core value for you?"*
>
> Client: *"Yes, very much so."*
>
> Coach: *"But this value seems to be leading you away from your other values of self-fulfilment and adventure that we identified last time."*
>
> Client: *"Yeah….but the family comes first for me, ultimately. I just couldn't imagine doing anything that would threaten that - that just wouldn't be me - I just wouldn't feel good about it.*

So we have some clues that this is an identity issue (*"that just wouldn't be me"*) **and** that there is some negative emotion connected to it (*"I just wouldn't feel good about it"*).

> Coach: *"Where do you think your Family Loyalty value comes from?"*
>
> Client: *"I don't know I guess it's always been there. It was definitely a big thing with my parents, I know that - and I really admire them for that"*

So now we have a clue that the Family Loyalty value is perhaps inherited from the client's parents.

> Coach: *"OK - so since you are going to make such a big decision about your sailing goals based on this value, would you like to test whether this value is really about you or what else might be involved with it?"*

(Note - the client is given the genuine choice whether to explore this or not).

> Client: *"Well I do feel pretty sure about it - but I can see it's in direct conflict with the Adventure value - so it would be good to really test it out".*

So why use EFT here? It would be quite possible simply to continue the coaching by asking the client to clarify what both values mean (Family Loyalty and Adventure) and come to a resolution that way.

We know as coaches that when clients are faced with the possibility of actually achieving goals, they can often magically discover all sorts of really solid reasons why they can't proceed. Clients quickly learn the language of values and can often appeal to other values in order to avoid what they really want.

They may not be doing so consciously or with intention to subvert the course of coaching. But a client who is "cornered" into getting on with his goals may try **any means** - especially means which look so logical to him (and to the coach!) that even he will not question or notice whether it is an avoidance tactic. Such is the nature and power of Psychological Reversal at work. Of course a valid response from a coach in this situation may be to decide the client is uncoachable (they are not committed to making the necessary changes in their lives) and to terminate the coaching. But the EFT Coach has alternative possibilities available.

The testing procedure here is as follows:

Ask the client to give a rating out of 10 for both values where the rating is how "correct" or "strong" each value feels. The two ratings indicate the intensity of each value individually as well as indicating the intensity of the conflict between the two. For instance, if the client rates both values as a 10, this implies not only that both are strong values by themselves, but that the conflict is intense - the client is being pulled equally hard in both directions.

If the client rates the values as a 10 and a 6, this suggests immediately that one value is dominant over the other and that the value rated as a 6 seems to have significant doubts or objections around it in any case.

The format for the test is again a Non-Judgement Conflict pattern. It can look at the values as a pair of concepts in isolation:

> "I value Family Loyalty and Adventure, and I deeply and completely accept myself."

Or it can test the relativity of importance of the values with respect to the particular goal at issue:

> "I value Family Loyalty and Adventure, and I really want to sail round the world, and I deeply and completely accept myself."

This format narrows the remit of the test to the current goal rather than requiring the client to think about the conflict at a wider level. So we may not find out everything there is to know about both these values and where they come from, even though the client may achieve resolution with respect to the goal. This is perfectly adequate within a coaching context.

Related sections:

6.1.9      Coachability ⇧

6.2.15    Tailenders ⇧

8.2.11    The Non-Judgement Pattern ⇧

9.1.12    Validating Goals ⇧


## 9.5.9.5    The Heresy of Values Testing

I realise I may be committing some kind of deep heresy by suggesting that clients may not want the goals they say they want or may not really value what they say they value.

Whether the client above really has a Family Loyalty value that is core to his Real Self, or whether it is a good reason to avoid achieving his goal of sailing round the world, probably neither coach nor client can really know or prove.

All we know is, having this value is causing the client to feel bad about his goal - a goal that he previously identified as something that would make him feel good. Clearly **something** is amiss, even though we don't yet know what. When you are in this situation (i.e. you have evidence that the identity value isn't quite as clean and pure as it needs to be to constitute a valid reason for dropping a long-cherished goal), then persisting with asking the client about his values and what they mean or which ones are more important, is unlikely to produce a resolution, since you will simply be triggering the current set of beliefs and Tailenders that have stopped him getting on with his goal.

The second that coaches buy into the perceived constructs of their clients as the total truth of the matter, is the second that the coach stops being an effective facilitator of the client's truth and starts being a collaborator in the client's self-construct.

EFT offers a way to test the emotional truth of any client value, belief or goal - without having to make a judgement about the client, or having to question the client's integrity or level of self-delusion (which we are all prey to in different ways). Where there are incongruities or negative emotional roots, EFT with reveal them quite naturally - and suggest that which is closer to the client's truth along the way.

Second-hand, inherited values can be dropped completely. Values which are partly truth and partly accumulated emotional debris (e.g. Loyalty which has become an excuse for domestic martyrdom), can be cleaned up and refreshed. And values which are genuinely true and essential to the client can be strengthened, felt and experienced as the truth that they are. Which in turn makes acting on those values - free of the Tailenders that used to accompany them - easier to do, leading to more congruent action and ultimately more Fulfilment.

Related sections:

6.1.5        Fulfilment Coaching ⇧

6.2.15      Tailenders ⇧


## 9.5.10  The Universal Belief Antidote Pattern

The above has shown how working with beliefs can lead to extensive work on many layers, uncovering memories, working through Aspects and so on in order to shift, modify or synthesise a client's belief.

But within coaching the most important reason for dealing with a belief is in order to proceed to a new, preferred future. Ultimately we are only interested in the characteristics of a belief as a way of getting it out of the way of achieving the client's goal(s).

I therefore offer a Universal Belief Antidote pattern, based on the Choices pattern, and which can be given to all clients to use on any belief they choose, by themselves, during and after the coaching.

> *"Even though I have this belief, I choose to notice what **else** is possible."*

This pattern has the following deliberate features:

- It accepts without judgement the existence of the belief

- It does not attack, question or threaten the belief - "what else" implies "as well as" not "instead of"

- It allows for the possibility that the belief may turn out to be wrong and be dropped.

- It allows for the possibility that the belief may be partly true and may be modified.

- It allows for the possibility that the belief may remain completely intact and be expanded on.

- It inhibits the action of the belief as a data filter and allows the client to notice and gather new evidence (which in turn may result in modifying the belief).

- It is fundamentally focussed on the future and on finding solutions.

The only necessary precursor to using this pattern successfully is a willingness to acknowledge the mutability of beliefs. If beliefs are assumed to be a reason to prevent further thinking, then it's unlikely that this pattern will have very much impact, since it will trigger a very obvious Tailender: *"But there **isn't** anything else possible".*

It is most effective therefore to introduce this pattern after you have done some more detailed belief work with a client and they have experienced how beliefs can be altered using EFT. This will provide them with the "evidence" they need for their "belief" that beliefs don't have to be set in stone.

Related sections:

6.2.8        The Choices Technique ⇧

6.2.12      Aspects ⇧

6.2.15      Tailenders ⇧

## 9.5.11 Key Points

- People generally aim to keep their behaviour and choices consistent with their conscious or unconscious beliefs. A departure from internal consistency generally produces a feeling of unease or "something feeling wrong", which immediately prompts a desire to return to consistent action. Therefore, attempting to effect client change simply by altering their behaviour is doomed to failure - and altering beliefs is therefore crucial in the process of achieving client change.

- Beliefs usually come with a "reason" attached, either explicitly or implicitly, and either consciously or unconsciously. And it is usually this "reason" which is the key to altering the belief.

- Clearing limiting beliefs involves addressing both the belief itself and the "reason" supporting it. If the reason is consciously known (or can be guessed at with intuition) then this is a good place to start applying EFT. If not, EFT can be applied to the belief directly.

- Most people's sense of self is based on a complex structure of beliefs. Taking something away from their identity - even if it is negative - can still produce a sense of loss, especially if it relates to the structure of their daily life. Fortunately there is an inbuilt safety mechanism when using EFT. EFT tends not to release any belief structure until its emotional roots (the client's emotional reasons for having the belief) have also been released along the way.

- It is hard to achieve behavioural flexibility and resourcefulness unless there is a belief flexibility underlying that i.e. the ability to question beliefs. Using EFT to examine beliefs about beliefs can be a useful way forward if the client's beliefs are proving to be obstacles towards achieving the client's goal(s) and the goals themselves are resisting modification.

- As with any coaching goal, the client gets to say not only what the goal is, but the timeframe over which he wants to make progress. Client beliefs about the "correct" rate of change is therefore one area of beliefs that you probably shouldn't start attacking with EFT, at least not while progress is going along at a reasonable rate. But if rate of change does become an issue, EFT can be used to address beliefs about how fast things could or should occur.

- The variety of beliefs, like Reversals, is infinite. But some of the most common that arise in a coaching context are Self-limiting beliefs (telling the client what they can do), Hand-me-down Beliefs (inherited from family or others), Identity Beliefs (who the client thinks they are), and Conflicting Beliefs.

- Goals which are perceived as being believable have a better chance of actually being achieved than goals which are not. The subjective believability of a goal (from a client's point of view) is a product of the client's current belief system and is amenable to change using EFT.

- EFT can be used to strengthen existing positive beliefs. This can be less unsettling to a client than the idea of removing beliefs, although by removing the Tailenders that are limiting the positive belief, they are probably chipping away at one or more negative beliefs in the process.

- Although values are used as a reference point within coaching, they also need to be treated with caution and questioned. Values are intricately bound to beliefs. In fact they are beliefs about Who the Client Believes They Are. So a client can have valid values, but also have limiting beliefs arising from them. It's also possible to have "pseudo-values" which are not expressions of the client's true self at all.

- Values (or pseudo-values) can be tested in isolation to look for any Tailenders or objections that arise. Values can also be tested against a goal, or against other Values, as a way of testing relative validity but also as a way of looking for conflict resolution or synthesis.

- Ultimately we are only interested in the characteristics of a client's belief to the extent that it affects the achievement of the client's goal(s). The Universal Belief Antidote pattern offers a way to approach any problematic belief in a non-judgemental way and to focus on the desire to move past it to a new solution.

# 10 A-Z of Coaching Specialities

Many coaches specialise in particular areas of coaching - and many coaching institutions and associations are springing up to support coaches specialising in a particular area. Having covered how EFT can help with specific coaching situations and specific coaching techniques, it is now useful to look at broader domains of coaching to see how EFT might be applied in those areas.

This section doesn't contain any significant "how to" information beyond what has been presented above. Instead it is intended to broaden the reader's awareness of different coaching specialties and give some ideas about how the techniques and patterns described above could be applied in these specific domains. For existing EFT practitioners thinking of adding coaching to their practice, I hope this section may be useful in suggesting possible areas in which to specialise. For existing coaches who have no particular specialism or niche, this section may serve as a way to start noticing to which areas you feel "drawn".

Since I believe one of the best ways to learn about the power and range of EFT is to see it applied in many different ways, I deliberately include as many examples and suggestions for setup statements as I can for each area. These are structured roughly around the key coaching tasks identified above: goals; fear and blocks; beliefs and values.

There are probably as many potential specialisms within coaching as there are life circumstances encountered by human beings. There are therefore probably many more areas that I could have covered. But these are the ones which are seen most commonly and all of them are specialisms which I have seen offered by real coaches or coaching organisations.

Nor do I intend the following to be complete or through representations of each specialism. Readers who do specialise will know far more about the issues involved in each area. But I do hope to trigger some insight into how EFT may be applied within the specialism. I look forward to seeing specialist coaches produce even more detailed presentations of how EFT may be used within their domain.

# 10.1 Bereavement Coaching

Nothing makes a person ask the question *"What does my future look like now?"* more than the experience of bereavement. But this question can be asked from a state of total despair or from a state of hope and excitement. Bereavement coaching offers to help the client make the transition from one to the other. Even if the person had a clear view of their life and goals before the bereavement, the chances are that those goals and that future assumed the presence of the departed loved one in some way or another. When that assumption is questioned, the associated life goals may come into question also.

Bereavement coaching is not a substitute for grief counselling. It is appropriate for the point where the client decides they want to start rebuilding and want to focus more on the future, but would like some help doing so. Bereavement coaching generally deals with the stage following the initial shock and grief, when the person is starting to re-create a life without the loved person involved.

And although the idea is that the initial intense stage of grief may be over, the process of focussing on the future can itself re-trigger feelings of grief. Often the process of planning a future without the departed person can trigger intense feelings of guilt, or issues of "permission" can arise - which can be experienced as blocks to planning a new life.

Sometimes the bereavement has resulted in a financial legacy or independence which allows the client to consider options they could never have considered before. This in turn can cause feelings of conflict and the idea that their good fortune is somehow being bought at the "expense" of the person who died. This can make bereaved people reluctant to use the money because it "means" they are profiting by the death.

Anniversaries (birthdays, Christmas, "when we met") can also be particular trigger points that can interrupt the rebuilding progress or even result in a relapse into grief, as can specific locations that had meaning for the people involved.

In other words, even though the initial grief stage may be over, there are many opportunities for emotional issues to arise during the process of rebuilding and getting on with a new and positive life. And therefore, EFT can legitimately be used as a support tool as part of the coaching process.

**Examples:**

### Goals

*"Even though I can't really imagine life without him,..."*

*"Even though, if I take that trip that would have been our 20th anniversary,..."*

*"Even though I have to totally rethink what my goals are now,..."*

*"Even though that was really her goal more than it was mine,..."*

### Fear and Blocks

*" Even though if I start enjoying myself it must mean I never loved them properly,..."*

*" Even though, it's not allowed/fitting/seemly to start living again so soon,..."*

*"Even though it doesn't seem right to be spending the money he worked for all his life,..."*

*"Even though I'm terrified at the thought of travelling by myself,..."*

### Beliefs and Values

*"Even though I don't believe it's right for me to be enjoying this by myself,..."*

*"Even though it feels disloyal to be starting to see new people,..."*

*"Even though I think not feeling grief will mean I didn't love her,..."*

# 10.2 Business Coaching

*"It's no overestimation to say that success in business has everything to do with the person's attitudes, values and beliefs"* [3]

Business coaching (including executive coaching, corporate coaching and organisational coaching) is perhaps one of the biggest - and most lucrative - coaching sectors. In fact the content of Business coaching is not really what defines it - since it can include Performance coaching, Creativity coaching, Leadership coaching, Stress coaching and many other types of coaching along the way.

What usually defines Business coaching is not the self-development goals that individual clients within an organisation may have, but the "bottom line" goals of the sponsoring organisation i.e. issues such as turnover, market share, customer perception, brand image, employee productivity and so on. Ultimately no organisation is going to pay for its executives to have coaching unless it believes it will reap these kinds of rewards from its investment.

Immediately we can observe the potential for conflict in this type of coaching - which boils down to the tension between the goals of the individual and the goals of the organisation. And these conflicts apply as much to individual entrepreneurs and small businesses as they do to larger corporations.

Even if the individual feels complete commitment to the job and to the goals of the organisation, there will be times when personal circumstances come up against job requirements. This includes issues such as hours worked, pay issues, balancing family commitments and work commitments, health issues possibly including stress, and so on.

So we can instantly see a value for EFT in this domain, simply helping the individual deal with these kinds of emotional conflicts.

**Examples:**

### Goals

*"Even though I don't think I agree with my company's goals this year,..."*

*"Even though I have this frustration over my company never setting proper targets,..."*

*"Even though I haven't been given clear objectives for my job,..."*

*"Even though I know my personal goals conflict with my company's goals,..."*

*"Even though I don't think I can achieve this goal,..."*

*"Even though I can't choose between the five different things that I want to do,..."*

### Fear and Blocks

*"Even though I'm afraid to talk to my boss,..."*

*"Even though there's this climate of fear around at the moment,..."*

*"Even though I can't see a way through this mess,..."*

*"Even though I feel totally trapped,..."*

*"Even though I can't think further than the second quarter results,..."*

*"Even though I have this block about cold calling,..."*

### Beliefs and Values

*"Even though this policy is against everything I believe in,..."*

*"Even though I feel torn between Loyalty to the company and Loyalty to my family,..."*

*"Even though no-one here really believes we can succeed with this plan,..."*

*"Even though I believe we have to put investors before customers,..."*

*"Even though I don't think I'm really cut out for this kind of job,..."*


# 10.3 Creativity Coaching

Artistic pursuits such as writing, painting, sculpture and musical composition are goals which particularly demand the need for both Doing and Being aspects to be covered. More and more artists - professional and amateur - are turning to coaching to give them that extra bit of support and non-judgmental guidance in what can be a very lonely occupation - and coaches are coming forward to fill this need.

Some of the particular issues that creatives - or would-be creatives - experience and which can be helped with EFT include:

- Identity issues (their beliefs about Who They Are)
- Their relationships to others or society generally (feeling different or separate to "normal" people)
- Blocks around the creative process itself (e.g. *"I can't think of anything original"*, *"I'll never be really creative."*, *"My mind's a blank"* etc).
- Stimulating ideas, insights, connections and generally providing material and impetus to the creative process.
- Integration of their creative existence versus their more everyday existence (e.g. resenting time spent on necessary but mundane activities, attitudes towards success and money)
- Issues around project initiation ("the blank page/canvas") and project completion.
- Ability and confidence issues (*"What makes me think I can do this?"*)
- Fear about audience reaction to their work.

Creativity coaching with EFT is likely to alternate between standard EFT to release obvious blocks, Choices EFT to stimulate positive feelings about the creative process, and SLOW EFT to stimulate ideas. The Doing and Being pattern is likely to be useful, as also are the Non-Judgement pattern and the Yes/No Commitment pattern.

**Examples:**

### Goals

*"Even though I don't really think of myself as an Artist,..."*

*"Even though I've been trying to finish this book for 5 years,..."*

*"Even though I don't know which book to write next,..."*

*"Even though I've wanted this since I was a child and I'm afraid what will happen to my dream if I get it now,..."*

*"Even though I need to spend time on my book synopsis, I choose to find it enjoyable and absorbing."* (Doing and Being pattern)

*"Even though I'm saying No to a safe job with a salary, I choose to say Yes to expressing myself with freedom"* (Yes/No Commitment pattern)

### Fear and Blocks

*"Even though I just go blank when I start thinking about this,..."*

*"Even though I just can't get started,..."*

*"Even though I can't see myself ever finishing this,..."*

*"Even though I'm afraid what people will think of my work,..."*

*"Even though I'll never be a Picasso so why am I bothering,..."*

*"Even though I shouldn't be spending my time on marketing myself,..."*

*"Ideas come to me when I'm least expecting it, and I deeply and completely accept myself."* (Non-Judgement pattern)

### Beliefs and Values

*"Even though I think only the really exceptional people have a chance of succeeding,..."*

*"Even though I think you have to suffer for your Art,..."*

*"Even though I think aiming to make a lot of money is wrong if you're a serious artist,..."*

*"Even though I can never be as good as X,..."*

*"Even though my father always said that artists were a burden on the state,..."*

# 10.4 Consciousness or Essence Coaching

Consciousness or Essence coaching has much in common with Spiritual coaching - but with less explicit emphasis on "the divine". Instead it focuses primarily on the expansion of consciousness of the individual. It is expressly interested in examining the client's belief systems and the client's understanding of himself.

Although these discoveries and re-evaluations may take place along the way within any particular domain of coaching, in consciousness coaching, they become the central goal. The focus is almost primarily on the Being aspects of the client, with Doing often taking the place of "mirror" or "feedback" to the client about the current state of their consciousness.

Consciousness coaching can also be a useful precursor to more traditional "Doing" coaching for clients who have no idea what goals to work towards but sense this should be decided as a result of becoming very clear about Who They Are and their purpose in life. Thus, consciousness coaching can serve to provide a space in which clients aren't under any pressure to "achieve" anything, except the task of connecting with their true selves, or their Essence.

As we know, EFT has the power to release any thought, feeling or belief which is not part of the client's True Self, but the result of life experience, conditioning by family or society, or emotional "neediness".

I believe that EFT can provide a vital tool in making the leap from identifying a belief or feeling as not being from the client's true self, and actually releasing it. In this view, the goal of the EFT is not so much to lose the unwanted thought or feeling, but to gain the state of consciousness that losing it allows. In other words, having the target belief may not be causing any direct intensity or obvious problem for a specific goal, but the client simply recognises that belief is preventing a higher level of consciousness to "come through".

And with this is mind, the uses I have outlined earlier involving testing beliefs, values and goals in a non-judgemental way seem to offer a particularly useful tool within this domain.

A potential risk of any sort of consciousness-evaluating experience (coaching, workshop or simply reading a book on the subject) is that the questioning of identity values and belief structures can be unsettling or even traumatic as the conscious mind (or "ego", if you like) comes under threat or otherwise has to come to terms with itself in new ways. EFT can clearly provide a support structure to the whole energy system to enable this process to occur with the absolute minimum of trauma and maximum insight.

**Examples:**

### Goals

*"Even though I feel this pressure to achieve consciousness,..."*

*"Even though I feel like I should be doing something,..."*

*"Even though I'm not sure where I'm really heading with all this,..."*

### Fear and Blocks

*"Even though I find really looking at myself scary,..."*

*"Even though seeing the world in this new way feels very weird,..."*

*"Even though I don't think I'm ever going to achieve full consciousnesses,..."*

*"Even though I'm not sure if I'm ready for this process,..."*

*"Even though I just can't seem to get to the next level,..."*

*"Even though I feel really confused about Who I Am right now,..."*

### Beliefs and Values

*"Even though I think true enlightenment takes time,..."*

*"Even though I don't think consciousness counts for much compared to what you Do,..."*

*"Even though I don't feel the way I expected,..."*

*"Even though I believe that everyone should work on their consciousness to help everyone else,..."*

# 10.5 Dating Coaching

Dating coaching - or Dating Support - is one of my own particular specialisms. It became clear to me as a result of my personal experience that the process of dating and relationships is a perfect crucible for learning about oneself. It also involves making decisions whose repercussions really will last a lifetime.

For most people past their teens and twenties, the process of Dating or looking for a new relationship and life partner can be a minefield of emotional obstacles and challenges. These include:

- Getting over past relationships (or "Love Pain" as Gary Craig calls it) in terms of lingering emotional attachments, or trauma arising from abusive relationships.

- How the client feels about themselves as a "catch" (e.g. age, appearance).

- The process of talking to new people, going on dates.

- Fear of rejection or of having to reject other people.

- Issues of general self-worth which can impact on how they think they deserve to be treated by a partner

- Other goals relating to relationships, such as the desire to marry, have children, acquire money or status. All these related goals can be tested for validity to enable the client to make "cleaner" choices based on their true wants rather their ideas of what a relationship "should" be.

EFT offers not only a tool to use within coaching sessions to address some of the above issues, but also a valuable self-support tool for clients (e.g. pre-date nerves, dealing with being rejected etc).

**Examples:**

### Goals

*"Even though I feel quite desperate to find a boyfriend/girlfriend soon,…"*

*"Even though I want to be married before I'm 35,…"*

*"Even though I feel pressure from my family to settle down,…"*

*"Even though I keep picking unsuitable people for me,…"*

### Fear and Blocks

*"Even though the idea of dating at my age is just terrifying,…"*

*"Even though I can't imagine ever finding someone as good as my ex,…"*

*"Even though I can't imagine ever finding happiness again,…"*

*"Even though I don't know if I can face all that heartache again,…"*

*"Even though I'm terrified of being alone,…"*

### Beliefs and Values

*"Even though I think I really need to be in a relationship before I can be truly happy,…"*

*"Even though I think there must be something wrong with me if I'm still single at my age,..."*

*"Even though a fortune teller once told me I'd be unlucky in love,..."*

# 10.6 Dream Coaching

Some coaches use the client's dreams as the primary material for coaching - on the basis that the client's dreams contain their wishes, their guidance and also their solutions. The aim is to help clients understand their dreams as a way of (for example) discovering life purpose, decision taking and generally getting in touch with what the client really wants.

Particular ways of using EFT to support the dream coaching process include:

* Obtaining insight from dreams or dream images.
* Working with the metaphors offered by dreams.
* Dealing with the fears or uncertainties presented by dreams.
* Assisting the client to have and be aware of their dreams.

**Examples:**

### Goals

*"Even though I don't dream as much as I'd like, I choose to have regular dreams and remember them clearly."*

*"Even though I have this issue, I choose to have a dream about it tonight."*

*"Even though I don't understand this dream,..."*

### Fear and Blocks

*"Even though I'm afraid of having scary dreams,..."*

*"Even though that dream left me feeling very unsettled,..."*

*"Even though I don't think it's possible to have useful dreams,..."*

### Beliefs and Values

*"Even though I wonder if I should really be putting so much store by my dreams this way,..."*

*"Even though I don't trust my dreams enough to really act on them,..."*

# 10.7 Exit Coaching

Exit coaching is coaching applied to the goal of getting away from a particular group or society of people. In an extreme case, it could involve freeing oneself from a religious cult. But one can imagine it being relevant to more everyday situations such as leaving a relationship, leaving a job that one dislikes or even freeing oneself from an over-powering or demanding family.

Initially this form of coaching seems to contradict the usual basic definition of coaching - that it should be about the future and "moving towards" what is wanted - not focussed on moving away from that which is negative.

But sometimes "the ties that bind" can be so strong that the sub-goal of safe extrication requires special attention before "what comes next" can even be considered.

When simply leaving the situation requires the client to develop in confidence and self-identity before leaving is possible, exit coaching is appropriate.

Specific uses of EFT to assist in this process could include:

- Fear of the reaction if one leaves, especially if explicit threats have been made.
- Overcoming conditioned beliefs about agencies which can be supportive such as police or social services.
- Overcoming self-identity beliefs or values which maintain the client in their existing situation
- Questioning and overcoming projected beliefs that have been deliberately planted by the controlling party.
- Controlling hopelessness or even thoughts of suicide.

Clearly some of these kinds of situation are extreme and are likely to require input from many other professionals or authorities apart from the coach, and any coach in this field needs to be fully trained in the legal implications before undertaking practice. But if a coach is already working in this field with appropriate support from the relevant authorities, EFT can add an additional tool to help break the cycles of control and emotional abuse that keep the client stuck in their situation.


**Examples:**

### Goals

*"Even though I have to leave for the sake of the children,..."*

*"Even though I want to find a way to get out without it becoming violent,..."*

*"Even though I need to find a creative way to get out of this job,..."*


### Fear and Blocks

*"Even though he said he'd kill me if I tried to leave,..."*

*"Even though he said he'd kill the kids if I tried to leave,..."*

*"Even though I don't trust the police / social services,..."*

*"Even though I can't imagine life on my own,..."*

*"Even though I don't believe I could get a job anywhere else,..."*

### Beliefs and Values

*"Even though I'm not strong enough to get away,..."*

*"Even though they'll always win because they always do,..."*

*"Even though I feel like a total nobody and no-one will listen to my side of the story,..."*

*"Even though I get this overwhelming feeling of shame anytime I really think about leaving,..."*

*"Even though I sometimes think the only way out is to die,..."*

*"Even though I think I should just wait until retirement rolls around so I don't have to face this,..."*

# 10.8 Illness Coaching

Some coaches specialise in coaching for people with chronic and/or terminal illnesses. For people in this situation, both coaching and EFT offer the same thing - not a cure for their illness, but the prospect of being able to handle it better and feel better about it.

As well as using standard EFT on emotions that are attached to the illness, use of the Choices pattern is a particularly useful tool here. Dr Pat Carrington writes about this use of EFT in her email newsletter of October 2003. In this article she talks about using EFT for issues such as anger at caregivers, anger at the illness itself, and discouragement or anger at being forced to be dependent on others, for example:

*"Even though I hate to have to depend on others this way, I choose to find an increasing number of small things that I can do for myself very satisfactorily."*

For people who want to go even further and use their illness as a route to personal or spiritual growth, coaching with EFT can provide that too.

### Examples:

#### Goals

*"Even though I just want to be able to walk one more step today than yesterday,..."*

*"Even though I want to be offering something not just receiving treatment all the time,..."*

*"Even though I think I must be mad wanting to run a marathon with my condition,..."*

*"Even though I'll never be able to fulfil my goal of X now, ..."*

#### Fear and Blocks

*"Even though I'm terrified of being in pain,..."*

*"Even though I can't seem to think of anything else than my illness,..."*

*"Even though I'm not sure who I'd be without this illness,..."*

*"Even though it's hard to feel gratitude for anything when I have this illness,..."*

**Beliefs and Values**

*"Even though I think I should have started getting over this by now,..."*

*"Even though I think my doctors should have started making progress by now,..."*

*"Even though I don't think my life can start until I beat this illness,..."*

*"Even though I think I need to demonstrate Courage when I'm around other people,..."*

*"Even though I think I must have done something bad to deserve this,..."*

# 10.9 Life Purpose Coaching

*"One way to bring a hidden life purpose to your awareness is to reflect on the patterns of your life so far. ... In our experience, people sometimes can't discover their purpose because they have learnt not to value or tune into themselves."* [5]

When someone wants to change their life but feels stuck, one of the biggest and most common obstacles is knowing what they want to do instead. Discovering and articulating a Life Purpose is, in my experience, one of the most powerful things that coaching can do for a client. With a well developed Life Purpose that feels solid, real and based on firm foundations of the person's essence, many other "problems" start to shift and disparate elements start to fall into place quite easily.

When you know your Life Purpose, the following things become much easier:

- Saying No to activities or demands that don't fit in with that Purpose

- Laying to rest ambitions or dreams which aren't related to that Purpose

- Leaving jobs or relationships which don't fulfil that Purpose, with a clear conscience.

- Choosing a new career with confidence.

- Being able to discern easily which battles are worth fighting and which you can just walk away from.

- Maintaining a sense of direction and mission.

- Making material or other "sacrifices" in order to achieve the Purpose.

- Letting attachments to material consumption fall away quite naturally - they just stop being interesting if they aren't supporting the Purpose.

- Finding extra energy and drive to achieve projects that are related to the Purpose.

- Maintaining a strong sense of meaning in one's life, no matter what crises or problems arise.

- Maintaining a strong sense of self-worth regardless of the apparent achievements, accomplishments, success or possessions of anyone else.

No wonder that many coaches emphasise or specialise in Life Purpose coaching - and EFT can be a wonderful aid in the process of discovering a client's Life Purpose.

For a start it can be useful for beginning the process of getting ideas and insights into what the client's Life Purpose might be. Or it can loosen any resistance or bad feeling the client has about not finding their Life Purpose yet.

Some coaches use visualisations to help a client contact their Life Purpose. This can give rise to images and metaphors that perhaps the client doesn't immediately understand. Or the client may start to have dreams which they feel are related to their search for a Life Purpose but they don't understand the symbols or events. EFT can be used to help unlock these metaphors, simply by tapping while focussing on the relevant image.

Sometimes the client will experience life events - such as meeting new people, visiting a place or finding a book or an internet site - which they feel somehow might be related to their Life Purpose, but they are having trouble really pulling the meaning of it into focus. Again, tapping while focussed on the relevant person, book or website can help the client make connections about how these events fit into the Life Purpose.

And when the client starts to generate possibilities for their Life Purpose, EFT can be used as a way to test the validity of the Purpose. For instance, it's possible for a client to have all sorts of beliefs around what a "proper" Life Purpose should entail. Tapping while focussed on the candidate Life Purpose can bring up objections, resistances, or incompletenesses. Making sure that the Life Purpose is clean and shiny, with all objections dealt with and nothing left out, helps to make the client's newly articulated Life Purpose extremely solid in their minds.

EFT can assist in the discovery of Life Purpose simply by encouraging and teaching the client to recognise and use their own internal responses as their benchmark - i.e. it teaches people how to tune into themselves in a very tangible way. A client who becomes used to noticing (and rating out of 10) their urges and responses to external triggers, also starts to become much more aware of when things in their lives are triggering them negatively or positively. And noticing what makes you feel good and bad is a key to noticing elements of your Life Purpose.


**Examples:**

### Goals

*"Even though I don't know if this goal fits my Life Purpose,..."*

*"Even though I haven't got a clue right now what my Life Purpose might be,..."*

*"Even though I don't know my Life Purpose, I choose to be totally open to any clues or information that will help me find it."*


### Fear and Blocks

*"Even though I'm so annoyed that after 45 years I still haven't found it...."*

*"Even though I'm angry at the education system that never helped me think about my Life Purpose..."*

*"Even though I hate myself for wasting so much time,..."*

*"Even though I'm afraid my Life Purpose might look really shallow or selfish to other people,..."*

*"Even though I'm embarrassed to tell people about my Life Purpose because they'll think I'm crazy,..."*

*"Even though I'm scared to know what my Life Purpose is because it might mean I have to give up things I don't want to give up,…"*

### Beliefs and Values

*"Even though I think my Life Purpose should be something really worthy like being the next Mother Teresa,…"*

*"Even though I think if God wanted me to know my Life Purpose it would just be revealed to me without having to do all this work,…"*

# 10.10 Leadership Coaching

Leadership coaching is a particular specialism within Business coaching and is aimed specifically at assisting those in an organisation who hold responsibility for providing direction and leadership for others.

Often the executives or leaders receiving Leadership coaching are themselves required to be effective coaches for their people - to know how to bring out the best in their people's performance, to know how to inspire and encourage, but also to provide clarity about what's expected. To be able to lead in this way requires not only high levels of competence regarding the actual job to be done, but also high levels of individual self-confidence, integrity, resilience to stress in the face of crises and more.

Demonstrating these qualities when one does not feel them or is hiding a whole set of stress and insecurities, is ultimately draining for the leader and must show up sooner or later, either in the organisation's bottom line results, in the responses he gets from his people (who somehow sense the incongruency even if they can't quite say what's wrong) or in a personal cost of stress or illness.

Leadership coaching may be seen as a combination of focussing on Business goals (Doing) and the personal qualities and needs of the leader trying to bring those about (Being).

In other words, as well as helping the leader clarify their business goals, create plans and so on, Leadership coaching also needs to ensure that the leader is able to Be the person who can lead the rest of the business while they deliver it. And that must include all and any source of doubt, insecurity or internal conflict.

Often, it's the leader who is the only person in the business without someone to turn to for help or support, even to discuss options openly and without judgement or fear coming into play, or to "make allowances" when personal difficulties mean he is having an off day. While coaching helps to rectify the problem of having help and support, EFT offers the prospect of making the leader much more self-sufficient emotionally even when the coach isn't around.

### Examples:

#### Goals

*"Even though I'm expected to be bloody Superman sometimes,…"*

*"Even though I need to come up with a really great mission statement for my people,…"*

*"Even though I need to believe this goal myself before I tell my people about it,…"*

### Fear and Blocks

*"Even though I feel my own people are conspiring against me sometimes,..."*

*"Even though I'm afraid I'll be found out one of these days,..."*

*"Even though I feel I have to keep being hard on them or it will all fall apart,..."*

*"Even though I can't imagine anyone else being willing to take some of this off my hands,..."*

*"Even though this business strategy is unproven,..."*

*"Even though I think we should just sit tight and wait for this downturn to blow over,..."*

### Beliefs and Values

*"Even though I believe a leader should lead and the workers should obey,..."*

*"Even though they hired me for my strong beliefs and now they want me to do a staff consultation exercise,..."*

*"Even though I know I'm right and I have to waste my time convincing everybody,..."*

*"Even though we've always based this company on Value for Money,..."*

# 10.11    Parenting Coaching

When you are a parent, your energetic system is open to additional challenges and sources of disruption. This is because parents (and particularly mothers) have literally shared an energy system during pregnancy, breast-feeding and the stages where the child is totally dependent for all physical and emotional needs. Parents will know that a change in their own mood can be picked up and reflected back in the mood changes of their young children; and changes in their child's state of health or emotion seems to have the power to affect the parents in turn.

Even if you don't like the idea of "shared energy fields" between different people, the power of parents and children to mirror and reflect each other's emotional state is self-evident. And parents are increasingly turning to coaching as a way to help them navigate the transitions in their children's lives and to establish or rediscover their own identities after a period of immersion in their children's concerns.

Indeed, many issues that parents have are exactly about the degree to which they and their children are independent energy systems with their own desires and ambitions, and the degree to which they are mutually connected reflections of each other. Since the problem is often at the level of interacting energy systems, EFT offers a gentle and powerful way to explore and define these, to the benefit of everyone concerned.

The acknowledgement of interacting energy systems between parent and child offer particular and profound ways for parents to be involved and directly contribute to the resolution of their children's problems. It's a fact that children often acquire their beliefs, their blocks, their ambitions and character traits from their parents or other people with whom they spend a lot of time. Issues like pressure to perform in exams, attitudes to food and feeding, or self-esteem regarding appearance, sociability or intelligence can be as much about the anxiety of parents as about the qualities, abilities or discipline of the child.

When you are part of any collective energy system (parent-child, husband-wife, brother-sister, lover-lover, business partner-partner etc) this puts you in a position of rather great power when it comes to transforming the dynamic between you. Of course this is a great responsibility and great integrity is required to carry out work of this nature - but really no more than is required to simply be the parent, the husband, the business partner etc. EFT is a powerful but very safe way to approach such changes, because it is impossible to intend or send anything harmful to the other part of the relationship. Tapping while holding any kind of negative thought or intention towards another person simply releases that thought. All tapping in relation to another person, if it produces any result at all, produces relaxation, calm, release of painful or negative feelings and promotes connection, compassion and very often forgiveness.

Thus EFT offers parents two ways to regain control over the parent-child relationship issues. Firstly, it allows the parent to take full responsibility for their own feelings, rather than seeing themselves at the mercy of their children. Secondly, it gives the parent a way forward to deal with aspects of their child's behaviour that are causing them anxiety.

The way in which this is used will vary depending on the age of the child, the degree to which the child is amenable to co-operating with the parent and the degree of relative independence appropriate to the child's maturity. For example, very young children (babies and pre-schoolers) may enjoy doing "play" EFT with their parents or enjoy being tapped by the parent. In contrast, adolescents who are quite naturally and properly experimenting with how to be separate people from their parents may not wish to co-operate physically, but can be tapped "about" or "for" as an assistance to the troubled parent. Either way, the Both of Us pattern is likely to be particularly useful in this context.

### Examples:

#### Goals

*"Even though I'm worried about Amy passing the SATS test today, I deeply and completely accept both of us."*

*"Even though Bob doesn't seem to be reading as fast as the other children, I deeply and completely accept both of us."*

*"Even though we don't have the kind of relationship I imagined when she was born,…"*

*"Even though he doesn't seem to want to take over the family business,…"*

#### Fear and Blocks

*"Even though I'm terrified every time she goes out on that bike,…"*

*"Even though I worry what kind of world my kids are growing up in,…"*

*"Even though she wants to be an artist and I don't want her to end up poor,…"*

*"Even though I'm terrified to stand up to the teachers at his school,…"*

*"Even though I'm scared I'm losing her,…"*

#### Beliefs and Values

*"Even though I think she should be giving more attention to her education,…"*

*"Even though he doesn't seem to share our religious values,…"*

*"Even though the only thing that seems to matter to him is acceptance by his peers,…"*

*"Even though he doesn't seem to care about anything,..."*

*"Even though I can't understand how someone like her could have come from people like us,..."*

# 10.12    Performance Coaching

Performance coaching covers many domains of activity - sales, sports, academic tests and more - but they all have one thing in common - they are activities where there is something significant at stake depending on how well the person performs. Failing to meet a sales target may mean losing a bonus that you need to pay the mortgage, or even losing your job. Failing an exam may mean not going to university. Failing to make the next shot may mean your team losing the final or losing your place on the team.

Whenever there is pressure to perform, there will be fear. And where there is fear (or stress, or nerves or whatever you happen to call it), there is usually a drop in performance. Fear produces effects in the brain and body that make good performance at anything, just that much harder. Adrenaline makes it difficult to focus and think clearly, and in extreme cases blood is diverted away from the brain and into the body which also reduces the ability to think clearly.

Meanwhile, the body is more tense than usual, possibly even trembling and sweating. All of which makes any activity requiring fluidity and co-ordination (such as sports or driving) much harder to perform well. So, fear is a performance killer - and where there is fear, EFT can help.

But EFT can also help performance in cases where the client hasn't yet achieved the standard they are seeking. In these cases, the issue is often one of blocks and beliefs (see below for examples). We've seen how EFT can undo these kinds of beliefs - and so it's not hard to see what a difference EFT could make to a client's performance in a wide range of areas.

I would like to finish this section by talking about what I call "leisure performance" - that is, performance at activities where perhaps there isn't a job or a career at stake, but where the client's goal is Fulfilment - i.e. getting more out of life and generally enjoying life more. There's nothing more unfulfilling than taking up a hobby or activity in order to expand one's sense of fulfilment, only to find that you find it so hard or you're so bad at it to start with that you dread the idea of continuing with it.

This kind of "failure" has worse repercussions than simply giving up the activity and going back to where you started. These kind of experiences can be enough to prevent you trying any more hobbies for fear of the same thing happening again. The effect can be especially devastating if the chosen activity is one that the person has waited 20 years to get round to trying. Using EFT to release any initial bad experiences and addressing any beliefs or blocks around the activity can help to make the whole activity enjoyable again - as well as quite possibly assisting in accelerated learning performance.

Even if you don't specialise in "Performance Coaching" in your practice, you may well find some of these issues relevant to more general coaching clients. For instance, clients seeking work/life balance may look around for new activities to achieve greater fulfilment outside work; or retired people who may be looking for ways to create meaning and enjoyment in their retirement.

**Examples:**

### Goals

*"Even though I need to make the next 3 shots count to get through to the next round,..."*

*"Even though I have to pass this aptitude test or I'll be locked out of this profession forever,..."*

*"Even though I need to be able to speak clearly in interviews,..."*

*"Even though my whole life is depending on the answer to this question,..."*

*"Even though I had my heart set on playing lots of golf when I retired and now it turns out I'm rubbish..."*

### Fear and Blocks

*"Even though only other people get really high scores on tests,..."*

*"Even though I was terrible at this when I tried it 20 years ago and I'm terrified how I'll be now,..."*

*"Even though I'll be a laughing stock if I miss this,..."*

*"Even though I've always been lousy at this sort of thing,..."*

*"Even though I can't even imagine passing this,..."*

### Beliefs and Values

*"Even though I'll never get my handicap lower than this,..."*

*"Even though I'll always be worst player in the club,..."*

*"Even though It's impossible to pass a driving test first time round,..."*

*"Even though I've always been a second eleven kind of guy,..."*

# 10.13    Relationship Coaching

Relationship coaching seems to be extremely fashionable at the moment - whether it be for new "pre-committed" couples, couples who are already committed via marriage or other means, or couples who are separated but have ongoing shared commitments such as children or business.

Relationship coaching is different to Dating coaching in that it is assumes there is already a relationship in existence. Relationship coaching can involve just one party, or both working together. The goal shifts from *"How do I find a good relationship?"* to *"How do we stay in one"* or *"How can we improve things even further?"*

Relationship coaching - in contrast to relationship counselling - is aimed not simply at resolving problems between couples - but at assisting couples who want to deepen and expand their relationship. Fundamentally the assumption is that the couple are committed to each other and the relationship is functioning.

The sorts of things that that relationship coaching can include are actually much the same as those for individual coaching, except that the goals concern the relationship itself, or goals from a relationship perspective. For example:

- Shared life goals - including financial, travel, career, living location etc
- Shared values or belief systems preventing progress

- Conflicting values or belief systems between the parties
- Priority differences e.g. how to spend time, relative importance of different issues
- Intimacy and communication issues
- Valuing each other and self-care issues

**Examples:**

### Goals

*"Even though we need to agree some financial goals,..."*

*"Even though we can't agree where to live,..."*

*"Even though we keep saying we want to spend more time together but it doesn't happen,..."*

*"Even though we don't give our relationship enough attention compared to our jobs and the kids and the house,..."*

### Fear and Blocks

*"Even though I'm scared to combine my finances with him,..."*

*"Even though I'm afraid of getting lost in the relationship unless I keep all my stuff separate,..."*

*"Even though I can't imagine us ever not being together so why do we need to go through all this,..."*

*"Even though every time we start to try and talk about this we just get distracted somehow and can't focus on it,..."*

### Beliefs and Values

*"Even though I think if we love each other all these issues should sort themselves out,..."*

*"Even though I think looking at stuff like this is unromantic,..."*

*"Even though I value Family and he values Career,..."*

*"Even though I'm torn between valuing Family and Career,..."*

*"Even though I have no idea what she even means by "more intimacy" - I thought we were doing just fine,..."*

# 10.14    Self-esteem Coaching

Which "I" is easier to have esteem for? The "I" that has a clear life purpose, knows and honours the values it stands for and believes it's goals are achievable? Or the "I" that never knew what it wanted in life, holds the identity of "not a BMW driver" or "just a housewife" and doesn't even have goals because no-one told it that it could and it believes it couldn't achieve them anyway?

Obviously the first "I" magnetises esteem - either from the self who owns it, or from other people who come into contact with it. The second "I" radiates "lack" and "not enough".

Self-esteem coaching is often about redefining the client's "I" to herself - by bringing her into conscious awareness of her values and Life Purpose and hence to generating achievable plans for goals that fulfil that purpose.

As such, the task within Self-esteem coaching is to assist the client to drop "What I Am Not" and reveal "Who I Really Am". Thought of this way, Self-esteem becomes the thing that is spontaneously revealed or arises when the client's negative identity issues are resolved and they fix on something worthwhile to do (that is, worthwhile in their **own** terms, not worthwhile according to someone else).

And as we have seen there are many ways of using EFT to assist in that process, including validating values, eliminating pseudo-values, eliminating self-limiting or hand-me-down beliefs, reducing fear and blocks and generating and validating goals that inspire the client and gives them a fulfilling direction in life. In addition, techniques such as Mirror Tapping, and the Celebration pattern may be useful in targeting self-acceptance directly and embedding positive self-esteem feelings when they begin to occur.


**Examples:**

### Goals

*"Even though I don't believe my goals are achievable,..."*

*"Even though I don't see much point setting goals,..."*

*"Even though that goal is too much for me,..."*

*"Even though I haven't found a goal that fulfils my Life Purpose yet, I choose to be open to ideas about that."*


### Fear and Blocks

*"Even though I can't really imagine a fulfilling future from here,..."*

*"Even though I'm afraid to think about a lovely future because I'll just be disappointed,..."*

*"Even though it's impossible for me to improve my self-esteem because of what happened to me,..."*

*"Even though I think my self-esteem stops me being someone I don't like,..."*

*"Even though I'm afraid if I lost my low self-esteem I'd end up proud instead, which is a sin,..."*


### Beliefs and Values

*"Even though I'm useless and I always will be,..."*

*"Even though I can't really accept myself, I'd like to accept myself more."*

*"Even though I think my self-esteem is a trivial thing compared to all the suffering that goes on in the world,...*

Related sections:

# 10.15    Spiritual Coaching

I once went to a remarkable talk by a spiritual coach in which he said something that totally resonated with the fundamentals of EFT and Energy Psychology. He was talking on the subject of gurus and of people's response to them. He said (and I paraphrase based on my memory):

*"You need to understand that when you respond with love and feel your heart opening in the presence of a guru, **you** did that - not the guru. Your response is created **by** you and **in** you. If you can feel it in his presence, then it's possible for you to feel it **away** from his presence too - and that's why you don't really need gurus to experience your Oneness."*

Looked at this way, spiritual coaching is about not only improving the client's ability to experience their own Oneness (divinity, universal connection, what you will), but doing it in such a way that the experience and their ability to recreate it is handed straight back to them, complete and intact and independent of the coach.

Although all coaching should be about assisting a client to find their own truth, there is no field where this is so true as the field of spiritual coaching - anything else would simply be greater or lesser degrees of indoctrination. A client who seeks out a spiritual coach is saying rather explicitly: *"I want to experience deeper connection with the divine, and I know I need help, but I don't want anyone telling me what to think or what to feel."* And EFT offers a way to fulfil that contradiction - for the coach to stay completely out of the way while the client travels their own path of enquiry and growth.

Although someone who seeks out spiritual coaching or spiritual development of any kind is probably seeking (negatively) some kind of relief from emotional issues or (positively) to experience a kind of peace of mind, bliss or oneness, the fact is that people have as much negative baggage, conditioning, memories, blocks and beliefs around the subject of Spirituality as they do around any other aspects of their lives. Not least because Spirituality has been so often hi-jacked by religions and cultures down the ages.

As with Consciousness or Essence coaching discussed above, one of the key tasks here is simply to remove what stands in the way and allow the client's true nature and spiritual response to be revealed. And the key element to be removed is fear - fear of really looking "into the void" of the self. As John O'Donohue writes in Anam Cara:

*"Spirituality becomes suspect if it is merely an anaesthetic to still one's spiritual hunger. Such a spirituality is driven by fear of loneliness. **If you bring courage to your solitude, you learn that you do not need to be afraid.** The phrase, do not be afraid, recurs three hundred and sixty-six times in the Bible. There is a welcome for you at the heart of your solitude. When you realise this, most of the fear that governs your life falls away. The moment your fear transfigures, you come into rhythm with your own self."* [12]

We could equally say: "If you bring EFT to your solitude, then you do not need to be afraid".

This is probably the appropriate section to make some observations about what I call "The Spiritual Mechanics of EFT". By which I mean, the inherent structural elements of the EFT protocol which implicitly invite and encourage a spiritual approach to dealing with client experience.

- The acceptance phrase ("*I deeply and completely accept myself*" or equivalent) expresses the unconditional acceptance (or love) that is usually attributed to God. It acknowledges the fundamental worth of the human being in question, regardless of the "problem" currently being experienced. It emphasises the existence of a part of the person (their essence) which is independent of any trauma, abuse, thought, feeling, anxiety or wish that may ever have occurred to them or may be going on at the same time.

- The contrasting of the "I" who is having the problem and the "myself" which is being accepted, immediately distinguishes and acknowledges the essential "I" from the "I" who has problems. To me this is a perfect summary of "God in all of us". Practically, this distinction between the "I" having the problem and the "I" observing the problem and accepting the problem-owner is very similar to the principle behind meditation and other "noticing" practices. It's completely compatible with Eckhart Tolle's observations on "The Pain Body" [13] and the use of "noticing and watching" as a method of starving it of the drama it feeds on.

- The physical action of EFT upon the body and the energy system has several implications and effects all of which I believe enhance a spiritual view of humanity. In a Western society, acting on the body and energy system as a route to consciousness change, is pretty radical, so identified are we with our conscious minds as "Who We Are". As well as bringing in awareness of the body and it's responses, it takes the focus away from the conscious mind as the seat of power and control, and places it somewhere "other". Not only that, the somewhere other is invisible and so far unprovable - and yet the effect of acting upon it through EFT causes noticeable and tangible effects on the experience of the client (intensity reduces and/or they experience a change in cognition). This strongly mirrors many people's understanding of God and/or their own spiritual nature and experience. They can't prove it to anyone, but they know what they know and they have experienced what they have experienced.

- Perhaps most spiritually liberating of all is the way that EFT is a content free technique, making absolutely no assumptions about "proper outcomes" for the EFT beyond the client's own internal benchmarks. The words used to describe the problem always come from the client, not the practitioner. The starting point for beginning EFT is defined by the client, not the practitioner. The client is required to connect and repeatedly re-connect with their own inner experience in order to asses progress and decide on the next step. This emphasises where the proper focus of attention should be for any type of spiritual work - and that is internal to the seeker.

It is perhaps no surprise to note that the developer of EFT, Gary Craig, is an ordained minister who makes frequent references to the spiritual nature of human beings in his workshops and writings. Whether he was consciously aware of the spiritual assumptions embodied in the EFT protocol I cannot say.

Finally, I believe EFT has the possibility of allowing those who wish to do so to examine what lies beyond our current understanding of our own experience i.e. our beliefs. I showed above how EFT can be used to examine beliefs, and help resolve conflict between beliefs, for the purpose of achieving specific coaching goals.

But sometimes it's the awareness of the conflict between one or more beliefs that is the uncomfortable part, rather than having a problem with either belief separately. In other words, the problem may not be in any particular goal or life situation, but in the awareness that one is being internally inconsistent. This gives rise to questioning that may be part of a search for spiritual meaning or understanding. The sort of belief conflict I'm talking about and which are normally considered to be in the realm of spirituality, or at least philosophy, include:

> "*How come there's so much suffering if God loves us?*"

> "*How can I turn the other cheek and be a protective father to my family?*"

*"How can we all be created in God's image if we were also born with sinful natures?"*

*"How can I experience Oneness in a world full of dualities?"*

Rather than seeking for one of the beliefs to "win" (which simply buys further into the power we give our beliefs to run the show and to be the referee for our feelings and actions), or seeking synthesis (which is another way of asking our "referee" to make up its mind), it's possible to take a spiritual leap.

Many spiritual traditions would regard all beliefs as being illusions of the conscious mind. In a spiritual coaching context therefore, one could imagine taking the approach of not aiming for any resolution of the conflict whatsoever, but for acceptance of oneself for having the delusion of beliefs at all:

*"Even though I have conflicting beliefs, I deeply and completely accept myself for having them."*

*"Even though this looks like a paradox I deeply and completely accept myself for not understanding it and not being able to resolve it."*

This approach invites the thought: if having lots of Reversals can be described as Global Reversal, can having lots of beliefs be thought of as a similar systemic level problem? And would the treatment for Global Delusion look like this?:

*"Even though I have all these beliefs and delusions, I deeply and completely accept myself."*

Releasing the need to consciously understand, might perhaps be a useful tool in the process of "surrender", a common spiritual goal.

I am not a spiritual coach and do not claim to have any particular skill or expertise in this area. I present the above thoughts purely on the basis of someone who does know EFT very well and who asks themselves the above sorts of questions from time to time. In presenting these thoughts I do not claim to be suggesting a good method for spiritual coaching - but I do hope to whet the appetites of some practising spiritual coaches out there who perhaps might be inspired to develop more well thought out ways to apply EFT to their area. I'd love to hear from you!


**Examples:**

### Goals

*"Even though I've been praying for salvation all my life and I just feel exactly the same no matter what,…"*

*"Even though I'm probably being arrogant even presuming to be closer to God,…"*

*"Even though I don't like having spiritual goals because they might not be God's will,…"*


### Fear and Blocks

*"Even though I'm afraid of going to Hell,…"*

*"Even though I feel having normal sort of human fun must be wrong because it doesn't look spiritual,…"*

*"Even though I'm a bit afraid of suddenly being taken over and not being me any more if I surrender to the divine,…"*

**Beliefs and Values**

*"Even though I think only Jesus/Buddha were capable of true connection with the divine,..."*

*"Even though I think I should be getting some kind of tangible vision if I were really spiritually enlightened,..."*

Related sections:

6.1.15     Accepting the Client Without Judgement ⇧

6.2.7     The Self-acceptance Statement ⇧

9.5.6.4     Conflicting Beliefs ⇧

# 10.16     Stress Coaching

Stress can, of course, involve any negative emotion experienced by a client. Trauma, anxiety and panic are obviously stressful, as are fear, anger, frustration and pain. And clearing the client's triggers (with EFT) and programming new responses to ongoing triggers (e.g. with Choices) can make significant in-roads into a client's stress levels.

But one of the most neglected sources of Stress is lack of what I call "Self-alignment".

If a client is living in a way which contravenes his values or which does not allow his talents and Life Purpose to be expressed, he is out of alignment with himself - and this can create a constant "friction" between his "self" and his lifestyle which creates a background feeling of Stress.

Coaching can be used to bring clients into closer relationship with their real selves - their values, their goals and their Life Purpose - and to help them express this in the way they lead their lives.

In the Stress model to the right, I show how self-alignment (coaching) issues around Stress interact with more classic EFT Stress issues involving past and present Stress triggers.

EFT assisted Stress coaching offers not only to reduce actual and immediate Stress intensity, but to look also at a client's long term goals and create a life consistent with their values, thereby reducing the likelihood of future Stress.

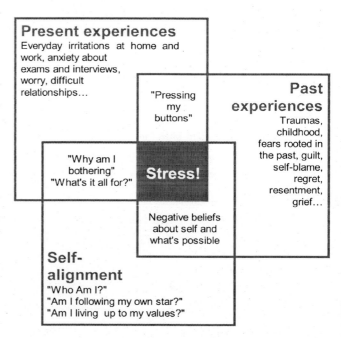

**Examples:**

### Goals

*"Even though I seem to have everything I thought I wanted but I still feel this Stress,..."*

*"Even though I want to have Happiness as a goal more than anything,..."*

*"Even though I don't know how to prioritise my life for the best to keep the stress down,..."*

*"Even though I'm too stressed to find time for these coaching goals,..."*

### Fear and Blocks

*"Even though I think I need some stress to keep me going,..."*

*"Even though saying No to my boss/family isn't an option,..."*

*"Even though I hate admitting I can't cope without getting stressed,..."*

*"Even though I'm scared what effect this stress might be having on my long term health,..."*

### Beliefs and Values

*"Even though I think some stress is good for you,..."*

*"Even though I think stress is a completely inevitable part of life,..."*

*"Even though I think stress is the price you pay for success,..."*

*"Even though this stress is stopping me from honouring my value of Family,..."*

*"Even though the conflict between Success and Happiness is causing me stress,..."*

# 10.17    Success Coaching

"Success coaching" is of course just like any other form of coaching, except that it takes it's name from the desired end result and feeling, rather than the starting problem. Success coaching is actually not a specific domain but can cover literally any subject area including Business, Relationships, Creativity, Spirituality and so on. Clients still need help identifying their values, getting in touch with their Life Purpose, and setting and achieving goals.

However, the focus on Success in the title does imply a particular focus from client and coach. Not only does the client want to achieve X, Y and Z, they want to feel **good** about it when they do. Success coaching could be renamed Fulfilment coaching and be conducted exactly the same way.

This "specialism" (if it is one) would be a particularly good place to make use of the Celebration pattern to maximise the client's experience of success whenever it occurs during the coaching.

In addition, this focus might also require the client and coach to examine the client's ideas around success (and therefore failure) as a route to enabling that experience.

**Examples:**

### Goals

*"Even though I want success and I don't know what it means,..."*

*"Even though I'm not sure if I deserve success,..."*

### Fear and Blocks

*"Even though I think true success is impossible,..."*

*"Even though I never really feel success even when I've completed a goal,..."*

*"Even though I'm scared how my family will react if I get really successful,..."*

### Beliefs and Values

*"Even though I think it's a very thin line between Success and Failure,..."*

*"Even though only one in three succeed at this game,..."*

*"Even though I should expect failure sometimes because that's just the way life is,..."*

Related sections:

6.1.5      Fulfilment Coaching ⇧

8.5.10.1   Failure to Feel Successful ⇧

8.5.10.2   The Celebration Pattern ⇧

# 10.18    Transition Coaching

Many coaches specialise in transition coaching - focussing on specific major life changes such as career change, divorce or retirement. In one key sense of course, all coaching is transition coaching - the client is transitioning from their current life to a new life. But often (although not always) an extra issue with transition coaching is that the choice to make the transition is largely or wholly out of the client's hands - such as with divorce, retirement, redundancy, children leaving home or other event or age-determined change.

This means that often the most prominent issue to be dealt with may be the client's attitude to change itself.

And the fact that the choice has not always been the client's means that there will be other potentially negative emotions surrounding the lead up to the change, including anger, fear, resentment or anxiety, as opposed to the hope, excitement and anticipation that are more like to be associated with client-originated change. The task is therefore to stop these negative emotions preventing what's positive about what's happening to be realised.

The typical sorts of coaching challenges that can occur in any transition can include:

- Dealing with fear of change generally - and changing the client's relationship with change.
- Learning new skills.
- Being in a new role.
- Envisioning new self-originated goals to replace the other-originated goals (corporate job, children, partner) that may have been dominating the client's life up till now.
- Seeing the future clearly and making any adjustments necessary to the client's Time Line so that the future becomes an easy place to see, to go to and to manipulate as desired.
- Resistance, or fear of resistance from others who may have expectations or their own change issues.
- Focussing on future opportunities and removing focus from the past.
- Building confidence that future changes can also be dealt with after the coaching.
- Making a start - at least beginning the process of taking action, not just considering possibilities.

**Examples:**

### Goals

*"Even though my goal of early retirement has been achieved, I can't see a goal past that,..."*

*"Even though my goals just feel too massive to really be feasible,..."*

*"Even though I'm not used to thinking about my own goals,..."*

*"Even though I don't know whether to start my own business or go back to college,..."*

### Fear and Blocks

*"Even though I'm afraid of the reaction of my family when I tell them my plans,..."*

*"Even though it's hard to even see the future clearly from here,..."*

*"Even though all this change is really unsettling,..."*

*"Even though I wish things could go back to the way they were,..."*

*Even though I didn't choose for this change to happen, I choose to make this change into something good."*

### Beliefs and Values

*"Even though I've always been a follower, not a leader,..."*

*"Even though I've always put my family first and so going off and doing this by myself just feels strange,..."*

*"Even though I've always valued Freedom, this is just a bit too much Freedom to handle."*

*"Even though I'm not sure if I have the ability to learn these new skills,..."*

*"Even though I never believed this would happen to me,..."*

# 10.19    Wealth Coaching

Wealth coaching is focussed primarily on financial goals. However, when people use the world Wealth they usually mean something more than what's in their bank account. It includes everything they think having money means and what it allows.

What money "means" to a client takes us into the area of identity, values and beliefs.

And what money "allows" takes us into the area of goals, dreams and life purpose.

Thus we are on familiar and broad coaching territory, even though the original subject appears to be extremely focussed.

But specific issues that are likely to come up here include attitudes to money, expectations of oneself and others around money, attitudes to success, the client's work ethic and beliefs about whether making money should be easy or hard, and so on.

Therefore EFT can help in this domain in virtually all the ways presented in this book. Any coach working in the area of wealth, money or success generally is advised to read the excellent section on "EFT and Money" in Adventures in EFT[3] for some very specific suggestions.

### Examples:

#### Goals

*"Even though being financially independent by age 50 seems impossible,…"*

*"Even though I want to be free to pursue my other dreams without money being an issue,…"*

#### Fear and Blocks

*"Even though I hate looking at financial stuff,…"*

*"Even though I never understand all that mumbo jumbo,…"*

*"Even though I'm terrified of being poor,…"*

*"Even though I don't like the idea of having money at someone else's expense,…"*

*"Even though I think that way of earning money is just too easy,…"*

*"Even though if I earn this amount it will mean I've done better than my own father,…"*

#### Beliefs and Values

*"Even though I think most rich people are very arrogant,…"*

*"Even though I come from a working class family and it would probably raise a few eyebrows back home if I became wealthy,…"*

*"Even though I think Family should come before Money,…"*

*"Even though I think getting wealthy means long hours and lots of stress,…"*

# 11 Integrating EFT into your Coaching Practice

In this section I assume that you have begun to see the benefits of using EFT for different types of issue within coaching. Even if you are totally convinced that EFT could be a great tool for your clients, there are various practical issues involved in actually using EFT within the coaching relationship.

## 11.1  Practice Integration Process

If you have worked through the self-management exercises above thoroughly and diligently and experienced the difference it can make to your levels of confidence, your ability to work fearlessly towards goals, not to mention your increased level of emotional happiness, I defy you to resist the urge to want to make these benefits available to your clients also.

In fact I strongly urge you to get extremely comfortable and familiar with using EFT on yourself before you even try using it with a client. It's all about congruency. When you know what EFT can do and how it feels, you will be able to integrate it seamlessly into your own ethics and principles for coaching. You will be able to answer the question "Is this in my client's best interests?" with total integrity.

Here is a detailed suggested procedure for learning and integrating EFT into your existing coaching practice.

### Step 1: Learn the basic EFT procedure…

…as a self-help procedure, following the basic recipe in section 12, or using one of the resources listed in section 13.

### Step 2: Apply EFT to yourself…

… for a range of your own real issues, taking care to document the rating levels at each stage and any other physiological or emotional changes that occur.

Start with highly specific and manageable issues rather than complex or extreme issues.

Since it is estimated that beginners following just the basic procedure and without additional training achieve approximately 50-80% success, do not be concerned if not every single issue that you choose to work on responds instantly. As you will discover later if you undertake more thorough training, there are a variety of reasons for this to happen which when known can be effectively addressed using EFT in particular ways.

When you do these test applications of EFT, make sure that you are feeling generally well (i.e. don't try it in the middle of a heavy cold), that you are reasonably alert (i.e. not after a long commute or at 2am), that your system is not under the heavy influence of medication or alcohol, and that you are well hydrated. Illness, fatigue, dehydration and some substances all interfere with the general functions of the energy system - which is why we feel so "scrambled" and generally "not with it" when these things are going on.

If you are already objecting that these are a lot of requirements to put on the test, simply ask yourself whether you would expect a coaching client to respond well to a coaching session if they were ill, tired, under the influence of alcohol or dehydrated.

### Step 3: Apply EFT to at least one other person...

...who is not in a client relationship with you. Ask a friend or relative. Again, pick a reasonably manageable and highly specific issue to work on. And again, document your results, noting down start ratings and what wordings you used on each round - plus any observations from your volunteer about how they feel before, during and after.

There are two reasons for working with at least one volunteer as well as trying it on yourself at this stage.

Firstly, even if you have been diligently documenting your own reactions to EFT, there is a chance that you might decide to dismiss the effects as being due to something else, or even believing that the issue you picked to work on wasn't really a problem. This is a known phenomenon and is called the "Apex Effect". Obviously, if this happens to you, it is going to be very hard for you to objectively assess whether EFT had an effect on you. Seeing the effects on other people however does not carry this risk.

Secondly, there is a small percentage of people who do not respond to EFT immediately or easily due to more general energy disruptions affecting them temporarily or permanently. (You will learn more about this if you take practitioner training.) If you happen to be one of these people, then trying it out with other people will give you a greater range of evidence to look at.

### Step 4: Get additional training in EFT...

... using the training resources listed in section 13.

The important thing here is to see expert EFT practitioners applying EFT to other people. This gets you over any doubts such as "Am I doing it right?" or "Am I saying the right thing?".

It also expands your idea about the range of issues it can help with. This will be stimulating your creativity about how you'd like to use it in your practice later on.

This stage may take several weeks or months (e.g. to work through books and CD training material). Increasing numbers of EFT practitioners run one or two day intensive trainings for beginners which can help shorten the learning experience if that's important to you. However, if you eventual aim is to become a practitioner then I would still recommend obtaining the CD training and reading as much as you can.

### Step 5: Get as much experience as you can of applying EFT yourself...

... for as wide a range of issues as you can and for more complicated issues.

The aim here is for doing standard EFT to become second nature to you so you no longer have to look at any diagrams, or even think too hard about what setup to use. This stage is about "getting fluent" as a self-help user.

### Step 6: Arrange to receive EFT from an experienced practitioner…

…so that you get to experience a different style of delivery and to see how practitioner guided EFT feels from the client perspective.

This is the same kind of thinking behind coaches having coaches - you need to know how it feels at the other end of the interaction as a way of properly relating to your clients.

### Step 7: Get as much experience as you can applying EFT to other people…

… for a wide range of issues and for more complex issues.

This stage is about building your confidence at using EFT. Assuming that after all this you are convinced of the value that EFT can offer to your clients, then:

### Step 8: Take a practitioner level training…

… e.g. through the AMT in the UK or the best available level of qualification available to you in your location.

AMT practitioner training will assume you know the EFT protocol and have seen Gary Craig's basic training CD's. The focus is on handling specific types of situation with clients, safety and ethical issues, and specialised applications of EFT for specific problems (e.g. addiction, phobias).

The important thing at this step is to satisfy yourself that you feel confident to recognise and handle pretty much any eventuality that might occur in a client session. There is nothing more off-putting for a client than a nervous coach or practitioner.

### Step 9: Examine the code of ethics…

…of the professional bodies and training schools you belong to, and any legal requirements that you are bound by in your country or state. Get clear how adding EFT to your practice will affect how these ethical and legal requirements apply to you and your practice (e.g. how you describe your coaching practice, what claims you make, any changes necessary to your professional insurance, and so on).

It's also useful to decide if there are any types of clients or any types of issue you will or will not deal with in the light of these legal or ethical requirements. For instance, if you are worried about dealing with "medical" cases you can decide not to work with clients on physical issues.

### Step 10: Introduce EFT into client sessions!

# 11.2 Tracking Notation

In order to "Hold the Client's Agenda" while doing EFT for a coaching issue, you need to keep track of progress with reference to the issue you started with, even if the EFT leads on to other related Aspects or issues.

All EFT practitioners and self-help users need to keep this kind of track, whatever the overall context of using EFT - but I believe it's especially important within a coaching context because there are **two** goals to be held in mind:

- The overall coaching goal that is being worked on; and
- The specific issue that you are applying EFT to.

For instance, suppose a client's overall coaching goal is to achieve better Work/Life balance.

Then suppose that as part of the coaching, you identify that the client has a limiting belief that *"If I'm not working, I'm wasting time."* which you both decide to use EFT to help undo.

The following is a suggested method of tracking what happens in an EFT session, what aspects you have worked on and the ratings for each aspect and the overall issue.

You may use any different form of notation that suits you, provided it lets you keep track and always know that any rounds of EFT you spend time doing are genuinely relevant to the chosen issues.

The key elements of my notation method are:

- Writing down each issue and the key words used in the setup (I don't normally have time to write down the full setup statement while I am working)
- Indenting Aspects or other rounds which occur within an issue
- Writing down one rating after each round of EFT - so each number indicates one round of EFT performed
- Arrows to show the flow and order of rounds

You may find that after some experience of using this notation it starts to be internalised more and more, so that it doesn't have to be written down for you to know where you are.

But this internalisation can only occur if you regularly use the same notation system for a considerable time.

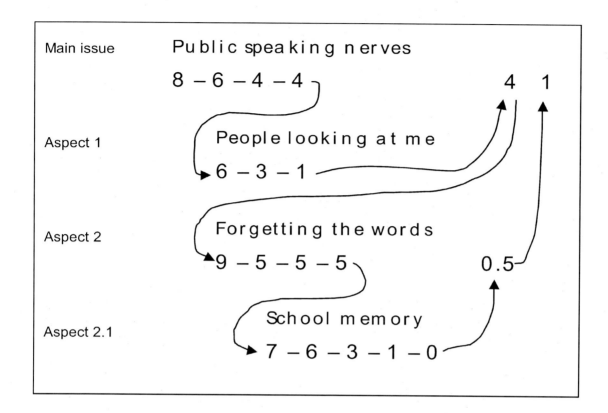

## 11.3 When to Use EFT for the First Time

Assuming an extended coaching relationship of several weeks or months, you need to decide at what stage to start using EFT on client issues. It's not necessarily at the first session, since it is but one more tool in your toolbox - so when is the right time?

The short answer to this is: when you have enough trust and rapport between you that the client feels safe to start working on emotional issues with you.

For any type of emotional work, whether it be "official therapy" or coaching towards goals, your client will always be pacing the degree to which they open up to you and are willing to go on an emotional journey with you. My feeling is that this occurs further down the road than in a "therapy" relationship - probably because when the relationship is a therapeutic one from the start, the client has already achieved a significant level of trust simply to have made an appointment with you.

In a coaching relationship, the fact that significant emotional issues might be dealt with along the way is rarely advertised by "straight" coaches and is not top of the client's agenda when they begin. Their official "reason for being there" is to achieve some goal. Diving into deep emotional issues on the first session, whether or not you use EFT, is therefore unlikely to be an appropriate pace for the work - and may even scare them off. The exception to this is if the client knows you are an EFT Coach and your client begins the work with an awareness that their goal has emotional issues attached to it.

So where should you begin, if not with EFT?

Begin where all coaching needs to begin - with finding out what the client's goals are for the coaching, what success will look like for them, and what type of alliance they want to create with you. Ensuring you are fully clear on the goals for the coaching is **the** best thing you can possibly do to build rapport and demonstrate your interest in the client's life.

Your first session with a client is your best shot at demonstrating your skill at tuning into the client, maintaining focus on them and their goals and giving them their first experience of you "being there" with them as a steadfast ally and loyal guide. You can't do all this if you are thinking about *"How can I get an EFT demo into this session somehow?"*.

However, if your client is completely new to EFT, and you intend to use EFT as part of the coaching, you do need to introduce the client to EFT in the first session somehow, in order to fulfil the requirement of accurately describing your working methods.

You could fulfil these requirements by giving a short description and perhaps some written materials (e.g. I give all new clients a paper or electronic copy of my QuickStart manual). This makes your intention to use EFT explicit, even if it isn't used straightaway. But, in my experience, nothing really describes EFT adequately to clients except actually **doing** it.

Written descriptions don't work for many people - because most people can't be bothered to read a manual unless they already know they are interested - and perfectionists (who tend to be well represented amongst coaching clientele) won't start reading something unless they have time to read it "properly" - which means they never do.

Verbal descriptions aren't idea either, because even if you start with your carefully planned spiel, people always have questions you haven't thought of. But more importantly it invites a dialogue **about** EFT (*"Is it like this?", Does it work for that?"* etc) which is usually fairly pointless and needs to be limited.

But, even a content-free physical demonstration of EFT (i.e. only showing where the points are and how to tap and say setup statements), doesn't fully convey the benefits of EFT because then they get to find out how weird and strange the process is but without actually feeling the positive effects. A totally content-free demo can be worse than no demo at all because after doing all the weird moves and saying all the weird statements - they feel the same!

The **only** thing that truly conveys what EFT does is experiencing it directly - and that means applying it to a real issue and having their rating fall.

I therefore suggest the following as a way of introducing and pacing the use of EFT from the first session:

- Don't aim to **use** EFT for coaching related issues in the first session unless it's what the client explicitly wants and expects. Focus instead on goals, getting to know the client and establishing trust and rapport (i.e. standard coaching practice!)

- Do **introduce** EFT to the client as part of explaining how you work and designing the alliance. Don't spend too much time on the theory or background, but get on to doing a familiarisation exercise as quickly as possible. Choose a neutral, non-coaching issue such as the breathing constriction exercise. Ensure the client has an accurate expectation of when EFT might be used and what for, success rates, and so on.

- Provide good quality materials which have at least a diagram of all the points, the basic setup statement format, and the sequence of events for the client to take away. It's also a good idea to put in writing what you have said in your introduction, such as success rates, the kinds of issues you will be using it for and so on.

- Consider setting some simple EFT **homework** after the first session to get the client used to it - perhaps using the Wheel of Life / Ecology template given in Ecology Testing. Whether you want to do this will depend on the client, their goals and whether you think they can do this on their own.

- The first time you use EFT should be driven by the flow of the coaching and occur when it is clearly and genuinely appropriate to use it. This might not be for two or three sessions - or even six.

- Make sure you know how to guide a client quickly and efficiently through an EFT sequence for the first time, such that you keep charge of the process and it doesn't take much time. (See next section for the method I have developed myself which you may wish to copy or adapt to fit your own style.)

Ultimately, the choice of when and how to introduce EFT will depend on the coaching/EFT mix you decide to use in your practice, your client's expectations and prior experience, and of course, client need.

Related sections:

11.4      Breathing Constriction Exercise ⇩

11.6      The Coaching/EFT Mix ⇩

# 11.4 Breathing Constriction Exercise

This is a useful demonstration exercise for familiarising new clients to the mechanics of the EFT process. It allows the client to feel actual effects of the EFT, but without risking getting into any emotional work before the client is familiar and able to use the technique.

The following gives only the very basic steps. How to embed this exercise into a full instruction sequence is given in the next section.

**Step 1:** Ask the client to take one or two full deep breaths as a warm up. Then ask them to take a "test breath" as fully and deeply as they can.

**Step 2:** Ask them to rate how deep the breath was, 0-10, where 10 is the fullest deepest breath they know they can take.

**Step 3:** Do the setup statement based on their rating:

*"Even though it was a 6, I deeply and completely accept myself."*

Make sure they can find the sore spot, or if they can't, switch to the side of the hand point instead. Ask the client to repeat the setup statement after you and say it 3 times.

**Step 4:** Guide the client through the EFT points, showing the location, speed of tapping and repeating a reminder phrase on each one - in this case "breathing".

**Step 5:** Do the gamut sequence (if you use it).

**Step 6:** Ask the client to take another full deep breath and to give you another rating.

# 11.5  Using EFT over the Phone

Most coaches work over the phone, as this is more time efficient for busy clients and allows coaches and clients who don't live close to each other to form relationships based on a good match of interests and skills rather than on who is available locally.

Since EFT is a physical technique, it if often asked whether it is possible for EFT to be effective over the phone, and whether it is hard for a client to learn EFT over the phone.

It is absolutely possible to do EFT effectively (i.e. producing the desired reduction in intensity levels etc) over the phone. Many of my phone clients can verify this.

As to the process of learning over the phone, it **is** possible and need not be a particular obstacle. However, be prepared for the fact that some clients will prefer to have a face-to-face session with you for the first session. Such clients tend to have worries about "whether I'm doing it right" and want to see you tap the correct points, see the speed of tapping and so on. You need to decide early on whether you can accommodate such clients or whether you will insist on phone sessions only.

## 11.5.1  Sequence for phone instruction

The following procedure is based on many phone calls with new EFT clients who had not done or seen EFT in action prior to the first call.

### Step 1: Provide written materials prior to the session.

This should include a good diagram of the points with text descriptions of their locations. This can be sent by email or post prior to the call, or can be made available online for the client to view or download.

Ask the client to look at the diagram before the call so that they have some familiarity with the location of the points when you begin. Emphasise that any uncertainty will be clarified on the phone call. This stops anxious or perfectionist types worrying about whether they will know what to do.

Try to have multiple versions and file types available. If a client can't read a pdf file, they might be able to read a Word file; if they can't read a Word file, they can probably view a JPEG file - and there is always fax or postal mail if none of these work.

If time or circumstances don't allow the client to see a diagram then you will need to resort to describing the points verbally. Aim to make such an event the exception - i.e. only where there is really no other option. For the sake of both you and your client, try not to make purely verbal EFT instruction your default method for phone work - it's time consuming and can be frustrating.

### Step 2: Say something about the general principles of EFT.

For instance, mention that it uses the meridian system just like acupuncture, that it works by correcting disruptions in the energy system. Use whatever description or analogies work for you based on the information you've received from training or your own words.

Asking the client if they have ever had acupuncture, kinesiology, acupressure, shiatsu etc can provide them with a point of reference. Don't linger on this stage - a couple of minutes at most - but it is good to give a client the opportunity to have some sort of understanding about where this technique comes from.

An alternative is to provide this type of explanation as part of your written materials.

**Step 3: Identify a problem to work on.**

Unless the client really wants and expects to start doing EFT straightaway on their actual issue (and some might), use the Breathing Constriction Exercise described above as a neutral example but which can allow effects to be experienced.

If the client does want to get started straightaway, choose a very specific and bounded issue to start with - such as a specific memory, or current anxiety level or craving for something.

**Step 4: Introduce the 0-10 rating scale.**

Don't call it a "SUDS" scale with clients as this introduces jargon which takes more time to define and explain. I prefer to use everyday words in sentence form which focuses clients on tuning in to their current level of intensity, not on wondering what words mean. Ask them to give you a rating in such a way that it is clear what 0 and 10 signify:

> *"So on a scale of 0 to 10, how deep was that breath, where 0 is nothing and 10 is the maximum it could be".*

Notice we didn't need to say SUDS or define what that is, or use other terms for it like "intensity rating" or "rating scale". Terms like "SUDS" and even "intensity rating" are ways for practitioners to talk to each other **about** what's happening with clients.

Clients don't want to talk **about** what's happening - they just want to focus on their issue and the more we can use language which doesn't distract from that, the more in tune the client will feel with the whole process of instruction.

**Step 5: Do the set up stage.**

Get the client to find the sore spot. This is one of the hardest spots to explain and for the client to find. Give them time to poke around and find it. Explain that the area is quite large and as long as they have found some area that feels tender that is fine.

Use this time to emphasise that this point is different to all the rest in that it is rubbed instead of tapped, and that it is always on the left side, while all the others are symmetrical - this sets up learning for later.

You may get an "ouch" response initially, so emphasise that they should not bruise or hurt themselves - rub just enough to feel it.

If they really can't find it, use the Karate Chop point (Side of Hand) instead.

Once they have found the sore spot (or karate chop point), ask them to repeat after you as you say an appropriate setup statement 3 times. Base it on the issue you are working on, making it as simple and straightforward as possible, with no frills or variations between the three repetitions.

Even if you have already detected or intuited some underlying causes or roots to the issue, now is not the time to bring them into play, as you want the client to focus on the **structure** of what is happening, not the **content** of the language you're using.

For the breathing constriction example:

> *"Even though my breath was a 6, I deeply and completely accept myself. Even though my breath was a 6, I deeply and completely accept myself. Even though my breath was a 6, I deeply and completely accept myself."*

After the 3 statements, say explicitly: *"We've now done the setup stage"*.

This creates a structural boundary in the client's mind and signals that what is to follow is going to be a new thing.

### Step 6: Do a complete sequence of 14 points and gamut sequence.

This sequence is going to be **very slow** - do not rush.

The goal is for the client to be confident about the **location** of every point, to learn **how to tap** (speed, number of fingers), and to get used to saying a **reminder phrase** on each point.

It does not matter how long this sequence takes to complete, or whether the client is properly tuning in to the issue - this sequence is about learning the mechanics and the structure.

Signal the start of the sequence by saying *"Now we're going to do the main sequence"*.

Ask them to find the first point (Eyebrow), checking that they have the right place. This is a good point to say that they can tap on either side and with either hand. Say:

> *"Use either one or two fingers. Now we tap the point, at this kind of speed: tap tap tap tap tap tap tap tap. We tap about seven or nine times, but it can be more if you want"*.

Tap the relevant point yourself, even if they can't see you. By saying *"tap tap tap..."* at the same speed as you are actually tapping, you get across the required rhythm very easily and without the need for more complex verbal explanation. As they tap, you say

> *"On each point we say a reminder phrase, in this case we'll say Breathing"*.

You choose the reminder phrase rather than having a discussion about it. Since the setup statement was deliberately simplified, so will the reminder be. Keep the reminder phrase the same on each point, regardless of what other words or intuitions come to mind.

Move the client onto the next point by saying *"Side of the eye"* following by a description of the location *"on the bony ridge"*, and check that that the client is happy with where that is.

As soon as you are confident they have found the right spot, say: *"Tap tap tap tap tap tap tap tap, Breathing"*.

Move the client onto the next spot by saying *"Under the eye, on the bony ridge"*, check they have it and then say *"Tap tap tap tap tap tap tap, Breathing"*.

Repeat this for each point in the sequence.

I tend to rarely use the gamut sequence these days, but I do include it in my instructions so I can put it back in if needed. This can also be described and learned over the phone. Finish the sequence by saying:

> *"That's one full sequence of EFT. Obviously all the future rounds will be much quicker."*

### Step 7: Re-take the rating.

Ask the client to think about the issue again (or take a new breath) and to give you a new rating.

You are less interested in the actual value of the rating than ensuring that the client gets the idea that they will be asked for a rating after every round of EFT.

**Step 8: Continue to provide verbal support for future rounds as needed.**

On subsequent rounds, use repetition of the reminder phrase as the cue to move onto the next point. An intermediate step is to say the name of the point and the reminder phrase together

> *"Eyebrow, Angry"*

> *"Side of eye, Angry"*

> *"Under eye, Angry" etc*

When you sense that the client is confident about the sequence, you can drop the point label and simply use the Reminder phrase itself as a cue to move on to the next point:

> *"Angry"*

> *"Angry"*

> *"Angry" etc*

When you make these transitions, do check that your client is doing what you think they are doing. You can do this by asking or simply stating what you are going to do *"I'm just going to say the Reminder phrases from now on, but feel free to stop me if you want to"*.

Clients do vary. Some clients can go to the minimal support stage (i.e. only saying the reminder phrase) within a few rounds. Others seem to want each point enumerated indefinitely. Your goal is to give whatever support they need to maximise the degree to which they are tuned into their issue (rather than being worried about where the next point is, or what to say next).

## 11.5.2 Tapping along with your client

Tapping along with your client is advisable even when working face to face, since it means you don't take your clients issues into your system. Any client issues that do resonate with you or which you feel empathy for, then get automatically dealt with as you go along.

But it is especially advisable when working on the phone, because it serves two additional purposes:

- It keeps you on track with where the client is up to in their sequence. If you just repeated the reminder phrase you could potentially lose track of which point they are on and say too few or too many. Trying to count to fourteen while also repeating a reminder phrase and probably processing your own thoughts about the issue or the next round, is hard - so don't do it.

- It can allow you to tune in to what's happening with your client energetically. I often notice some points producing more release than others in myself, while I am tapping along with the client, and get intuitions to spend more time on some points than others. This all helps to increase and maintain energetic rapport with someone you can't see.

At no stage should you intend to do surrogate or proxy tapping for your client for reasons I give in Principle of Client Responsibility.

Related sections:

5.4.6     Principle of Client Responsibility ⇑

8.2.2     Co-active Tapping ⇑

### 11.5.3 Finding out the client's "state"

Practitioners and coaches are trained to be alert to changes in client state and to use this as feedback to inform the next stage of the session. Although working over the phone inevitably focuses attention on audible indications like breathing and "emotionality" of voice (e.g. calm, angry, upset), there are other ways to find out what's happening to a client who is invisible to you.

It is especially useful to ask the client what is happening in their body to accompany an intensity rating. Clients are often aware of things like burning sensations in their stomach, heaviness in the chest, tension in the back, shoulder or head - or any other physical sensation unique to them.

When I note down ratings as we progress, I also write down any accompanying physical symptoms. These are useful as a check back when intensity levels start to get very low.

For instance, if after a few rounds a client is telling you that *"it's hard to think about"* or *"it seems very distant now"*, it can be **very** hard to get an actual number out of them. Of course these statements are good evidence of EFT working - but we need a number to know what to do next.

The first resort is to ask explicitly *"Is it a zero?"* Often it is not a true zero but the drop has been so dramatic that for some reason they find it hard to notice a 1 or a half when it was an 8 or a 10 just a minute before. Instead they are focussed on the **lack** of intensity and are busy saying **"***Wow, where did the feeling go?***"**.

As a practitioner it's important to be thorough and not stop at a 1 or half if a 0 is possible and you need to somehow establish whether you have a zero situation or not.

If a client is finding it hard to say whether it's a zero or not, you can refer back to the physical feelings they identified earlier and ask about those. Clients seem to find this **much** easier to do. As well as indicating more work to be done, physical sensation also provides a direct focus for the next round of EFT if the issue itself (a memory or emotion) has "gone blurry" and is hard for the client to focus on. It is frequently the case that by doing EFT on the remaining bodily symptom (e.g. *"Even though I still have this heart feeling,..."*) the remaining issue can be cleared.

# 11.6 The Coaching/EFT Mix

There are (at least) three different ways of combining EFT and coaching in terms of which dominates or "leads". Which mix you prefer depends on your personal style, but also on the needs of different clients. There is no right or wrong about this. These differences are enumerated here simply to make you aware of the differences and the pros and cons of each.

### 11.6.1 Coaching with added EFT

In this "light" style, EFT is truly just "one more tool in the coach's bag". In this style, conventional coaching leads the interaction and EFT is brought out when clear blocks or EFT-able issues arise during the course of coaching.

In this style of coaching, the coach will tend to use his conventional coaching tools as the first port of call. EFT may be used sporadically and perhaps not at all in some sessions if the required progress to achieving goals is being made via other means.

This mix may be more appropriate when the emphasis is on the Doing aspects of a client's goal (i.e. making plans, problem solving etc). The primary use of EFT here would be not necessarily to do too much

Being work involving generating insights or questioning beliefs, but to keep the client's energy good and to clear any fears or blocks sufficiently to allow action to be taken.

Related sections

| | |
|---|---|
| 9.2.1 | Clearing Fears ⇑ |
| 9.3.1 | An Energy View of Blocks ⇑ |
| 9.3.4 | Shortcut Reversal Correction ⇑ |

## 11.6.2 EFT-led coaching

In EFT-led coaching, EFT dominates the coaching interaction. As soon as the client has stated a goal, EFT can be used almost all the way through the remaining interaction as problems, blocks and solutions to achieving the goal are discussed and worked through.

Where EFT dominates the coaching, the emphasis is likely to be on the Being aspects of the goal (how the client feels about the goal, how they feel about themselves in relation to the goal etc)

I have stated above that EFT should always be in the **service** of the coaching, rather than dominating it and being the primary tool used. I would no more want to dominate my coaching with EFT than I would want to dominate it with visualisation exercises. However, I can imagine particular and occasional sessions being EFT-dominated, just as occasional sessions may be devoted just to a Future Self or Life Purpose visualisation exercise, for instance.

The main thing to watch out for is that even though the interaction may be dominated by EFT, that it does not become "EFT with coaching added", but remains "EFT-assisted coaching".

## 11.6.3 Homework only EFT

A third option is to have virtually no EFT occur within the coaching session itself, but to have the client do EFT in his own time either as formally agreed homework or under his own supervision.

This style will suit a coach who finds the prospect of using EFT within coaching just too much like "therapy" to deal with. But just as it is perfectly acceptable for a coach to suggest a client seeks out a therapist to deal with an emotional problem from the past, it is equally as valid for the client to use self-help EFT as their chosen form of emotional support in between sessions.

Clients who are already familiar with using EFT will appreciate being able to work with a coach who understands what EFT can do and can work with EFT as one of the **client's** own resources. This makes EFT just a resource that the client may use to support himself, just as some clients may use meditation, prayer, exercise, mind-mapping or whatever else that works for them.

Even if the regular style of coaching is to use EFT in a coaching context, there is always the option to fall back to this option for issues which the coach feels fall on the side of "therapy" rather than coaching (i.e. assisting progress towards the client's goals). Again, this exactly parallels what might happen if a client wants to do some physical exercise to help towards one of his goals. The coach may agree it as a Homework item and encourage the client to do so, without worrying about whether he has over-stepped his role as coach by becoming a fitness trainer.

Related sections:

| | |
|---|---|
| 5.1 | EFT isn't (Psycho)therapy ⇑ |

# 12 EFT QuickStart

This section describes the basic EFT procedure and tapping points for those who wish to try EFT for the first time. It is based on my own EFT QuickStart manual[9]. Following this procedure will familiarise you with the basic mechanics of how to apply EFT, and allow you to try it out on some personal issues. It is not a thorough training in self-help EFT although it is estimated that beginners using this basic information can get success rates of 50-80%. Readers who want to use EFT either for more complex personal issues or as a practitioner are referred to the training resources listed below (section 13). The easiest way to get started with EFT is to follow these steps:

- Familiarise yourself with the location of the points and how to tap.
- Learn how to "tune in" to the problem with Setup Statements and Reminder Phrases.
- Learn how to measure progress using the rating scale.
- Put the tapping and statements together in a few practice rounds, using the guide below, until you feel used to doing the basic sequence.
- Read the "What to do if…" section in the full QuickStart manual[9] which covers issues like how to tackle complex issues, what to do if the problem "changes" part way through, etc

## 12.1 The Points

The points are shown in the diagram below. Descriptions of the points are in the table.

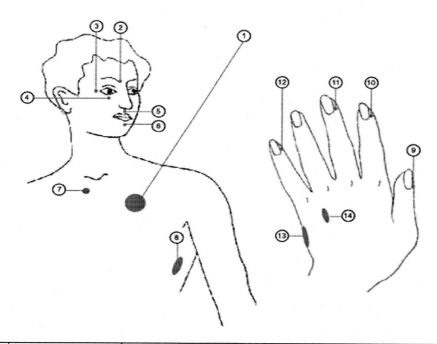

| No. on diagram | Name of point | Location of point |
|---|---|---|
| 1 | Sore spot | Left hand side of chest, midway between armpit crease and centre of chest. There may be several sore spots in this region. |
| 2 | Eyebrow | Beginning of the eyebrow, above and slightly to the side of the nose |
| 3 | Side of eye | Outer corner on the bony ridge |
| 4 | Under eye | Directly beneath on bony ridge |
| 5 | Under nose | Centrally between nose and upper lip |
| 6 | Chin | Centrally under bottom lip |
| 7 | Collarbone | One inch to side of central indent |
| 8 | Underarm | Four inches below armpit on side of body |
| 9 | Thumb | Side of thumb at base of nail |
| 10 | Index finger | Side of index finger at base of nail |
| 11 | Middle finger | Side of middle finger at base of nail |
| 12 | Little finger | Side of little finger at base of nail |
| 13 | Side of hand | Halfway down side of hand |
| 14 | Back of hand | One inch behind 3$^{rd}$ and 4$^{th}$ knuckles |

# 12.2 How to Tap

- Tapping is done using the index and middle finger tips together. If you have long nails, use the finger pads.
- You can use either hand and tap on either side of the body. (Except for the Sore Spot which is only on the left side of the body)
- For the Collarbone, Underarm and Side of hand points, using several fingers helps ensure the right point is covered.
- Tap about 7 times on each point. It does not have to be exactly 7 times. You may tap longer on one or more points if they "feel good".
- Speed of tapping is approximately 2-4 taps per second.
- Tap firmly enough to feel the vibration in the surrounding skin, but not hard enough to hurt or bruise.

# 12.3 The Setup Statement

While you rub the Sore Spot you say a "Setup Statement" which tunes you into the problem. The basic form of a Setup Statement is:

**"Even though < X >, I deeply and completely accept myself"**

where < X > is a description of the issue you want to solve (see table below for examples).

- If you find the Sore Spot hard to find or too painful, tap the Side of Hand point instead - using the Sore Spot is considered to be slightly better but both are effective.
- There is no right or wrong about Setup Statements. Think about the problem and how you would describe it to someone else - and use those words.
- Use the words that you really use with yourself everyday - not the "official" or "clean" words you think you should use. e.g. Don't say "gastrointestinal pain" if what you would usually say is "gut ache".
- The Setup doesn't have to be grammatical or logical or even have proper words for how you feel. If you have an "eugh feeling" you can say "Even though I have this eugh feeling,..."
- You don't have to say "I deeply and completely accept myself" if that feels uncomfortable or false. Pick equivalent words that indicate in some way that you accept yourself e.g. "I accept myself", or "I'm an OK person", or, "I'm an OK bloke", or "I'm OK".

# 12.4 The Reminder Phrase

Each time you tap on a point you say a Reminder Phrase - a word or short phrase which keeps you tuned into the issue. The phrase is typically taken from the Setup Statement.

The following table gives examples of Setup Statements and corresponding Reminder Phrases.

| Setup Statement | Reminder |
|---|---|
| *Even though I have this problem, I deeply and completely accept myself* | This problem |
| *Even though I'm angry about what happened, I deeply and completely accept myself* | Angry |
| *Even though I'm embarrassed, I deeply and completely accept myself* | Embarrassed |
| *Even though I feel all this guilt, I deeply and completely accept myself* | This guilt |
| *Even though she said I was ugly, I deeply and completely accept myself* | Said I was ugly |
| *Even though my shoulder hurts like hell, I deeply and completely accept myself.* | Shoulder |
| *Even though I really want a fag, I deeply and completely accept myself* | Really want a fag |
| *Even though I feel like I've got the world on my shoulders, I deeply and completely accept myself* | World on my shoulders |

# 12.5 Rating the Problem and Measuring Progress

To see how you are doing you need to take before and after measures of the problem you are working on. This is done using a 0-10 rating scale as follows.

## For issues involving emotional intensity
(e.g. Fear of heights) or physical pain (e.g. Headache):

- Ask yourself "On a scale of 0 to 10, how bad/intense is it right now?".
- Zero means no intensity or discomfort at all; 10 is the worst it has ever been or could be.

## For issues involving beliefs
(e.g. "I'm no good at maths"):

- Ask yourself "On a scale of 0 to 10, how much do I believe this?".
- Zero means you don't believe it at all; 10 means you believe it completely.

Don't think too hard about it - what number pops into your head?

# 12.6 The Full Sequence

A full sequence of EFT is achieved by carrying out the following actions using the following points and saying the following phrases in the order given below.

Remember to get a 0-10 rating of the problem before you start and again at the end.

| Action | Point | Say |
|---|---|---|
| Rub (OR Tap | Sore spot Side of Hand) | "Even though I have <this problem> I deeply and completely accept myself" |
| Rub (OR Tap | Sore spot Side of Hand) | "Even though I have <this problem> I deeply and completely accept myself" |
| Rub (OR Tap | Sore spot Side of Hand) | "Even though I have <this problem> I deeply and completely accept myself" |
| Tap | Eyebrow | "This problem" |
| Tap | Side of eye | "This problem" |
| Tap | Under eye | "This problem" |
| Tap | Under nose | "This problem" |
| Tap | Chin | "This problem" |
| Tap | Collarbone | "This problem" |
| Tap | Underarm | "This problem" |
| Tap | Thumb | "This problem" |
| Tap | Index finger | "This problem" |
| Tap | Middle finger | "This problem" |
| Tap | Little finger | "This problem" |
| Tap | Side of hand | "This problem" |
| Tap | Back of hand | "This problem" |
| Keep tapping while you: Close eyes, Open eyes, Point eyes hard down left, then hard down right, Roll eyes right round, then back the other way, Hum a few notes, Count to five, Hum a few notes* | Back of hand | NB - This part can be omitted if the rest of the sequence is working. If you omit it and the main sequence does not work, reintroduce it.

*e.g. "Happy Birthday to you" |

# 13 Information and Training Resources

As EFT spreads, so do the number of practitioners, books, organisations, workshops and trainings all increase. The following therefore cannot be a complete guide to all available resources on EFT. I have limited it to the resources that I have personally used and can vouch for. These offer the reader a safe starting point for their own learning - but you may well come across other good resources yourself.

Exclusion of any organisation, book, person or training resource from this list should not be taken to imply any negative judgement on my part - it simply means that I do not have personal knowledge of it and therefore cannot personally vouch for it.

Up to date resource links are maintained at The EFT Coach website (www.eftcoach.com).

## 13.1 Manuals and Books

**Emotional Freedom Techniques: The Manual.** The original EFT manual, by the developer of EFT Gary Craig. 79 pages, available as a free ebook download from www.emofree.com. An easy to read but thorough starting point for learning how to apply EFT for self-help. Required reading for Gary's CD training course.

**EFT QuickStart manual.** My own beginner's manual, 7 pages. Free ebook download from www.thefuturestartsnow.com/downloads/EFTQuickStart.pdf. Also available in A5 paper format from the author, cost £2 including postage.

**Adventures in EFT.** By Silvia Hartmann, co-founder of the Association for Meridian Therapies. Thorough and easy to read survey of many different uses for EFT. Suitable for the beginner and practitioner alike. Available as ebook (£12.50) or hardcopy (£16.95) from www.dragonrising.com. ISBN: 1-8734836-3-5

**Advanced Patterns of EFT.** By Silvia Hartmann. Aimed at the serious therapist and practitioner, covers deeper therapeutic uses of EFT. Perhaps optional reading for the EFT Coach, I believe the additional depth it provides is still useful as training for the serious practitioner in any context. Available as ebook (£20.00) or hardcopy (£26.95) from www.dragonrising.com. ISBN: 1-8734836-8-6

**EFT & NLP.** By Silvia Hartmann. A shorter book covering the relationship between NLP and EFT. May be of interest to coaches with existing NLP background. Special Report on EFT as a module for use by practitioners of Neuro-Linguistic Programming. Topics include TimeLine Applications, EFT as the missing kinaesthetic quadrant, integrating EFT into NLP corporate presentations and the Energy Healing Progression Model. Available as ebook (£9.99) from www.dragonrising.com.

**The Choices Method.** By Dr Pat Carrington. Describes a powerful variant of EFT used extensively in this book and highly recommended in all contexts but especially coaching. Available as ebook ($30) from www.eft-innovations.com/Choicesmanual.htm.

**Getting Thru to Your Emotions with EFT.** Phillip and Jane Mountrose. Aimed at the beginner, but quickly gets into deeper material. Includes subject areas relevant to coaching such as improving performance and fulfilment. ISBN: 0-9653787-6-4

# 13.2 Gary Craig's CD training

Probably the cheapest, easiest and most convenient way to learn EFT is to watch it being applied by an expert while they explain what they are doing as they go along. Obtaining CD training provides you with a permanent resource which you can return to again and again, and which you can view at your own pace. I still watch mine years later, and continue to get more out of them every time. They are a crucial bridge between the theory you can read about in books and manuals, and the practice of applying EFT to yourself or others. In my opinion these are a "must buy" whether you want to learn EFT for self-help or as a stepping stone to becoming a practitioner. They are also an excellent and very good value alternative to attending a live workshop.

There are currently four training sets available, with more on the way:

**The EFT Course** - The Basic Training course covering all the basics and including many case studies on issues such as PTSD, phobias, anxiety etc. Detailed knowledge of this course is a requirement to achieve the EFT Certificate of Completion (EFT-CC) and to take the AMT Practitioner training.

**Steps toward becoming The Ultimate Therapist:** Shows other therapists using EFT in combination with their own discipline. While still firmly in "therapy" territory there are glimpses of coaching applications. Detailed knowledge of this course is a requirement to achieve the EFT Advanced certificate (EFT-ADV).

**From EFT to the Palace of Possibilities:** Highly relevant to the coaching context. Gary covers how EFT can be used for issues such as beliefs about money and success, plus practical ideas for building a practice which uses EFT.

**EFT Specialty Series 1:** Specialists present the use of EFT for business, addictions/overweight, relationships, sexual trauma and severely emotionally disturbed children. Excellent for expanding and deepening understanding of how EFT can be applied. The relationship coaching section is great viewing for any coaches working in this field.

All the CD courses can be ordered from www.emofree.com, where you can also see much more detailed contents descriptions.

# 13.3 Live Events

More and more practitioners are running introductory trainings. These vary from a couple of hours for an evening to a whole weekend.

They also vary in focus. Some are straightforward introductions to EFT, while others focus on specific issues such as stress or weight loss.

Many events are listed at:

- www.emofree.com - Live Workshops
- www.theamt.com - Trainings and Courses

These listings include beginner, intermediate and practitioner events, so check with the organiser before booking.

Alternatively, contact a practitioner in your area and see if they are planning any workshops in the near future. Practitioners also sometimes announce forthcoming workshops on the web discussion forums.

Several organisations run conferences on the subject of Energy Psychology at which you may be able to take introductory trainings, practitioner trainings or specialist seminars. In particular:

- AMT - Association for Meridian Therapies - runs a UK-based summer conference. See: www.theamt.com for details.

- ACEP - Association for Comprehensive Energy Psychology - runs conferences in the US and Canada. See: www.energypsych.org for details of upcoming events.

# 13.4 Practitioner trainings

**EFT-CC - The Basic EFT Certificate of Completion.** EFT-CC is obtained by sitting an open book exam in your own time, and is based on the content of "The EFT Course" (see above). This certificate does not prove competence as a practitioner but does ensure that the person has thoroughly studied and understood the basic EFT CD training course. Visit www.eftcertificate.com for details and to order exam. Completion qualifies someone to be included in the online practitioner listing.

**EFT-ADV - The Advanced EFT Certificate of Completion.** EFT-ADV is obtained by sitting an open book exam in your own time, and is based on the content of "Steps toward becoming The Ultimate Therapist" CD course (see above). This certificate does not prove competence as a practitioner but does ensure that the person has thoroughly studied and understood the Ultimate Therapist CD training course. Visit www.eftcertificate.com for details and to order exam.

**AMT Certified Practitioner.** This is a formal practitioner training designed and run by the Association for Meridian Therapies, UK. It assumes an existing high level of familiarity with the basic EFT protocol either by having attending a introductory training or having studied the basic EFT training course on CD. The practitioner training is available either as a two day live event with an approved AMT trainer, or as a correspondence course, which may be of interest to non-UK people. The training involves assessment by an AMT trainer, and completion of an open book examination and includes documentation of case studies with a clients. Successful completion includes AMT membership and online practitioner listing. Visit www.theamt.com for details of live and correspondence trainings.

**AMT Advanced Practitioner.** This extends the knowledge gained at the basic practitioner training, advanced variations of EFT, and basic introduction to other meridian therapies such as TAT, BSFF and EmoTrance. It assumes successful completion of the basic practitioner certification.

Other organisations or individual practitioners may offer practitioner level trainings in your area. Check what completion gives you access to in terms of membership, ongoing support and so on, and ensure it gives you what you want in terms of professional development, before you sign up.

# 13.5 Websites

www.emofree.com - This original EFT website by Gary Craig, the developer of EFT. An excellent resource for beginners and practitioners alike. Gary's original and comprehensive beginner's manual is available for download, along with many case histories in a well organised archive. Also includes international practitioner listing and training materials for those who want to learn EFT more thoroughly. Also available is an excellent email list which you may subscribe to for free, to receive regular case histories and thoughts by Gary.

www.theamt.com - Website of the AMT - Association for Meridian Therapies - UK. As well as practitioner listings, contains articles, bookshop, notice of workshops and trainings. Includes information about many types of meridian-based techniques, not just EFT. Also has many documents for free download.

www.thefuturestartsnow.com - My own website which includes free QuickStart manual. Includes an expanded resource guide for both coaching and EFT, free downloads and a free email newsletter including articles relevant to coaching and EFT. Check here regularly for upcoming workshop dates and events.

www.eft-innovations.com - Dr Patricia Carrington's website which includes articles and information, newsletter signup and links to books and other training materials. It also contains a practitioner listing for people who have achieved EFT-CC and EFT-ADV.

Many other practitioners also have their own websites which often contain additional information, training resources or workshop information.

# 13.6 Discussion forums

To get in touch with other people learning and practicing EFT and other energy therapies, you might want to check out the following newsgroups where there are many people willing to answer questions, share experiences and offer support:

http://groups.yahoo.com/group/MT-newbies - Run by the AMT UK, this a good place to start with basic questions. It is moderated and frequented by trained practitioners who are very willing to answer questions and give advice. Very friendly and positive atmosphere. Not limited to EFT, but also other types of meridian-based techniques.

http://groups.yahoo.com/group/EmotionalFreedomTechniques - More US focussed but with a large (over 1700) international membership - which makes for varied and interesting discussion. It is moderated (assisted by myself) and is a very friendly group. Membership varies from complete beginners to highly experienced practitioners. It also includes discussion of therapies other than EFT.

# 13.7 Finding a practitioner

Practitioner listings are available on the following websites:

www.theamt.com - This lists mostly UK practitioners, although a few are overseas. All practitioners on this listing are required to have completed the AMT practitioner training in order to be listed. AMT training requires assessment by an AMT trainer and completion of a written exam, including case studies.

www.eftsupport.com - International Practitioner listing. All those listed are required to have achieved EFT-CC (EFT Certificate of Completion) which involves completing Gary Craig's video training program and passing a written examination. Some will also have achieved EFT-ADV which means they have passed an exam based on Gary Craig's "Ultimate Therapist" CD training.

www.emofree.com - International Practitioner listing. Practitioners are asked to declare their level of training, but this is not guaranteed.

There are many EFT practitioners who are not listed in these places. A web search is likely to produce details of other practitioners who may be self-taught or who have taken different forms of practitioner training. Ultimately, you need to assess the competence of a practitioner yourself.

# 14 References

Up to date links to suppliers are maintained at The EFT Coach website (www.eftcoach.com).

[1]     Emotional Freedom Techniques™. A universal aid to healing. The Manual. 3rd Edition. 1999. Gary Craig. Free download from www.emofree.com

[2]     Coactive Coaching: new skills for coaching people toward success in work and life. Laura Whitworth, Henry Kimsey-House & Phil Sandahl. Davies-Black publishing, Palo Alto California. 1st Edition, 1998. ISBN 0-89106-123-1

[3]     Adventures in EFT. Silvia Hartmann. DragonRising.com, Eastbourne. 6th Edition, January 2003. ISBN: 1-8734836-3-5

[4]     The Advanced Patterns of EFT. Silvia Hartmann. DragonRising.com, Eastbourne. Version 1.0, January 2003. ISBN: 1-8734836-8-6

[5]     The NLP Coach. Ian McDermott and Wendy Jago. Piatkus publishing, London. 2001 ISBN: 0-7499-2277-X

[6]     EFT & NLP. Silvia Hartmann. DragonRising.com, Eastbourne. Version 3.0, May 2001.

[7]     Choices Training Manual: How to creative positive choices in energy psychology - a new approach to EFT and related methods. Dr Pat Carrington. Pace Educational Systems Inc, New Jersey. Ebook: http://www.eft-innovations.com/Choicesmanual.htm

[8]     Living Your Best Life. Laura Berman Fortgang. HarperCollins. 2001. ISBN: 0-007111-83-5

[9]     The EFT QuickStart manual. Mary L.R. Jones. The Future Starts Now. 2003. Ebook: http://www.thefuturestartsnow.com/downloads/EFTQuickStart.pdf

[10]   Taming Your Gremlin: A guide to enjoying yourself. Richard D. Carson. HarperPerennial, New York. 1983. ISBN: 0-06-096102-3

[11]   A Return to Love: Reflections on the Principles of a "Course in Miracles". Marianne Williamson. HarperCollins. 1996. ISBN: 0-722532-99-7

[12]   Anam Cara: Spiritual Wisdom from the Celtic World. John O'Donohue. Bantam. 1999. ISBN: 0-553505-92-0

[13]   Living the Liberated Life and Dealing with the Pain Body. Eckhart Tolle. Audiobook. ASIN: B0000645HJ

# 15 About the Author

Mary L.R. Jones BSc MSc is a Personal Coach, Advanced Practitioner and Trainer of Meridian Therapies, Advanced Practitioner of EmoTrance and NLP Practitioner.

She is a member of the International Coaching Federation and the Association for Meridian Therapies in the UK.

Originally trained in Experimental Psychology (BSc) at Durham University and Information Systems (MSc), she spent 13 years in industry as a User Interface designer and Human Factors consultant. As a telecommunications researcher and manager she specialised in human communication and behaviour, and authored and co-authored several research papers and presented at national and international conferences. In her role as team leader she began her interest in coaching and personal development, before leaving to pursue a career as a professional coach and author.

Mary's own coaching specialisms of Dating Support and Stress, both combine coaching and EFT.

Mary writes and runs her own workshops, publishes a free monthly e-newsletter and is an active member and co-moderator of the largest EFT discussion group on the web.

She is available for private consultations, private and corporate training and speaking engagements.